INTRAVENOUS THERAPY

The Jones and Bartlett Series in Nursing

INTRAVENOUS THERAPY

A Comprehensive Application of Intravenous Therapy and Medication Administration

Phyllis Fichtelman Nentwich, RN, MF

JONES AND BARTLETT PUBLISHERS
Boston

Editorial, Sales, and Customer Service Offices

Jones and Bartlett Publishers
20 Park Plaza
Boston, MA 02116

Printed in the United States of America
10 9 8 7 6 5 4 3 2 1

Library of Congress Cataloging-in-Publication Data

Nentwich, Phyllis Fichtelman.
    Intravenous therapy : a comprehensive application of intravenous therapy and medication administration / Phyllis Fichtelman Nentwich.
       p.   cm.
    Includes bibliographical references.
    ISBN 0-86720-419-2
    1. Intravenous therapy. 2. Nursing. I. Title.
    [DNLM: 1. Drugs—administration & dosage—nurses' instruction.
2. Infusions, Parenteral—nurses' instruction. 3. Parenteral
Feeding—nurses' instruction. WB 354 N437i]
RM170.N45 1990
615'.6—dc20
DNLM/DLC
for Library of Congress   89–71687
                                            CIP

ISBN 0-86720-419-2

Production: Editing, Design & Production, Inc.
Production Services Coordinator: Judy Salvucci
Cover Design: Rafael Millán

Contributors

CHARLINE CATT, RNC, MS
Head Nurse, Metabolic/Endocrine
Children's Hospital
Columbus, Ohio

ELAINE GLASS, RN, MS, CNA, OCN
Clinical Nurse Specialist
The Ohio State University Hospitals
Columbus, Ohio

NAOMI HAUTALA, RN, BSN
Intravenous Therapy Nurse Clinician
Children's Hospital
Columbus, Ohio

MARCIA MILLER, RN
Nurse Researcher, Infectious Disease
Children's Hospital
Columbus, Ohio

MERRI LYNN DREIER OSBORN, RN, BSN, CCRN
Education Coordinator
Riverside Methodist Hospital
Columbus, Ohio

CARLA POWELL, RN
Nutritional Support Service
The Ohio State University Hospitals
Columbus, Ohio

Contributing Editors

PAUL CERRATO
Associate Editor
R.N. Magazine
Oradell, New Jersey

LAUREL R. TALABERE, MS, RN, CPNP
Associate Professor
Capital University
Columbus, Ohio

Contents

Preface

PURPOSE

Nursing today is a discipline of high technology coupled with a wealth of complex information. The nurse's role is to apply that knowledge in an efficient and cost-effective manner. Intravenous therapy is an example of such a technical application. The purpose of this book is to provide a practical and concise reference manual for the IV practitioner or student nurse in the neonatal, pediatric, or adult setting. Included is all the information needed to administer a drug safely via a peripheral or central venous catheter in the acute care environment or at home.

ORGANIZATION OF THE TEXT

The text is organized into several units. Units I through V contain detailed chapters on the technical and theoretical aspects of intravenous therapy. Upon completion of these units, the reader will have a step-by-step understanding of peripheral and central venous IV therapy, proper IV medication administration, and IV therapy in the home setting.

Unit VI applies this knowledge base to the administration of over 250 IV medications. Specific technical information is provided on each drug so that the nurse can refer to the text and administer the drug in the most therapeutic manner in any situation.

Each concise drug profile includes the following:

Generic Name: Medications are listed alphabetically by generic name.
Trade Name: The trade name is identified on the second line of each drug profile, just under the generic name. Both generic and trade names are listed in the index.
Classification: Each drug profile is identified by its major drug classifica-

tion. The index also lists each classification and the drugs that fall within it.

Action: Physiological and pharmacologic actions are identified for each drug, based on the manufacturer's research.

Indications: A concise listing of each drug's indications is included to assure the reader that the appropriate drug is administered for the appropriate indication.

Dosage: Neonatal, pediatric, and adult dosages are provided based on milligram per kilogram of weight when appropriate, or on the standard accepted dosage range. If the information is not available or not applicable, this notation is made.

Preparation: This section includes information on how the drug is supplied, and the method of dilution when appropriate. Each medication should be assessed prior to administration for discoloration, separation, or precipitation. If any of these conditions are present, the drug should be discarded.

Home Stability: Since intravenous medication administration has spread into the home setting, home storage has become a necessity. This section identifies where, and for how long, each drug is stable.

Compatibilities: Every IV solution, including TPN, that is compatible with the medication is listed. If the solution is incompatible with the drug, flush thoroughly with a compatible IV solution prior to administration.

Administration: The intravenous site of administration is identified for each medication based on the client's age. Neonatal, pediatric, and adult administration is based on the differing IV rates appropriate for the client's size.

Contraindications: All contraindications, derived from a variety of sources (including the manufacturer), are identified. A medication should never be administered that is contraindicated for that client.

Side Effects: Primary and secondary adverse reactions are listed in a systematic manner. Prior to administering any drug, the client should be assessed for drug allergies and hypersensitivty reactions.

Nursing Implications: Drug-specific nursing actions are listed for each drug. This information assures that appropriate assessment and planning are done prior to administration of the drug and that, following administration, the proper evaluation of effectiveness and side effects is once again made.

Prior to the administration of any medication, the nurse must remember the basics: to assess that the right drug is being administered to the right patient. The information presented applies to intravenous medications only, and the IV site should be assessed for patency prior to, during, and following drug administration.

As a handy, pocket-sized guide to IV medications, the *1991 Handbook of Intravenous Medications*, published annually by Jones and Bartlett, provides the nurse or IV practitioner with a quick, yet comprehensive, source for administering IV therapy medications in an efficient, therapeutic, and cost-effective manner.

UNIT I

INTRODUCTION TO INTRAVENOUS THERAPY

Chapter 1 FLUID AND ELECTROLYTE OVERVIEW

CHAPTER 1

Fluid and Electrolyte Overview

Phyllis Fichtelman Nentwich, RN, MS

Body Water Content
Osmolality of Intravenous Solutions
Fluid and Electrolyte Regulation Mechanism
Fluid Volume Deficit
Fluid Volume Excess
Electrolyte Imbalances
    Sodium Imbalance
    Potassium Imbalance
    Calcium Imbalance

Fluid and electrolyte balance is a fundamental principle of intravenous therapy. This chapter will provide an overview of the fluid compartments of the body and the organs of fluid and electrolyte regulation.

BODY WATER CONTENT

Water, the primary fluid of the body, has two major functions: transportation of nutrients to the cells and removal of waste products. Water content varies with age, lean body mass, and sex.

The adult body is about 60 percent water, whereas the water content of an infant is 70 to 80 percent of total body weight. Body fluid content decreases with age. The body of a premature infant of 13 to 14 weeks gestation is 95 percent water, compared to 78 percent for a full-term infant. This is in marked contrast to the gerian whose water content averages 45 to 55 percent of body weight.

Since muscle tissue contains more water than adipose tissue, males, who have more lean body mass, have greater water content. Thus, based on total body water, neonates, infants, and the elderly are more prone to fluid volume imbalances than are adults.

There are two main fluid compartments in the body: intracellular and extracellular. Intracellular fluid (ICF) is located within the cells. In the adult, it constitutes about 40 percent of total body weight or 70 percent of total body water.

Extracellular fluid (ECF) is of three types—interstitial, intravascular, and transcellular. Interstitial fluid exists between the cells. Intravascular fluid is the plasma within the blood vessels. Transcellular fluids include cerebrospinal fluid, intraocular fluid, and gastrointestinal secretions. In the adult, extracellular fluid constitutes about 20 percent of body weight or 30 percent of total body water. Of that 20 percent, plasma accounts for 5 percent and interstitial fluid 15 percent.

Each fluid compartment has a primary cation (an electrolyte with a positive charge) and a primary anion (an electrolyte with a negative charge). The primary cation of the extracellular compartment is sodium; the primary cation of the intracellular compartment is potassium. The primary extracellular anion is chloride; the primary intracellular anion is phosphate. Calcium, a cation, is found only in the extracellular fluid. All other electrolytes are found in varying concentrations in both compartments. Electrolytes have several functions in cellular metabolism: regulation of water distribution, transmission of nerve impulses, clotting of blood, generation of agenosine triphosphate, and regulation of acid-base balance.

The processes that control the movement of fluids and electrolytes are diffusion, osmosis, and active transport. Diffusion is the movement of molecules from an area of higher concentration to an area of lower concentration. This passive process, which does not require energy, occurs in liquids, gases, and solids. Diffusion ends when the concentrations in both areas are the same.

Osmosis is the flow of water between two compartments separated by a semipermeable membrane. The membrane is permeable to water but not to a solute. Water moves from an area of low solute concentration to an area of high solute concentration. As with diffusion, osmosis is a passive process that does not require energy.

Osmolarity, or total milliosmoles of solute per unit of total volume of solution, is used to measure solutions of equal weight and volume. An example of such a solution is an intravenous solution. Osmolality, the osmotic force of solute per unit of weight of solvent, is used to compare body fluids that do not have the same weight for equal volumes, such as plasma and urine.

The osmolality of body fluids is regulated by the kidneys. Normal osmolality of body fluids is 275 to 295 mOsm. The normal range for urine osmolality is 300 to 1090 mOsm/kg.

Active transport is the process by which electrolytes are pumped into and out of cells using energy. Active transport regulates sodium and potassium within the cell. As sodium passively diffuses into the cell and potassium out of the cell, sodium is being actively pumped back into the extracellular compartment and potassium to the intracellular compartment. Thus, active transport, which reverses the passive process of diffusion, is an important mechanism in the maintenance of fluid and electrolyte balance.

OSMOLALITY OF INTRAVENOUS SOLUTIONS

The osmolality of the fluid that surrounds a cell affects the cell. Isotonic solutions are fluids that, when added to the body, have the same osmolality as the interior of the cell. Solutions with a different osmolality contain either more water than the cell and are called hypotonic, or less water than the cell and are called hypertonic. Extracellular and intracellular fluids are isotonic to each other, resulting in an equal exchange of fluids and solutes between these compartments. When a cell is surrounded by a hypotonic solution, water will move into the cell. The effect will be one of swelling. Hypertonic solutions will cause water to move out of the cell. The effect will be one of shrinking.

FLUID AND ELECTROLYTE REGULATION MECHANISM

The organs of fluid and electrolyte regulation include the hypothalamus, posterior pituitary, adrenal cortex, gastrointestinal tract, kidneys, lungs, and skin. The thirst center is located in the hypothalamus. A dry mouth, decreased cardiac output, and intracellular and extracellular dehydration will signal the need to drink, even in the absence of a measurable body water deficit.

Antidiuretic hormone (ADH), which regulates water retention by the kidneys, is secreted by the posterior pituitary gland. ADH increases the permeability of the distal tubules and collecting ducts of the kidneys. Therefore, more water is reabsorbed into the blood stream, resulting in urine that is more concentrated.

Glucocorticoids and mineralocorticoids are secreted by the adrenal cortex. The anti-inflammatory effect of the glucocorticoids and the enhancement of sodium retention and potassium excretion by the mineralocorticoids assist in the maintenance of extracellular fluid volume. A naturally occurring adrenocortical steroid is cortisol; aldosterone is the naturally occurring mineralocorticoid.

While the kidneys are responsible for fluid excretion, through reabsorption by the glomerular filtrate, the gastrointestinal tract is responsible for most fluid ingestion.

Table 1.1   NORMAL FLUID BALANCE IN THE ADULT

Intake

Fluids	1200 ml
Solid food	1000 ml
Water from metabolism	300 ml
	2500 ml

Output

Insensible loss	900 ml
Feces	100 ml
Urine	1500 ml
	2500 ml

The lungs and skin account for the excretion of approximately 900 ml of fluids per day through vaporization, called insensible water loss. The main function of this excretion is the regulation of body temperature. Only water is lost through this process (Table 1.1).

FLUID VOLUME DEFICIT

A fluid water deficit can be defined as "the state in which the individual experiences or is at risk of experiencing vascular, cellular or intracellular dehydration" (Carpenito 1985). Fluid water deficit, or dehydration, may be precipitated by several causes, which are listed in Table 1.2.

The nursing interventions for a client with a fluid volume deficit focus on correction of the cause of the imbalance and prevention of further dehydration. Such nursing actions include observation of the client for signs of insensible water loss from hyperventilation and diaphoresis; weighing the client daily or twice a day on the same scale with the same or similar clothing; accurate monitoring of intake and output; careful assessment of laboratory data, especially electrolytes and osmolarity; and monitoring of associated electrolyte imbalances. Intravenous fluids should be administered cautiously: during rapid administration the client may experience signs and symptoms of fluid volume excess.

FLUID VOLUME EXCESS

Fluid volume excess can be defined as "the state in which the individual experiences, or is at risk of experiencing, peripheral edema." Fluid volume

Table 1.2   CAUSES AND CLINICAL MANIFESTATIONS OF FLUID VOLUME DEFICIT (CARPENITO, 1985: LEWIS AND COLLIER, 1983).

Causes	Clinical Manifestations
Excessive use of diuretics	Decreased skin turgor
Administration of osmotic agents	Dry, sticky mucous membranes
Fever with excessive diaphoresis	Rough, dry tounge
Excessive gastrointestinal drainage	Weight loss
Diuretic phase of renal disease	Fever
Diabetes insipidus	Agitation
Burns	Restlessness
Dialysis	Weakness
Vomiting and diarrhea	Orthostatic hypotension
Inadequate fluid replacement during medical or surgical procedures	Decreased urine output
	Specific gravity > 1.030
Impaired thirst center	Increased sodium
Dysphagia	Increased protein
	Increased hematocrit
	Increased serum osmolality
	Increased urine osmolality

Table 1.3   CAUSES AND CLINICAL MANIFESTATIONS OF FLUID VOLUME EXCESS

Causes	Clinical Manifestations
Renal failure	Weight gain
Decreased cardiac output	Edema
Varicosities of the legs	Confusion
Liver disease	Lethargy
Excessive IV fluid intake	Weakness
Overtransfusion	Seizures
Excessive sodium intake	Full, bounding pulse
Inappropriate secretion of ADH	Jugular distension
	Nausea, vomiting
	Liquid stools
	Increased urinary volume
	Specific gravity < 1.010
	Decreased sodium
	Decreased protein
	Decreased hematocrit
	Decreased serum osmolality

excess, or overhydration, can be caused by several factors: acute or chronic renal failure, administration of excessive intravenous fluids, decreased cardiac output, or excessive antidiuretic hormone secretion. Table 1.3 presents the signs and symptoms of fluid volume excess.

The nursing interventions for the client with fluid volume excess also focus on correcting the cause of the excess. An assessment of the imbalance can be made by strict monitoring of the client's intake and output, weight, and laboratory data. Accurate administration of IV solutions will prevent situational overhydration. Diuretics may be ordered to correct the excessive state.

ELECTROLYTE IMBALANCES

Electrolyte imbalances can occur with the administration of diuretics in clients with fluid imbalances. Table 1.4 defines each electrolyte imbalance, associated clinical manifestations, and appropriate nursing action.

Table 1.4   CLINICAL MANIFESTATIONS AND NURSING INTERVENTIONS OF ELECTROLYTE IMBALANCES

Electrolyte Imbalance	Clinical Manifestations	Nursing Interventions
Hypernatremia ($Na+$ > 135 mEq/L)	Dry, sticky mucous membranes Flushed skin Intense thirst Oliguria or anuria Elevated temperature Rough, dry tongue Edema Weight gain Weakness Lethargy Restlessness Increased central venous pressure Distended veins Decreased specific gravity Decreased hematocrit Decreased serum protein	Record 24-hour fluid intake and output Monitor weight daily Provide frequent skin and mouth care Turn every 2 hours Assess IV rate hourly Assess electrolyte values closely Offer oral fluids frequently Monitor urine specific gravity Monitor level of consciousness Restrict sodium intake
Hyponatremia ($Na+$ < 135 mEq/L)	Headache Anxiety, apathy Confusion	Record 24-hour fluid intake and output Monitor weight daily

Table 1.4   continued

Electrolyte Imbalance	Clinical Manifestations	Nursing Interventions
	Anorexia	Assess IV flow rate closely
	Nausea, vomiting	Assess electrolyte values
	Diarrhea, cramping	Monitor level of con-sciousness
	Clammy skin	
	Weakness	Avoid rapid changes in position
	Stupor, coma	
	Rapid, thready pulse	
	Postural hypotension	
	Decreased central venous pressure	
	Muscle weakness	
	Lower extremity muscle cramping	
	Decreased specific gravity	
	Increased hematocrit	
	Increased serum protein	
	Increased urine osmolality	
Hypokalemia (K+ < 3.5 mEq/L)	Cardiac arrhythmias	Monitor EKG
	T wave inversion	Administer potassium supplements per physician's order or administer potassium chloride IV slowly
	Fatigue	
	Leg cramps	
	Anorexia	
	Vomiting	
	Paralytic ileus	Monitor potassium levels closely
	Drowsiness, confusion	
	Postural hypotension	Monitor urine specific gravity
	Increased serum pH	
	Decreased specific gravity	Monitor level of con-sciousness
Hyperkalemia (K+ > 5.5 mEq/L)	Cardiac arrhythmias	Monitor EKG
	Peaked T waves	Restrict potassium intake
	Decreased deep tendon reflexes	Administer glucose and insulin IV per physician's order
	Paresthesias	
	Decreased serum pH	Administer Kayexalate orally or per rectum per physician's order
	Apathy, confusion	
	Abdominal cramping	Assess for signs of hypo-kalemia
	Nausea	
		Monitor serum potassium levels

Table 1.4   continued

Electrolyte Imbalance	Clinical Manifestations	Nursing Interventions
Hypocalcemia (Ca+ < 4.5 mEq/L)	Muscle tremors Tetany, twitching Cardiac arrythmias Anxiety, irritability Depression, fatigue Colicky abdominal discomfort Hyperflexia Muscle cramps Numbness and tingling in extremities Carpopedal spasms Chvostek's sign Trousseau's sign	Monitor EKG Monitor serum albumin levels Administer calcium gluconate or calcium chloride per physician's order Assess calcium level
Hypercalcemia (Ca+ > 5.8 mEq/L)	Lethargy Weight loss Dehydration Malaise Confusion, coma Increased thirst Hypertension Anorexia, nausea Constipation Decreased muscle strength Depressed reflexes Increased urinary output	Monitor serum calcium level Administer loop diuretic per physician's order Administer normal saline to hydrate client

Sodium Imbalance

Sodium imbalances are usually associated with fluid volume deficit or excess. Hypernatremia, or excess sodium in the extracellular fluid, is also called hypertonic dehydration or salt excess. The client's serum sodium will be greater than 135 mEq per liter. The causes of hypernatremia include decreased water intake, excessive sodium intake, watery diarrhea, and saltwater near-drowning. Hyponatremia, or sodium deficit of the extracellular fluid (less than 135 mEq per liter), is also called hypotonic dehydration. It can be caused by near exhaustion, excessive excretion of sodium via the kidneys, gastrointestinal suction, repeated administration of water enemas, administration of diuretics, parenteral infusion of an electrolyte-free solution, or freshwater near-drowning.

Potassium Imbalance

Hypokalemia, a deficiency of potassium (serum potassium levels less than 3.5 mEq per liter), is associated with the administration of potent diuretics such as the thiazides, vomiting, ulcerative colitis, diarrhea, or kidney disease. Other causes of decreased serum potassium include potassium-free intravenous fluid therapy and excessive gastrointestinal fluid losses from nasogastric suctioning, vomiting, diarrhea, or intestinal fistula. A potassium loss may also occur in a client with severe burns or diabetic acidosis.

Hyperkalemia, excess potassium at the extracellular level (greater than 5.5 mEq per liter), can be caused by kidney disease, excessive infusion of potassium solutions, adrenal insufficiency, and crushing injuries.

Calcium Imbalance

Hypocalcemia, a deficiency of calcium (plasma calcium usually below 4.5 mEq/L), is associated most frequently with a hypoactive parathyroid gland or its removal, excessive administration of citrated blood, sprue, massive quantities of subcutaneous injections, or generalized peritonitis.

Hypercalcemia, an excess of calcium (plasma calcium greater than 5.8 mEq/L), may be caused by a tumor or hyperactivity of the parathyroid gland, excessive administration of vitamin D, or multiple myeloma.

BIBLIOGRAPHY

Carpenito, L. 1985. *Handbook of nursing diagnosis.* Philadelphia: J. B. Lippincott Co.

Lewis, S., and I. Collier. 1983. *Medical-surgical nursing: assessment and management of clinical problems.* New York: McGraw-Hill Book Co.

UNIT II

PRINCIPLES OF PERIPHERAL IV THERAPY

CHAPTER 2

Peripheral Intravenous Insertion

Phyllis Fichtelman Nentwich, RN, MS

Peripheral IV insertion presents a unique challenge to the nurse. A thorough understanding of the rationale for client and family preparation, the anatomy of the venous structure, and the IV insertion procedure is a prerequisite for safe and successful IV insertion. This chapter will explore all of these elements.

PURPOSE OF IV INSERTION

Prior to the insertion of an IV the purpose for the infusion must be assessed. The implications for intravenous therapy are multiple. No matter what the client's age, an IV may be necessary to administer medications, to replace fluids and electrolytes, or to increase caloric intake when the gastrointestinal route is not a viable choice. Insertion in the hospital setting is required for emergency administration of medication for example, during a cardiac arrest, for restoration of electrolytes, or for blood or blood product administration. In the home, an IV may be inserted for antibiotic or chemotherapy administration or for total parenteral nutrition. The purpose of the infusion has implications for equipment and site selection and patient teaching.

PSYCHOSOCIAL DEVELOPMENT

The second factor to be assessed prior to IV insertion is the psychosocial development of the client. The preparation of the family and client, as well as the diversional techniques used during insertion, are based on this assessment. An understanding of normal growth and development cues the practitioner to the expected client response during insertion. Two noted theorists, Erik Erikson and Jean Piaget, define normal psychosocial development through the age span.

According to Erikson, an infant from birth to 1 year of age is in the oral-sensory stage. The infant is developing trust in the world. If the newborn is supported and basic needs are met consistently, then a sense of trust is developed. However, if the infant experiences a lack of support and deprivation of basic needs, mistrust develops (Salkind 1985, 111).

Piaget describes the first stage of infant development as reflexive in nature. The reflexes (sucking, grasping, crying, and movement of the arms, trunk, and head) are responses to any stimulus. The 1-month-old cannot differentiate among objects (Wadsworth 1973, 36). Therefore, according to Lutz, the infant will respond to the pain of an IV insertion with generalized body movements, withdrawal of the extremity, and irritability in the form of crying (Lutz 1986, Table 1).

To meet the developmental needs of the newborn during IV insertion, the infant should be held by another staff member. This provides a sense of support and also immobilizes the extremity that will respond in a reflexive manner. The assistant can satisfy the infant's need to suck by providing a pacifier during the procedure. Wrapping the infant in a blanket will facilitate the restraining process as well as keep the infant warm. Warming lights should be considered if the infant's temperature is unstable. To prevent possible vomiting and aspiration, avoid feeding the infant immediately prior to the IV insertion.

Preparation for IV insertion at this stage of life is focused primarily on the family. The family should be instructed on the purpose of the IV, possible site placement, and care of the IV after the procedure. Family members should be encouraged to continue the role of supporter after the procedure by providing the infant with visual and tactile stimuli. The family should be shown safe ways to hold and feed the infant (Guhlow 1979, Care Guide). Clarifying any misconceptions about the procedure and providing written information will reinforce the teaching.

The 1- to 8-month-old infant, who is developing hand-mouth coordination, will grasp and manipulate all objects within reach. Infants at this stage will repeat pleasurable experiences, for example by grasping and manipulating the IV tubing. During the insertion process, the IV should be secured well yet provide for visualization of the site. Methods for securing the IV include taping a paper or plastic cup over the needle or catheter or covering the catheter with stockinette with a hole cut for visualization of the site. Both allow the infant to pull or suck on the IV without interfering with the IV site itself. Taping the tubing to the IV board and adding additional tubing to the IV setup will allow the infant to manipulate the IV tubing without disrupting the IV flow. Taping the IV site and tubing securely eliminates the need for extensive restraining of extremities.

Visual and auditory acuity are also developed during this stage as evidenced by the infant's moving in the direction of visual and auditory stimuli. Therefore, effective diversional techniques during the IV insertion procedure include shaking a rattle or playing a lullaby. The infant will focus on brightly colored objects such as a picture or a toy. Thus a brightly decorated treatment room will divert the child's attention.

The 8- to 12-month-old infant clearly shows the ability to anticipate events. Prior to this stage, infants feel that all of their actions cause a response, but now they are aware that actions independent of themselves can have an effect (Wadsworth 1973, 50). Now when the infant enters a treatment room in which the child has experienced a painful event, his or her immediate reaction will be to cry: the treatment room is associated with pain. When the IV site is prepared with iodine, the nurse can expect a similar response. Anticipatory fear is noted when a child's eyes widen and its body becomes stiff or tense. Explaining this to the family ahead of time may decrease their anxiety as they wait for the completion of the procedure.

During this stage the infant begins to search for objects that disappear. Playing peek-a-boo may distract the child during the preparation phase of the procedure. A firm restraining hold during the procedure is necessary for a successful venipuncture. A papoose board may prove helpful in securing the infant. Upon completion of the procedure, the infant should be rocked and cuddled by the family or the nurse to foster the feeling of trust and security.

Toddlers, who are in the muscular-anal stage according to Erikson, are experimenting with their ability to control their own behavior. Careful permissiveness and support on the part of adults result in the child's developing autonomy. Overprotection and lack of support result in self-doubt on the part of the child (Salkind 1985, 111). The toddler reacts to a painful procedure by withdrawing the extremity or by hitting, biting, or kicking and screaming and may use the entire body to resist the caretaker (Lutz 1986, Table 1).

Preparation of the child should be done in simple terms immediately before the procedure to prevent anxiety. Allow the child to explore the equipment such as the tape or armboard. Another person will be required to restrain the child and more importantly to provide reassurance during the procedure. Providing the child with toys to hit or throw allows for expression of anger. This should be done immediately after the procedure and throughout hospitalization. Again, thoroughly securing the IV site and adding additional tubing allow the toddler to explore the environment without interrupting IV therapy.

According to Piaget, the child 3 through 7 years of age is in the preoperational phase. This stage is characterized by the onset of sophisticated language and reasoning (Salkind 1985, 196). Erikson states that the developmental task of this stage is initiative. Encouragement and opportunity foster initiative. Negative feelings and lack of opportunity result in guilt (Salkind 1985, 111). The child is learning to share while attempting to master new skills and independence. Magical thinking is also in operation at this age. Castration fears are common, adding to the fears of intrusive procedures (Guhlow 1979, Care Guide).

The preschooler may attempt to postpone the painful procedure by pretending to be another person or hiding. Aggression is goal-directed. It is not uncommon for the preschooler to push the nurse away, proclaiming "I hate you. Go away!" (Lutz 1986, Table 1).

The preschooler should be prepared for IV therapy just prior to the procedure. It is important to provide the child with as much sense of control over the situation as possible. The nurse can demonstrate the procedure on a doll with play tubing and needles and allow the child to open packages and cleanse the site. The child should be told that crying or even screaming is permitted but that it is important to hold still and that an assistant will help the child do this (Guhlow 1979, Care Guide). Appropriate diversional techniques for this age group include focusing on a cartoon character on the wall, making the sound of a choo-choo train, and cutaneous stimulation (Lutz 1986, Table 1). The speed of the choo-choo train and the strength of rubbing the extremity should increase as the pain of the insertion increases.

The school-age child, aged 6 to 11, is in the stage of industry versus inferiority, according to Erikson. Adequate training supports the ability to solve concrete problems and results in industry. Poor training and lack of direction result in feelings of inferiority (Salkind 1985, 111). The child is struggling between mastering new skills and failing to master them (Guhlow 1979, Care Guide). Relationships with peers are of great importance to the child at this stage. Competition is a key part of life.

The child may act bravely, responding to the painful procedure with passive resistance: the body may become rigid, with clenched teeth or fists. The child may also regress during hospitalization (Lutz 1986, Table 1).

The child and family should be prepared together so that the family can reinforce the teaching. The child's anxiety will be decreased if preparation is done ahead of time on the day of the procedure. Information should be given clearly, using demonstration and allowing an opportunity for questions. The child should be given as much control as possible by being offered realistic choices, including whether or not the parents are to be present during the procedure. The insertion should be performed in the absence of peers so that the child can express discomfort freely. The child should be told that it is acceptable to cry, but ways to control pain, such as relaxation, should be taught in advance.

The 12- to 18-year-old is going through puberty and adolescence. Questions such as "Who am I?" and "What are my beliefs?" are common during this stage. Internal stability and continuity, well-defined sex models, and positive feedback result in the child's developing a clear identity. Confusion of purpose, unclear feedback, and ill-defined expectations result in role confusion (Salkind 1985, 111). The adolescent vacillates between needs for independence and dependence. This age group is particularly concerned with body image, as body changes with maturing sexuality become increasingly evident (Guhlow 1979, Care Guide).

Preparation of the teenager should be at the adult level, allowing time for absorption of the information and as much control over the procedure as possible. Parents need to encourage independence by allowing the youngster to make as many decisions as possible, including whether the parents will be present during the IV insertion. The nurse should offer an in-depth explanation of the reason for the IV therapy, the mechanics of insertion procedure, and what can be expected during IV therapy. The adolescent should be given privacy during the IV insertion so that pain may be expressed openly.

Multiple distraction techniques can be taught ahead of time to both the school-age child and the adolescent. For example, the nurse can use guided imagery or suggest that the child use it to imagine becoming limp like a rag doll, floating on a cloud, or sinking into a soft chair. The technique of positive self-talk through the insertion can also prove successful: the client states, "I can make it. I'm doing great." Progressive relaxation and rhythmic breathing are additional methods of achieving a state of relaxation. Both age groups can be taught to alternate the tensing and relaxing of selected groups of muscles or to take a deep breath and then release it very slowly (Lutz 1986, Table 2). Allowing them to choose a record or tape of background music will not only facilitate relaxation but also enhance their feeling of control over the situation. All of these techniques are also appropriate for adult and gerian clients.

The adult's fears and anxieties can be minimized through teaching. The client should be instructed in the purpose of the IV, the mechanics of the insertion process, and the degree of discomfort to be expected. If the client is agitated or in pain, the procedure should be postponed if possible. If the client is taking a pain medication, the procedure should be done during the drug's peak effectiveness to minimize the pain. Consideration of the client's psychosocial needs prior to insertion will facilitate a successful IV insertion.

SITE SELECTION

An understanding of the anatomy of a vein (Figure 2.1) and the venous system (Figure 2.2) will assist the nurse in selecting the most appropriate IV site.

A vein consists of three layers. The *tunica adventitia* is an outer layer of connective tissue that surrounds and adds support to the vein. The *tunica media* consists of muscle and elastic tissues that constrict and distend the vessel. If your client is relaxed or tense, this is the layer that will dilate or constrict. The third layer, the *tunica intima,* is endothelium. This layer can be injured if traumatized during IV insertion. Injury to the tunica intima will result in roughened endothelial edges and possible adherence of platelets, which may form clots. Semilunar valves (part of the tunica intima) are directed toward the heart and prevent blood from flowing toward the extremities (Masoorlie 1981, 22). Therefore, the direction of the IV needle should always be toward the heart, with the flow of circulation.

Proper venous site selection is the key to a successful venipuncture. The purpose of the IV, duration of therapy, age of the client, condition of the veins, and patient preference are just a few of the factors that must be considered in site selection. Table 2.1 presents guidelines for peripheral IV site selection.

The major peripheral superficial veins may be used for any IV solution or

Figure 2.1   Anatomy of a vein.

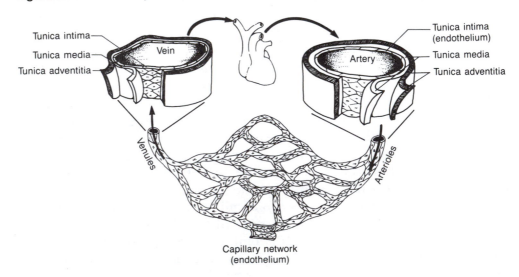

Tunica intima

Tunica media

Tunica adventitia

Vein

Venules

Tunica intima (endothelium)

Tunica media

Tunica adventitia

Artery

Arterioles

Capillary network (endothelium)

Figure 2.2   Anatomy of the venous system.

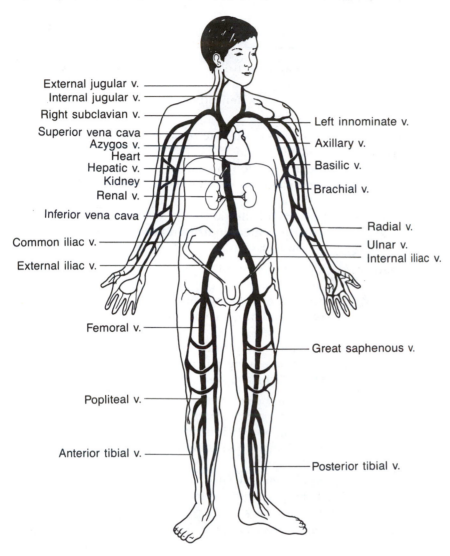

External jugular v.
Internal jugular v.
Right subclavian v.
Superior vena cava
Azygos v.
Heart
Hepatic v.
Kidney
Renal v.
Inferior vena cava
Common iliac v.
External iliac v.
Left innominate v.
Axillary v.
Basilic v.
Brachial v.
Radial v.
Ulnar v.
Internal iliac v.
Femoral v.
Great saphenous v.
Popliteal v.
Anterior tibial v.
Posterior tibial v.

medication preparation except those that are extremely caustic to the venous system. Caustic medications need increased blood volume to dilute them. IV solutions that are *not* recommended for peripheral IV use include dextrose concentrations of greater than 12.5%. Medications such as antilymphocytic globulin may also require central venous access. Irritating drugs such as the penicillins require venous rotation to prevent phlebitis and sclerosis of the veins. The site should be changed every 24 to 36 hours to prevent complications.

Table 2.1   GUIDELINES FOR PERIPHERAL IV INSERTION

Site	Age	Purpose of Therapy	Needle Recommendation
Digital	Neonate–gerian	Fluid and electrolyte replacement Medication administration Heparin lock	Over-the-catheter needle
Metacarpal	Neonate–gerian	Fluid and electrolyte replacement Medication administration Blood and blood component therapy Specimen collection Total parenteral nutrition heparin lock	Over-the-catheter needle Stainless steel needle
Cephalic	Neonate–gerian	Fluid and electrolyte replacement Medication administration Blood and blood component therapy Specimen collection Total parenteral nutrition Heparin lock	Over-the-catheter needle Stainless steel needle
Accessory cephalic	Neonate–gerian	Fluid and electrolyte replacement Medication administration Blood and blood component therapy Specimen collection Total parenteral nutrition Heparin lock	Over-the-catheter needle
Median ante-brachial	Neonate–gerian	Fluid and electrolyte replacement Medication administration Blood and blood component therapy Specimen collection Total parenteral nutrition Heparin lock	Over-the-catheter needle
Basilic	Neonate–gerian	Fluid and electrolyte replacement Medication administration Blood and blood component therapy	Over-the-catheter needle Stainless steel needle

Table 2.1   continued

Site	Age	Purpose of Therapy	Needle Recommendation
		Specimen collection Total parenteral nutrition Heparin lock	
Antecubital fossa	Neonate–gerian	Fluid and electrolyte replacement Medication administration Blood and blood component therapy Specimen collection Total parenteral nutrition · Heparin lock	Over-the-catheter needle Stainless steel needle
Frontal	Neonate–infant	Fluid and electrolyte replacement Medication administration Blood and blood component therapy Specimen collection Total parenteral nutrition Heparin lock	Over-the-catheter needle Stainless steel needle
Superior temporal	Neonate–infant	Fluid and electrolyte replacement Medication administration Blood and blood component therapy Specimen collection Total parenteral nutrition Heparin lock	Over-the-catheter needle Stainless steel needle
Posterior auricular	Neonate–infant	Fluid and electrolyte replacement Medication administration Blood and blood component therapy Specimen collection Total parenteral nutrition Heparin lock	Over-the-catheter needle Stainless steel needle
Great saphenous	Neonate–infant	Fluid and electrolyte replacement Medication administration Blood and blood component therapy Specimen collection	Over-the-catheter needle

Table 2.1   continued

Site	Age	Purpose of Therapy	Needle Recommendation
		Emergency medication administration	
		Heparin lock	
Small saphenous	Neonate– infant	Fluid and electrolyte replacement	Over-the-catheter needle
		Medication administration	
		Blood and blood component therapy	
		Specimen collection	
		Total parenteral nutrition	
		Heparin lock	
Anterior tibial	Neonate– adolescent	Fluid and electrolyte replacement	Over-the-catheter needle
		Medication administration	
		Blood and blood component therapy	
		Specimen collection	
		Total parenteral nutrition	
		Heparin lock	
Dorsalis pedis	Neonate– infant	Fluid and electrolyte replacement	Over-the-catheter needle
		Medication administration	
		Blood and blood component therapy	
		Specimen collection	
		Total parenteral nutrition	
		Heparin lock	

Begin the site selection process by searching for a vein, using a systematic approach. Begin distally and work proximally. If repeat venipunctures are anticipated, *always* choose the most distal site so that the more proximal sites will be available in the future. The ideal vein is one that is long and straight, easily palpated, and easily visualized.

Methods of dilating a vein for palpation and visualization include tourniquet application, heat therapy, and cutaneous stimulation. Apply a tourniquet approximately 2 to 6 inches above the vein to be assessed. The tourniquet should be tight enough for venous distension without occluding arterial flow. Apply the tourniquet for only a few minutes. If the tourniquet does not distend the veins, apply a warm compress to the extremity for 10 to 20 minutes by wrapping it in a warm wet towel and covering it with a plastic wrap. A heating pad will have the same effect. Reapply the tourniquet after the heat therapy and again assess for venous distension. Rubbing the vein toward the tourniquet or patting the vein may allow visualization. Other techniques to dilate the veins include having the client open and close the hand or dangle the extremity below the level of the heart. An infant can be stimulated to cry or placed with the head lower than the trunk to improve visualization of the scalp veins.

Veins of the Upper Extremities

Knowing the location of the major superficial veins can assist the nurse when visualization is not possible. The veins most commonly used in the upper extremities are the digital, metacarpal, cephalic, accessory cephalic, median antebrachial, and basilic veins (Figure 2.3) (Masoorlie 1981, 22). The digital veins can be assessed along the lateral and dorsal segments of the fingers, especially in clients with increased collateral perfusion, as in cystic fibrosis or a cardiac anomaly. A flexible catheter is indicated, and usually the digital veins are large enough to accommodate a large-bore needle. A tongue blade can be used to stabilize the digital vein.

The metacarpal veins are located on the dorsum of the hand proximal to the knuckles. They are formed by the union of the digital veins. This union, or bifurcation, contains a valve, which is the strongest part of the vein. The bifurcation is the best insertion site, because the valve should be able to handle the trauma of venipuncture without infiltration. Either an over-the-catheter needle or a steel needle may be inserted in the metacarpal veins.

Figure 2.3   The major veins of the upper extremities.

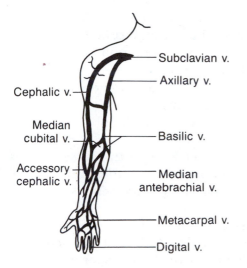

Subclavian v.
Axillary v.
Cephalic v.
Median cubital v.
Basilic v.
Accessory cephalic v.
Median antebrachial v.
Metacarpal v.
Digital v.

The cephalic vein is a continuation of the metacarpal vein of the thumb. It parallels the radial bone and inserts into the antecubital fossa. The advantage of this vein is that it is immobilized by the radial bone; therefore, an arm board is not necessary. Both the cephalic vein and the accessory cephalic vein, which branches off the cephalic vein, can accommodate a large-bore IV catheter.

The median antebrachial vein begins in the palm and travels along the ulnar side of the inner forearm. Venipuncture in this area is extremely painful. However, this vein is easily visualized, especially in children. The size and anatomical position of the vein dictate the use of a small, flexible catheter.

The basilic vein can be visualized along the ulnar bone. It empties into the antecubital fossa. The position of this vein makes it easy to miss and dislodge, since it is located on the underside of the forearm. In order for the nurse to access the site, the client must lie prone, either with the arm at the side or with the elbow bent.

The brachial and cephalic veins travel up into the upper arm and can accommodate a large-bore catheter without the need of an arm board. Use of these veins should be limited to blood specimen collection and emergency medication administration. They should be used for IVs only when other sites are not available. Immobilization of the antecubital space is a necessity but can result in a stiffened joint over a short period of time.

Veins of the Lower Extremities

Research indicates that the veins of the lower extremities should be used sparingly because of an increased complication rate when compared to veins of the upper extremities. The veins most commonly used in the lower extremities include the great and small saphenous, anterior tibial, and dorsalis pedis.

The great saphenous vein (Figure 2.4) is the longest vein in the body. It begins at the dorsal venous arch of the foot and empties into the femoral vein in the groin. The saphenous is easily palpable, but care must be taken not to mistake for it the tendon that parallels the vein. The great saphenous is used frequently in children for an emergency IV access route.

The small saphenous vein begins at the lateral end of the dorsal venous arch of the foot and empties into the popliteal vein in back of the knee. Because of the position of this vein, a protective device must be placed over the IV site.

The anterior tibial vein is the upward continuation of the dorsalis pedis vein and joins the posterior tibial vein to form the deep popliteal vein. Rarely is this vein used for venous access, but in clients with limited venous availability, this vein should be assessed.

The most common veins of the lower extremities are the tributaries of the dorsalis pedis. As with the digital veins of the hand, the dorsalis pedis can accommodate either a stainless steel needle or an over-the-catheter needle. An

Figure 2.4   The major veins of the lower extremities.

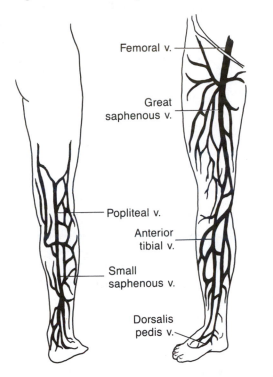

Femoral v.

Great
saphenous v.

Popliteal v.

Anterior
tibial v.

Small
saphenous v.

Dorsalis
pedis v.

arm board will stabilize the foot, but care should be taken to tape the foot in proper anatomical position.

Veins of the Scalp

Use of scalp veins should be limited to children less than 1 year of age. The superficial veins of the scalp are the superior temporal vein, the posterior auricular vein, and the frontal vein. The veins should be well visualized or palpated prior to shaving the scalp site. Shaving of the scalp is indicated for taping but is not necessary for infection control. The veins can be dilated by placing a rubber band around the scalp. A tab of tape will allow easy removal of the rubber band. The needle should be directed toward the heart upon insertion. A protective device such as a paper cup is usually indicated after insertion because of the child's age and activity level.

EQUIPMENT SELECTION

The types of needles most commonly used for peripheral IV insertion are the stainless steel needle, or butterfly, and the flexible over-the-catheter needle. The butterfly is a short metal needle coated with silicone. Metal is a deterrent to bacteria. Therefore, the infection rate associated with butterfly needles has proven to be less than that with plastic over-the-catheter needles. Despite this advantage, the stainless steel needle is indicated only for short-term therapy. The butterfly has a high infiltration rate with limited venous site selection. For example, experience indicates that a butterfly inserted over a joint penetrates the vein wall in a short period of time. Table 2.1 identifies the sites and corresponding needle selection.

Stainless steel needle sizes range from 27 to 19 gauge in order of increasing diameter. A 27-gauge needle is indicated when venous access is limited and IV push medications are prescribed. This needle size is contraindicated for blood and blood products and specimen collection, because blood cells hemolyze as they travel through a small-gauge needle. The 25-gauge butterfly is also indicated when venous access is limited, but it can be used for arterial blood sampling. A needle as small as 23 gauge can be used for fluid and electrolyte replacement, maintenance IV therapy, blood specimen collection, total parenteral nutrition, and administration of medications and blood products. A small-gauge needle is recommended especially with caustic medications such as those used for chemotherapy or antibiotic therapy. The small gauge (large size) allows sufficient blood to flow around the catheter to dilute the drug. Thus the potential for phlebitis is decreased. The optimal needle size for blood administration is a 21-gauge. A 19-gauge or larger should be used for phlebotomies. Both sizes allow for rapid blood administration or withdrawal.

An over-the-catheter needle is a metal stylette with a plastic catheter. The stylette is used for penetration of the skin and vein wall and removed after the catheter is threaded into the vein. Because of the flexibility of the catheter, it can be inserted into any venous site. Also, the infiltration rate appears to be lower than with the stainless steel needle. A disadvantage of the over-the-catheter needle is that frequent blood sampling is more difficult. The smallest over-the-catheter needle is the 24-gauge. Like the 27- and 25-gauge butterfly, a 24-gauge over-the-catheter needle is indicated when venous access is limited. A 22-gauge needle is used for fluid and electrolyte replacement, medication administration, and total parenteral nutrition. The optimal size for blood product administration is the 20-gauge needle. Larger gauges and longer catheters are available for rapid fluid or blood administration.

· The additional equipment needed for venipuncture includes a tourniquet, tape, povidone iodine, alcohol, IV tubing or a 3-ml syringe with normal saline for IV use, and a T-connector. Further equipment depends on the taping technique chosen during insertion.

VENIPUNCTURE PROCEDURE

The insertion technique varies with the client's age. Therefore the step-by-step procedure for IV insertion in a neonate, child, and adult will be discussed separately.

Neonatal Venipuncture Technique

The insertion procedure begins with the nurse and assistant thoroughly washing their hands, assembling all the equipment, and preparing the neonate. Preparation of the neonate begins with explaining the procedure to the family. The body area selected for IV insertion should be made warm—for example, under a warming light or in an isolette. The actual procedure is as follows:

1. Request the assistance of a helper and provide for adequate lighting.
2. Assemble all the equipment within easy reach of your dominant hand.
3. Apply a tourniquet if necessary. If the vein is easily visualized, a tourniquet is not recommended. A tourniquet increases the venous congestion of fragile neonatal veins. Therefore, the veins will tend to roll or infiltrate upon needle puncture. If a tourniquet is necessary for visualization, apply a rubber band approximately half the distance to the next joint. Upon tourniquet placement, palpate for arterial flow. The tourniquet should be tight enough to cause venous distension but loose enough to provide for arterial flow. It should be left in place for no longer than 3 to 5 minutes. The tourniquet should be released after site selection and reapplied after preparing the site.
4. Select the venipuncture site according to the criteria previously outlined.
5. Select the needle based on the criteria discussed. If a stainless steel needle is chosen, immobilize the neonate's extremity on a board prior to insertion. Then flush the tubing with normal saline: the initial blood flashback on a neonate may not be forceful enough for the blood to clear all the air in the tubing.
6. Cleanse the site with a povidone iodine swab and allow it to dry for 30 seconds to provide for antibacterial action.
7. Cleanse the site with alcohol to remove *all* the iodine. Povidone iodine may irritate or burn a neonate's sensitive skin. Allow the alcohol to dry. Alcohol burns as it enters the skin.
8. Holding the skin taut, insert the needle or catheter through the subcutaneous tissue, at approximately a 10- to 30-degree angle, beside or directly into the vein, with the bevel up. As the needle enters the vein, assess for a blood return. This indicates a successful venipuncture. Completion of the procedure is now based on the type of needle inserted.

Insertion of a stainless steel needle

9. Do not advance a stainless steel needle in a neonate. Since visualization of the vein is difficult, advancing the needle may result in tearing the vein.

10. Attach a syringe of normal saline for IV use to the tubing.
11. Release the tourniquet.
12. Gently flush the tubing with the saline while assessing for infiltration.
13. Place a piece of 1/2-inch tape slightly under the wings of the stainless steel needle, adhesive side up.
14. Fold the tape over the wings of the needle at a 90-degree angle in the direction of the needle. The taping will look like an "H."
15. Place a 1/2-inch adhesive bandage with povidone ointment over the insertion site.
16. Curl the remaining tubing on the side of the IV board and secure with tape.
17. Continue to secure the wings of the needle by adding 1-inch strips of tape over the wings but allowing for visualization of the site. Taping the site securely minimizes the need for additional restraining devices such as wrist restraints and allows the neonate freedom of movement.
18. Label the IV site with the type, gauge, and length of catheter; the insertion date; and your initials.

Insertion of an over-the-catheter needle

9. While holding the metal stylette still, advance the catheter hub approximately 1/4 inch with a twisting-pushing motion. This assures that the catheter is also through the vein wall.
10. Assess for continued blood flashback.
11. Continuing to hold the metal stylette still, advance the full length of the catheter into the vein.
12. Gently place pressure over the catheter tip to prevent bleeding while removing the metal stylette.
13. Release the tourniquet.
14. Connect a normal saline syringe, IV tubing, and T-connector with a normal saline syringe or T-connector with IV tubing, and flush the tubing to assure patency without infiltration.
15. Place a 1/2-inch piece of tape approximately 3 inches long under the catheter hub, with the adhesive side up. Fold both sides of the tape toward the center of the catheter to form "wings."
16. Place an additional piece of tape above the wings, adhesive side up, to form the "H" described previously. Fold the tape up at a 90-degree angle to secure the catheter.
17. Place a 1/2-inch adhesive bandage with povidone ointment over the insertion site.
18. Continue to secure the catheter by adding 1-inch strips of tape over the wings, allowing for visualization of the site. Tape the site securely to minimize the use of additional restraining devices such as wrist restraints and to allow the neonate freedom of movement.

19. Secure the neonate's extremity to an arm board if necessary to prevent needle dislodgement.
20. Label the IV site with the type, gauge, and length of the catheter; the insertion date; and your initials.

Pediatric Venipuncture Technique

As with the neonate, preparation begins with hand washing, assembly of the equipment, and preparation of the child and family. The nurse should instruct the child on the procedure at an age-appropriate level and should request the assistance of a helper to support the child emotionally and to restrain the child if necessary. A papoose board may be the restraint of choice for an older infant or toddler. A treatment room or procedure room should be used for the IV insertion. This allows the child to see the hospital room as a "safe" place and the treatment room as the room where all the "ouchy" things happen. Also, the procedure room offers additional lighting and equipment.

1. Assess for a venipuncture site, based on the criteria previously discussed.
2. Select the needle based on the criteria discussed. If a stainless steel needle is chosen, restrain the child's extremity on an arm board prior to insertion. Flush the tubing with normal saline unless a blood specimen is to be collected.
3. Cleanse the site with a povidone iodine swab in a circular fashion and allow it to dry for 30 seconds for antibacterial action.
4. Cleanse the site with alcohol if unable to visualize the vein. Allow the alcohol to dry. Alcohol burns as it enters the skin.
5. Apply tourniquet.
6. Holding the skin taut, insert the needle or catheter through the subcutaneous tissue at approximately a 10- to 30-degree angle, beside or directly into the vein, with the bevel up. As the needle enters the vein, assess for a blood return. This indicates a successful venipuncture. Completion of the procedure is now based on the type of needle inserted.

Insertion of a stainless steel needle

7. Do not advance a stainless steel needle in a child. This may result in tearing the veins, since visualization of the vein is difficult. Support the wings of the needle in the inserted position by placing a cotton ball or sterile gauze pad under the wings during taping.
8. Attach a syringe of normal saline for IV use to the tubing.
9. Release the tourniquet.
10. Gently flush the tubing with the saline while assessing for infiltration.

11. Place a piece of 1/2-inch tape slightly under the wings of the needle, adhesive side up. Support the wings of the needle with a cotton ball or sterile gauze if the needle is not parallel to the skin.
12. Fold the tape over the wings of the needle at a 90-degree angle in the direction of the needle. The taping will look like an "H."
13. Apply a transparent occlusive dressing over the site for ease of visualization.
14. Curl the remaining tubing on the side of the IV board and secure with tape.
15. A clear medicine cup, a paper cup with the bottom cut out, or a stockinette with a hole over the site are just some of the imaginative methods that can be used to protect the IV site, maintain visualization of the site, and minimize the need for restraint of the extremity.
16. Label the IV site with the type, gauge, and length of the catheter; insertion date; and your initials.

Insertion of an over-the-catheter needle

7. While holding the metal stylette still, advance the catheter hub approximately 1/4 inch with a twisting-pushing motion. This assures that the catheter is also through the vein wall.
8. Assess for continued blood flashback.
9. Continue to hold the metal stylette still, and advance the full length of the catheter into the vein.
10. Gently place pressure over the catheter tip to prevent bleeding while removing the metal stylette.
11. Release the tourniquet.
12. Connect a normal saline syringe, IV tubing, and T-connector with a normal saline syringe or T-connector with IV tubing, and flush the tubing to assure patency without infiltration.
13. Place a 1/2-inch piece of tape approximately 3 inches long under the catheter hub, adhesive side up, and fold both sides of the tape toward the center of the catheter to form "wings."
14. Place an additional piece of tape above the wings, adhesive side up, to form the "H" described previously. Fold the tape up at a 90-degree angle to secure the catheter.
15. Apply a transparent occlusive dressing over the site for ease in visualization.
16. Continue to secure the catheter by adding 1-inch strips of tape over the wings but allowing for visualization of the site. Taping the site securely minimizes the need for additional restraining devices such as wrist restraints and allows the child freedom of movement.
17. Secure the child's extremity to an arm board if necessary to prevent needle dislodgement.

18. Label the IV site with the type, gauge, and length of the catheter; the insertion date; and your initials.

Adult Venipuncture Technique

Again the insertion procedure begins with the thorough hand washing, assembly of the equipment, and preparation of the client. Preparation includes discussing the step-by-step procedure with the client and allowing the client to control the procedure as much as possible. For example, permit the client to choose the extremity in which the IV will be inserted. If the client is uncooperative as a result of disease or medications, obtain the assistance of a helper to provide emotional support to the client and to prevent movement during the procedure. The procedure is as follows:

1. Assess for a venipuncture site based on the criteria previously discussed.
2. Select the needle based on the criteria discussed. If a stainless steel needle is chosen, flush the tubing with normal saline unless a blood specimen is to be collected.
3. Cleanse the site with a povidone iodine swab in a circular fashion and allow it to dry for 30 seconds for antibacterial action.
4. Cleanse the site with alcohol if unable to visualize the vein. Allow the alcohol to dry. Alcohol burns as it enters the skin.
5. Inject lidocaine intradermally at the exact insertion site. Use a 25- or 27-gauge needle and 0.1 to 0.2 ml of 0.5% or 1% lidocaine, forming a wheal into which the IV needle will be inserted.
6. Apply the tourniquet.
7. Holding the skin taut, insert the needle or catheter through the subcutaneous tissue at approximately a 10- to 20-degree angle, beside or directly into the vein, with the bevel up. As the needle enters the vein, assess for a blood return indicating successful venipuncture. Completion of the procedure is now based on the type of needle inserted.

Insertion of a stainless steel needle

8. If the vein is easily visualized, carefully advance the steel needle into the vein.
9. Attach a syringe of normal saline for IV use to the tubing or the IV tubing.
10. Release the tourniquet.
11. Gently flush the tubing with the saline or turn the infusion on at a slow rate while assessing for infiltration.
12. Place a piece of 1/2-inch tape slightly under the wings of the needle, adhesive side up.
13. Crisscross the tape over the wings of the needle like a chevron.

14. Apply a Bandaid with povidone iodine ointment over the site and secure the wings with 1-inch pieces of tape.
15. Curl the remaining tubing and secure.
16. Label the IV site with the type, gauge, and length of the needle; the insertion date; and your initials.

Insertion of an over-the-catheter needle

8. While holding the metal stylette still, advance the catheter hub approximately 1/4 inch with a twisting-pushing motion. This assures that the catheter is also through the vein wall.
9. Assess for continued blood flashback.
10. Continuing to hold the metal stylette still, advance the full length of the catheter into the vein.
11. Gently place pressure over the catheter tip to prevent bleeding while removing the metal stylette.
12. Release the tourniquet.
13. Connect a normal saline syringe, IV tubing, and T-connector with a normal saline syringe or T-connector with IV tubing, and flush the tubing to assure patency without infiltration.
14. Place a 1/2-inch piece of tape approximately 3 inches long under the catheter hub, and crisscross the tape in a chevron pattern.
15. Apply a transparent occlusive dressing over the site for ease of visualization or a bandage with povidone ointment.
16. Continue to secure the catheter by adding 1-inch strips of tape over the catheter, allowing for visualization of the site.
17. Secure the extremity to an arm board if necessary to prevent needle dislodgement. Double-back the tape for easy and pain-free removal.
18. Label the IV site with the type, gauge, and length of the catheter; the insertion date; and your initials.

BIBLIOGRAPHY

Anthony, C., and N. Kolthoff. 1975. *Textbook of anatomy and physiology.* Saint Louis: C.V. Mosby Co.

Guhlow, L. J. 1979. Pediatric IV's: special measures you must take. *RN* (March): 40–51.

Jackson, E. 1981. *Nursing photobook: managing IV therapy.* Horsham, Pa.: Internal Communications.

Lutz, W. 1986. Children's responses to pain. *Journal of Pediatric Nursing* 1 (Feb.).

Masoorlie, S. 1981. Toward impeccable IV technique: trouble free IV starts. *RN* 2 (Feb.): 21–33.

Salkind, N. J. 1985. *Theories of human development.* New York: John Wiley & Sons.

Wadsworth, B. J. 1973. *Piaget's theory of cognitive development.* New York: David McKay Co.

CHAPTER 3

Peripheral Intravenous Therapy Maintenance

Phyllis Fichtelman Nentwich, RN, MS

MAINTAINING A PERIPHERAL IV

Intravenous therapy, a method of administering fluids, water, electrolytes, and medications directly into the extracellular tissue via the venous system, bypasses the gastrointestinal tract. It is indicated for clients who are NPO due to surgery, who are dysphagic, or who are unable to take fluids orally for any reason. Clients requiring rapid fluid and electrolyte replacement, as well as clients whose gastrointestinal tract is impaired, are also candidates for IV therapy. Other indications include clients requiring medications that will either be destroyed by gastric secretions or not be absorbed by the gastrointestinal tract and clients receiving blood or blood products. This chapter will describe the mechanisms and nursing implications of maintaining intravenous therapy.

Table 3.1 lists the major steps of maintaining an IV. The text describes each step in depth.

Table 3.1   MAJOR STEPS IN MAINTAINING A PERIPHERAL IV

1. Double-check the physician's order to verify the solution to be infused.
2. Assemble the infusion equipment.
3. Assess the infusing IV solution for clarity, cracks, leaks, and expiration date.

Steps 4–10 should be repeated hourly.

4. Assess the IV tubing for kinks and tight connections.
5. Assess the fluid level of the IV bag to determine the amount to count.
6. Validate that the ordered amount of IV solution has been infused.
7. Calculate the infusion rate.
8. Count the infusion rate hourly.
9. Assess the IV site for evidence of erythema, edema, tenderness, coolness, or exudate.
10. Document the procedure.

Verification of Physician's Orders

Before assembling the IV equipment, the nurse should check the physician's order to verify the solution to be infused. Appropriateness of the solution and rate should also be assessed.

IV additives should be clearly labeled. The manufacturer will describe the solution and specify the expiration date. The client's name, room number, additives with dosage, volume per hour, drip rate, date and time the solution was hung, and nurse's signature should be added to the label. The National Coordinating Committee of Large Volume Parenterals (NCCLVP) recommends that containers be numbered sequentially to decrease administration errors.

Assembling IV Equipment

The first step in assembling IV equipment is to assess the IV solution for clarity and the container for cracks, leaks, and expiration date. IV solutions should be clear and free from foreign substances. Check for cracks and leaks by gently squeezing the IV bag or holding the glass container up to the light and rotating it slowly. Cracks and chips in the glass will reflect the light. Check the expiration date and the medication additive label. The seal on the spike should be intact. The solution should be discarded if any of the following are present: (1) the solution is cloudy or contains particulate matter; (2) the container is cracked or chipped; (3) the expiration date has passed; or (4) the seal is broken.

Selection of the IV tubing is based on the client's infusion needs. According to Centers for Disease Control (CDC) guidelines, IV tubing should be changed every 24 to 48 hours and labeled to indicate the date and time of change.

Vented versus nonvented tubing

Vented tubing must be used in all nonvented IV bottles to allow air to enter the bottle and displace the solution as it flows out. Nonvented tubing should be used with bottles having a built-in air vent and with IV bags.

Macrodrip versus minidrip tubing

Macrodrip tubing is tubing with a large bore drip chamber and a drop factor of 10 to 15 drops per milliliter. It should be used when a large quantity of solution or a fast rate of infusion is required. Microdrip tubing is used when a small amount of solution is to be delivered or when a "keep open" rate is ordered. A microdrip chamber delivers 60 drops per cubic centimeter.

Volume control fluid chamber

A volume control fluid chamber is added to the delivery system when a small amount of fluid or medication is to be administered over an extended period of time. The chamber is graduated in milliliters for accurate assessment of the infusion rate. A volume control fluid chamber can be added to micro-drip tubing or may be manufactured with minidrip tubing attached. A filter may or may not be present in the chamber.

Filters

The first and best defense against contamination is strict aseptic technique. However, filters provide a second line of protection. The function of a filter is to allow fluid, but not particulate matter, to pass.

Filter membranes range in size from 5 microns, the largest bore, to 0.22 microns, the smallest. The smaller the bore, the more particulate matter will be filtered. Sizes 1 to 5 microns remove all particulate matter except fungi and bacteria. Filters of 0.45 micron remove fungi and most bacteria. Filters of 0.22 micron remove all fungi and bacteria. The disadvantage of the smaller bore filter is that the smaller the bore, the more slowly the IV infusion will drip when dependent on gravity.

This final filtration is a practice of controversy. The conclusions of research studies are mixed, with support both for and against the use of final filters. The National Intravenous Therapy Association (NITA), the CDC, and the NCCLVP have developed standards of practice in reference to these conclusions.

NITA recommends the use of 0.22 μm air-eliminating filters

> . . . to protect the patient from induced particles, possible air emboli, pathogenic bacteria (microorganisms) and to minimize the risk of I.V. related complications and sepsis.
>
> NITA's recommendations of practice: (1) the routine use of 0.22 μm air-eliminating filters is advocated in delivering routine I.V. therapy since these filters effectively remove particles and bacteria and prevent air from entering the system; (2) 0.22 μm air-eliminating filters should be routinely changed every 24–48 hours (Harrigan 1985, 428).

The CDC does not recommend the 0.22 μm air-eliminating filter as a routine infection control measure. The CDC categorizes final filtration as Category II, suggesting that studies support the clinical efficacy of these devices but that the rationale for their use may not be clear (Harrigan 1985, 428).

NCCLVP recommends that in-line filters that are microbe and/or particulate retentive be used for clients receiving total parenteral nutrition and for immunocompromised clients such as neonates, burn victims, and those with transplants or with leukemia. Additional recommendations include the use of final filtration for clients receiving infusions with increased particulated additives. The NCCLVP also recommends not infusing drugs through a filter in concentrations of less than 5 μg/ml or in quantities of less than 5 mg over 24 hours unless there are studies verifying that the medication will not bind to the filter (Harrigan 1985, 428).

The use of a filter needle is always recommended when drawing a medication into a syringe from an ampule to remove glass fragments. The needle should be removed or changed before injection into the IV system.

Determining Flow Rates

IV flow rates are determined by the physician. The order is based on several factors: the type and purpose of the solution; the client's hydration, renal, and cardiac status; the client's body size and age; and the size of the vein into which the IV device is inserted.

Several mechanical factors affect IV flow rates, including the type of solution, size and placement of the needle, height of the IV bottle, and patency of the needle. Viscous solutions such as fat emulsions are infused more slowly than 5% dextrose and water. Small-gauge needles (such as 24 or 25 gauge) infuse more slowly than larger gauge needles (such as 18 or 20 gauge). The flow rate will be decreased if the bevel of the IV needle is positioned against the vein wall. The height of the IV bottle affects the rate because of the principle of gravity: the higher the IV container, the faster the flow rate. Therefore, clients should be instructed to place the arm or leg with the IV at heart level when in bed and the arm with the IV across the abdomen when ambulating. The client should avoid combing hair or brushing teeth with the IV arm. Clients should also be instructed not to move the roller clamp or kink the IV tubing. Any of the following will slow the infusion: clot formation, infiltration, phlebitis, venous spasm, lying on the IV extremity, or a constricted BP cuff.

Calculating IV Flow Rates

Three questions must be answered prior to calculating the client's IV flow rate:

1. How much solution did the physician order?
2. How much time is allowed for delivery of this volume?
3. What is the drop factor of the IV tubing?

The volume and time are indicated in the physician's order (e.g., Infuse 400 ml of 5% dextrose and 0.2% NaCl over 8 hours). The drop factor is indicated on the IV tubing box. With this information, the flow can be calculated using the following formula:

$$\frac{\text{Volume (in ml)} \times \text{Drop factor}}{\text{Hour} \times 60 \text{ minutes} = \text{Minutes}} = \text{Drops}$$

Assuming the tubing of choice is a macrodrop (10 drops/ml), the physician's order above would be calculated as follows:

$$400 \text{ ml} \times \frac{10 \text{ gtts}}{\text{ml}} = 4000 \text{ gtts}$$

$$8 \text{ hours} \times 60 \text{ minutes} = 480 \text{ minutes}$$

$$4000 \text{ gtts}/480 \text{ minutes} = 8.3 \text{ gtts/minute}$$
$$\text{or } 8 \text{ gtts/minute}$$

The calculation should be rounded to the nearest whole number.

To insure that the ordered amount is infusing, the nurse should assess the IV container hourly, determine if the amount "to count" is the amount ordered by the physician, and adjust the roller clamp accordingly. A timing label (see Figure 3.1) allows the nurse to make this determination easily. A piece of tape is applied to the IV container and the expected level for each hour is indicated by marking the tape. The amount "to count" is the amount of solution actually remaining in the container upon assessment.

Hourly infusion records are also invaluable tools in assessing and documenting the amount of solution the client is receiving. Figure 3.2 is an example of such a record. The amount infused in the past hour is easily compared to the amount ordered by the physician.

Figure 3.1 Marked solution bottle.

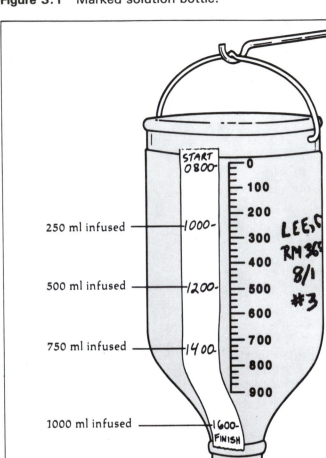

Infusion devices such as pumps and controllers are available when calculation and infusion by gravity flow will not meet the client's needs. Electronic flow devices maintain more accurate flow rates, and some notify the nurse of complications in the infusion. Cost, storage space, and the creation of a false sense of security are all disadvantages of the infusion devices. Several types of device are available, including nonvolumetric, volumetric, and syringe pump.

Nonvolumetric infusion devices deliver solutions in drops per minute. Peristaltic pumps and controllers are examples of such devices. Peristaltic pumps administer the drops per milliliter by milking the tubing. A controller, which works on the principle of gravity, is an electronic flow clamp that adjusts the rate of flow based on the height of the solution. A controller will not add pressure to the IV line and will set off an alarm if the rate cannot be maintained. The purpose of this device is to monitor IV rates only.

Figure 3.2 Infusion record.

DATE:

Time	IV solution	Rate	Amount infused in last hour	Running total of infusion	Comments and site assessment

Volumetric infusion pumps do not operate on the principle of gravity but exert their own pressure to overcome the resistance of the client's pressure. Some deliver a specific volume in a given time (e.g., a certain number of milliliters per hour). Many administer the volume as a continuous infusion. When administering medications, these pumps will maintain constant serum drug levels. Some volumetrics use a piston-cylinder or piston-diaphragm mechanism that acts like a syringe. Solution is drawn into the piston and then delivered from the chamber. Special tubing is frequently required.

Syringe pumps are infusion devices that operate with the use of a syringe or cassette. Minute amounts of medication can be infused slowly and continuously. Bolus amounts can be programmed into the pump to be administered every so many minutes in addition to the maintenance dose. For example, a client receiving patient-controlled analgesia can push the dose button and receive a bolus amount of analgesia as needed. Once a bolus is delivered, the pump will not deliver another until the programmed time has expired. Some pumps also have lock levels requiring code information to change the pump's program. This prevents client overdosing but allows the client the security of knowing that pain relief is available.

Some of the infusion devices currently on the market offer more than just delivery of IV solutions. They also provide digital displays, volume-delivered readouts, and a wide range of flow rates (0.1 ml/hour to 999 ml/hour). A variety of alarms with readout messages are also available, including infusion complete, air in line, occlusion, and low battery.

Additional factors to consider when working with an infusion device include (1) the possibility of RBC hemolysis when using peristaltic infusion devices, (2) the importance of checking the filter's package insert to assure proper functioning with the infusion pump, and (3) the need to add piggybacks or injections above the air-in-line detector to prevent air infusion.

As described, a variety of infusion devices are available for home and hospital use. Nurse and patient education is the most important factor in their safe and efficient use. As technology progresses, precautions must be taken to prevent the nurse from becoming "pump dependent"—that is, relying on the pump rather than nursing judgment to assess complications.

DISCONTINUING A PERIPHERAL IV

The peripheral infusion device should be discontinued if the physician orders it to be discontinued or if a complication of the site has occurred (e.g., phlebitis or infiltration). The IV should be changed routinely every 48 to 72 hours to prevent phlebitis.

To discontinue the IV, begin by checking the physician's order. Then turn the IV off at the tubing roller clamp. Stabilize the needle or catheter with one hand while removing one piece of tape at a time. Assure that all the tape is removed from the skin and remove the needle or catheter by gently withdrawing it at the same angle it was inserted. Immediately apply pressure over the site with sterile gauze until bleeding has stopped. Avoid using an alcohol wipe, because alcohol can reduce clotting time. Assess the site. Cleanse and apply a povidone ointment and a dressing or bandage. Document the procedure and the appearance of the site.

DOCUMENTATION

Documentation of the insertion, maintenance, and discontinuation of an intravenous infusion serves as a legal account of the hourly IV assessment. As discussed in Chapter 2, the date, time of insertion, type and gauge of needle, insertion site, and client's response to the procedure should be documented at the time of needle or catheter insertion. The example below demonstrates such documentation.

Example 1: May 24, 1989   1030   20-gauge angiocatheter inserted into the left antecubital space. Site without signs of erythema, exudate, or edema. Patient cooperated during procedure.

An hourly infusion record or shift graphics sheet should indicate the solution infusion hourly or per shift. The amount "to count" and the hourly rate of the infusion should also be documented on this form. The nurse's notes or other designated form should also include documentation of the appearance of the IV site. For example, upon assessment of the IV site or at discontinuation of the IV, the record will indicate if the IV site is free of signs of redness, swelling, exudate, or pain. When the IV is discontinued, the reason for the procedure and any relevant nursing actions should be documented as shown below.

Example 2: May 24, 1989   1400   IV site in left antecubital space appeared red with 2-cm area of edema. IV discontinued and a Williams wrap applied.

CONCLUSION

The National Intravenous Therapy Association and the Centers for Disease Control each publish standards of care designed to assist hospital and home care agency administrators in writing policies and procedures. Following these standards of care in the maintenance of intravenous therapy will assist in the prevention of IV complications.

BIBLIOGRAPHY

Harrigan, C. A. 1985. Care and cost justification of final filtration. *NITA* 8 (Sept./Oct.).

CHAPTER 4

Peripheral Intravenous Therapy Complications

Phyllis Fichtelman Nentwich, RN, MS

Infiltration
Thrombophlebitis
Catheter Embolism
Hematoma
Infection of the Venipuncture Site
Systemic Infection
Circulatory Overload
Air Embolism
Hypersensitivity
Speed Shock

In this age of technology, intravenous therapy is a major part of everyday nursing care. Though routine in nature, IV therapy presents several risks for the client. This chapter will discuss peripheral intravenous therapy complications, including their causes, clinical manifestations, and nursing management.

INFILTRATION

Definition

An infiltration, the most common peripheral IV complication, is a significant leakage of IV fluid or blood into the extravascular tissue.

Etiology

An infiltration occurs when the venipuncture needle penetrates through the vein or becomes fully or partly dislodged from the vein. This allows IV fluid to flow into the surrounding tissues until swelling blocks the IV needle or catheter opening. An infiltration may also occur if the infusing device has not been positioned correctly in the vein when initially inserted. An infiltration does not occur until there has been significant seepage of IV fluids. Tissue necrosis and sloughing may result if the infusing fluid is caustic to the tissue. Highly irritating fluids include total parenteral nutrition, chemotherapeutic agents, aminophylline, and antibiotics.

Clinical manifestations

An infiltration is characterized by pain and edema at the insertion site and coolness of the adjacent skin. Part or all of the limb may be swollen. An absence of blood backflow when the IV is lower than the limb or disconnected at the site is another sign of an infiltration. The gravitational flow of the IV may also be sluggish.

Nursing implications

If an infiltration is suspected, place a tourniquet above the IV site; if the IV continues to flow by gravity, an infiltration has occurred. Another way to test for an infiltration is to lower the IV bag below heart level: absence of blood indicates an infiltration.

Once an infiltration has been identified, the IV should be discontinued immediately. If the complication has been assessed within 1/2 hour of infiltration and the edema is minimal, ice will decrease further edema. Moist heat will facilitate the absorption of fluid at grossly infiltrated sites.

Prevention measures include stabilization of the site upon insertion, avoidance of insertion over joints, insertion of small-lumen catheters, and assessment of the IV site at least hourly.

THROMBOPHLEBITIS

Definition

Phlebitis is the inflammation of a vein, and thrombosis is the formation of a clot in the blood vessel. Therefore, thrombophlebitis is the inflammation of a vein caused by clot formation.

Etiology

Thrombophlebitis may be caused by an injury or irritation to the vein or by clot formation. The vein may be injured during venipuncture or by movement of the needle during therapy. Irritation to the vein may occur as a result of long-term IV therapy, irritating or incompatible IV additives, use of a vein that is too small for the IV flow rate, or use of a needle or catheter size inappropriate for the vein size. A sluggish flow rate may cause clot formation.

Clinical manifestations

Thrombophlebitis appears as a vein that is sore, hard, cordlike, and warm to the touch. A red line above the venipuncture site is the major sign of thrombophlebitis. Other symptoms include a sluggish flow rate and edema in the limb.

Nursing implications

Upon assessment of thrombophlebitis, the infusion should be discontinued and the needle or catheter removed. The application of a warm compress will increase client comfort.

Preventive measures include firm stabilization of the infusion device, adequate dilution of irritating additives, and infusion of compatible drug additives. A small-gauge needle is recommended for the infusion of caustic drugs. The small lumen allows the blood to circulate quickly around the catheter and dilute the drug. The catheter should be removed every 48 hours and reinserted in a different location. Insertion of IVs over joints, where movement of the catheter will occur, should be avoided.

CATHETER EMBOLISM

Definition

A catheter embolism is a free-floating or dislodged fragment of a catheter in the circulatory system. This usually occurs with flexible catheters rather than with needles.

Etiology

An embolism can occur upon insertion when the catheter is withdrawn before the needle, when the needle is rethreaded into the catheter, or when the catheter is not secured to the skin.

Clinical manifestations

The signs and symptoms of a catheter embolism include a decrease in blood pressure, a rise in central venous pressure, discomfort along the vein, a weak, rapid pulse, and cyanosis and unconsciousness.

Nursing implications

Upon assessment of these signs and symptoms, the IV should be immediately discontinued and the catheter inspected for rough edges that might indicate loss of fragments. A tourniquet should be applied above the site and an X ray obtained to determine if fragments are present. Surgical removal of the fragments may be necessary.

HEMATOMA

Definition

Hematoma is the seepage of blood into the extravascular tissue.

Etiology

A hematoma may occur when clients with coagulation defects are undergoing venipuncture or are being maintained on IV therapy or when anticoagulant therapy is being administered to a client.

Clinical manifestations

A hematoma is characterized by discoloration of the tissue at the IV site, with or without edema.

Nursing implications

Upon initiation of therapy, palpate the vein and slowly advance the catheter to prevent the needle from puncturing both vein walls. Assess the IV site hourly for signs of hematoma, and discontinue the device if edema appears. When discontinuing the IV, apply pressure for 5 minutes.

INFECTION OF THE VENIPUNCTURE SITE

Etiology

Infection of the venipuncture site is a result of a break in aseptic technique. The organisms most frequently involved are *Staphylococcus aureus, Klebsiella, Serratia,* and *Pseudomonas aeruginosa.* These organisms can be transferred to the infusion site through poor aseptic technique either during IV insertion or secondary to the use of contaminated IV equipment.

Clinical manifestations

An infected IV site appears red, sore, and edematous, and may contain discharge that is purulent and foul smelling. If the infection is not treated, septic phlebitis may occur. In this condition, purulent material collects in the infected vein, leading to a systemic infection.

Nursing implications

Upon assessment of a localized infection, the infusion device should be removed and the drainage and catheter tip cultured. The site should be cleansed with povidone iodine and bandaged. Treatment for septic phlebitis involves either stripping the vein surgically or a resection of the infected portion. Prevention measures include the following: restarting the IV every 48 to 72 hours, preferably in a different extremity; adhering strictly to aseptic technique when in contact with IV equipment; assessing the IV solution for evidence of contamination; changing the IV tubing every 24 to 48 hours; and changing the IV dressing whenever it becomes wet or moist.

SYSTEMIC INFECTION

Definition

A systemic infection is an infection of the blood stream.

Etiology

Like a local infection, a systemic infection is caused by poor aseptic technique. A break in asepsis can occur during insertion, maintenance, or drug infusion. Either contaminated equipment or a small clot dislodged by irrigating a clotted IV catheter or needle provide an excellent medium for bacterial growth in the bloodstream.

Clinical manifestations

A client with a systemic infection will exhibit a sudden rise in temperature and pulse with chills and shaking. Subsequently, the client's blood pressure will decrease.

Nursing implications

The appropriate nursing action is to discontinue the IV immediately and send all the equipment to the laboratory for culture analysis. The client should be assessed for other sources of infection by culturing urine, sputum, and blood. A broad-spectrum antibiotic should be administered as ordered.

CIRCULATORY OVERLOAD

Definition

Circulatory overload is an excess of fluid volume in the circulatory system.

Etiology

This complication can be caused by infusion of an excessive amount of fluid at a rate greater than the client can absorb or excrete.

Clinical manifestations

The client experiencing circulatory overload will exhibit the following clinical signs: a rise in blood pressure and central venous pressure, dilatation of the neck veins, shortness of breath, and tachypnea with rales. The client's intake and output will vary significantly.

Nursing implications

Upon assessment of circulatory overload, slow the infusion to a "keep open" rate, raise the client's head to 45 degrees, monitor vital signs, and administer oxygen if indicated. Keep the client warm to increase peripheral circulation. Circulatory overload can be prevented by calculating the client's IV rate accurately and closely assessing the client's intake and output.

AIR EMBOLISM

Definition

An air embolism is the entry of a bubble of air into the client's circulatory system.

Etiology

An air embolism can occur during intravenous therapy if the IV container becomes empty, if air enters the IV tubing or is not initially purged from the tubing, or if the IV connections become loose, allowing air to enter.

Clinical manifestations

A client experiencing an air embolism will have a sudden drop in blood pressure, a rise in central venous pressure with cyanosis, and a weak, rapid pulse leading to loss of consciousness.

Nursing implications

The client should be turned onto the left side with the head lower than the heart. Oxygen should be administered if indicated and the IV system assessed for the source of air.

An air embolism can be prevented by removing all the air from the IV line or syringe of IV medication prior to administration, securing all IV connections, and frequently assessing the IV fluid level so that an IV bottle, bag, or Volutrol does not become empty.

HYPERSENSITIVITY

Definition

Hypersensitivity is an allergic reaction.

Etiology

This reaction may be to IV solutions or additives, cleansers, tape, ointment, or infusion devices.

Clinical manifestations

A localized reaction is manifested by a wheal at the IV site with redness and itching. A systemic reaction produces a generalized rash with pruritus and shortness of breath. The most severe form of systemic reaction is anaphylactic shock, a rapidly occurring condition characterized by increased irritability, dyspnea, cyanosis, sometimes convulsions, unconsciousness, and death.

Nursing implications

A hypersensitive reaction can be prevented by assessing the client for all known allergies prior to IV insertion. Upon assessment of a local reaction, remove the source of irritation by discontinuing the infusion, changing the IV dressing to remove the antiseptic ointment, and applying a hypoallergenic tape. Nursing actions for a systemic allergic reaction include slowing the infusion to maintain a "keep open" rate, elevating the head of the bed, administering oxygen if indicated, and notifying the physician.

SPEED SHOCK

Definition

Speed shock is a rapid change in the venous system usually resulting in hypertension.

Etiology

Speed shock can be caused by administering drugs or bolus infusions too quickly.

Clinical manifestations

A client experiencing this complication may exhibit a flushed face, headache, tight feeling in the chest, and irregular pulse. Loss of consciousness leading to shock and cardiac arrest can occur if the situation continues unchecked.

Nursing implications

The drug infusion should be discontinued immediately. However, an IV solution of 5% dextrose in water should be maintained to keep the vein open. Notify the physician immediately for further treatment. Speed shock can be prevented by administering drugs and bolus infusions at the prescribed rate.

UNIT III

PRINCIPLES OF CENTRAL VENOUS CATHETER CARE

CHAPTER 5

Central Venous Catheter Insertion

Phyllis Fichtelman Nentwich, RN, MS

The insertion of a central venous catheter was once reserved for the acutely ill client in whom peripheral venous access was not available. Central venous catheter placement is now part of the protocol for long-term caustic drug administration, frequent blood sampling, or administration of total parenteral nutrition. This chapter will discuss the purpose and types of central venous catheters, site selection and insertion techniques, maintenance, and complications of central venous access.

PURPOSE OF CENTRAL VENOUS CATHETER PLACEMENT

A central venous catheter (CVC) can have multiple purposes. It may be inserted for physiological assessment of the acutely ill client; monitoring of central venous pressure, pulmonary capillary wedge pressure, or cardiac output; or rapid infusion of IV solutions or blood products. Long-term CVC placement is indicated for the client with limited venous access requiring caustic drug administration, such as chemotherapy, antibiotics, or total parenteral nutrition. Caustic drug infusion in a large vessel allows dilution of the drug, thus preventing phlebitis. Multiple-lumen catheters utilize CVC placement to the fullest by providing routes for a variety of solutions at the same time.

TYPES AND INSERTION TECHNIQUES OF CENTRAL VENOUS CATHETERS

Hickman Catheters

The Hickman catheter, introduced in 1979, is a modification of the Broviac catheter (Moore 1983, 35). Both are Silastic indwelling catheters with a small Dacron cuff approximately 25 cm from the end of the catheter (Figure 5.1).

The Broviac or Hickman catheter can be placed via the subclavian vein, cephalic vein, or femoral and inferior vena cava. Insertion is done under local or general anesthesia. Using sterile technique, a small incision is made, the vein of choice is located, and subcutaneous tunnel and exit site are created. The catheter is introduced through the tunnel and threaded into the vein. The Dacron cuff is placed approximately 25 cm from the exit site. Both sites are sutured closed. Placement is verified by radiography.

Advantages of this catheter are: (1) it is a flexible catheter and (2) the insertion site of the catheter is removed from the exit site. This assists in the prevention of systemic infection. Additionally, once the tissue adheres to the Dacron cuff, another barrier to infection is created, and the secured cuff prevents catheter dislodgement. The main disadvantage is that the catheter is outside the body and thus provides a vehicle for infection. Additional disadvantages are that it requires daily flushes and frequent dressing changes and creates limitations for swimming or bathing.

Figure 5.1 Anatomical placement of a central venous infusion line.

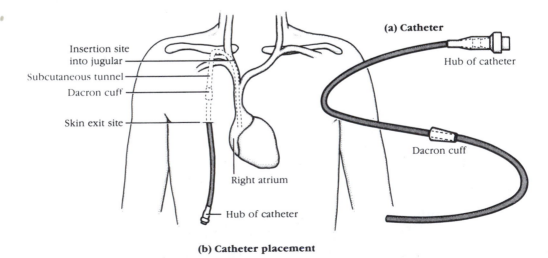

Insertion site into jugular

Subcutaneous tunnel

Dacron cuff

Skin exit site

Right atrium

Hub of catheter

(a) Catheter

Hub of catheter

Dacron cuff

(b) Catheter placement

Multiple-lumen catheters consist of two or three ports feeding into one insertion site. This allows for simultaneous infusion of incompatible solutions.

Implantable Catheters

Infuse-a-Ports or Port-a-Caths are infusion systems that contain a self-sealing injection port connected to catheter tubing implanted in the chest wall. Like the Hickman or Broviac catheters, the systems can deliver chemotherapeutic agents, total parenteral nutrition, antibiotics, and blood products, and blood samples can be obtained.

Insertion is completed under anesthesia using sterile technique. For placement into the subclavian vein, an incision is made on the anterior chest wall just medial to the shoulder. The catheter is inserted through the cephalic and subclavian veins terminating in the superior vena cava or right atrium. Verification is completed by radiography. The catheter is routed through a subcutaneous tunnel to a site prepared for the injection port. Preparation of the site is completed by surgically creating a large subcutaneous pocket. The unit is then sutured into place and heparinized (Sellu 1985, 40–41). Both incisions are closed and covered with a transparent dressing.

The main advantage of this system is that no part of it is exposed outside the body. Research has indicated that the infection rate is low and catheter displacement and venous occlusion are rare (Speciale 1985, 41). Ease of care is another advantage. When the port is not in use, it only requires flushing every 5 to 6 weeks and does not require a dressing after the incision heals.

Implantable catheters should be avoided in clients who have or might develop peritonitis or an allergic reaction or who are extremely susceptible to infections.

Prior to infusion, the implantable device should be palpated and the skin thoroughly cleansed with a povidone-iodine solution. A Huber point needle with a stopcock and extension tubing is primed with a heparin solution. The center of the device is palpated with sterile gloves and the Humber needle is inserted into the center of the port until the needle stops. To prevent cutting the septum by twisting or tilting the needle, a sterile gauze is secured under the needle and a transparent dressing is applied. Infusion can be bolus or continuous via the stopcock. Upon completion of the infusion, 6 ml of a heparin solution are infused and the needle is removed without twisting or tilting (Speciale 1985, 43).

Cutdown Catheters

A cutdown catheter is used when peripheral vein visualization is limited or in an emergency situation. Various types of catheters are used for the cutdown procedure. Whether a cutdown catheter or an over-the-catheter needle is used, the surgical procedure is the same. Using aseptic technique, the site is prepped with povidone-iodine and an incision is made over the vein site. The surgeon identifies the vein, punctures the site, and threads the flexible catheter into place. The incision is sutured and a dressing is applied. This procedure is rarely used with Hickman, Broviac, or implantable catheters. The main advantage of the cutdown catheter is that insertion can be completed on the client's unit or in an emergency setting. Since the catheter is inserted peripherally, its use is for short-term therapy only.

Jugular/Subclavian Catheters

An inside-the-needle catheter can be inserted via the jugular or subclavian vein. Like the cutdown catheter, this catheter can be inserted on the client's unit when emergency venous access is needed or when only the chest and arms are accessible, as in the case of burns. Though placed in a large-bore vein, the inside-the-needle catheter is associated with an increased incidence of occlusion, phlebitis, and infection. Catheter sensitivity due to the firmness of the catheter also occurs.

In the Trendelenburg position, the client is positioned on the back with the head down. This position exposes the sternal and clavicular portions of the sternocleidomastoid muscle. The client's head is turned away from the site. The site is prepped with a povidone-iodine solution and a local anesthetic is injected. The inside-the-needle catheter is advanced into the cervical space and fed into the subclavian vein or right atrium via the internal jugular. The obturator and needle are withdrawn and the plastic needle guard placed. Gauze or transparent dressing is applied, and placement is verified by radiography.

BIBLIOGRAPHY

Moore, D. J. 1983. Venous access using a Hickman catheter. *Irish Medical Journal* 76 (Jan.):35–36.

Sellu, D. 1985. Long-term intravenous therapy. *Nursing Times* (May 22):40–42.

Speciale, J. L., and J. Kaalaas. 1985. Infuse-a-Port: new path for I.V. chemotherapy. *Nursing 85* (Oct.):40–43.

West, R., ed. 1981. *Nursing Photobook: Managing I.V. Therapy.* Horsham, Pa.: Intermed Communications.

CHAPTER 6

Central Venous Catheter Maintenance

Phyllis Fichtelman Nentwich, RN, MS

Central Venous Catheter Dressing Change
Changing IV Tubing on a Central Venous Catheter
Heparinization of a Central Venous Catheter
Changing an Injection Cap on a Central Venous Catheter
Drawing Blood from a Central Venous Catheter

The goal of maintaining a central venous catheter is to prevent complications such as infection, occlusion, and air emboli. This chapter will discuss nursing measures to prevent these complications.

CENTRAL VENOUS CATHETER DRESSING CHANGE

The main site of infection of a central venous catheter (CVC) is the catheter exit site. The application of a sterile occlusive dressing will assist in the prevention of microorganisms at the site. Two types of dressing changes, transparent and gauze, will be discussed. Both types are based on the same principles of cleansing; only the dressing itself differs.

A CVC dressing in the hospital setting should be changed every 48 to 72 hours or more frequently if the dressing becomes wet or loosened. In the home setting, gauze and transparent dressings should be changed weekly. Masks and gowns are recommended for all people present during the dressing change in the hospital environment. The client should be instructed to wear a mask or turn the head away from the site. Masks and gowns are not necessary in the home setting.

The following steps outline the procedure for the dressing change:

1. After thoroughly washing hands, remove the old dressing cautiously. This prevents contamination of the area and avoids dislodging the catheter.
2. Don sterile gloves and place the equipment within easy reach.
3. Cleanse the area from the insertion site outward, using a circular motion and covering an area approximately 2 to 3 inches in diameter, with three acetone-alcohol swabs.
4. Repeat step 3 with three povidone-iodine swabs. Allow the povidone-iodine to dry approximately 30 seconds for antibacterial action.
5. Apply povidone-iodine ointment to the catheter insertion site.
6. For a gauze dressing, apply a slit 2 × 2 inch gauze pad around the catheter insertion site and cover with another gauze. Apply an occlusive dressing covering with tape. For a transparent dressing, apply an occlusive dressing with the transparent sheet.
7. Secure the remaining catheter and tubing with tape to prevent dislodgement. Avoid occluding or kinking the tubing.
8. Label the dressing with the date, time of dressing change, and your initials.
9. Document the procedure and appearance of the insertion site in the nursing record.

CHANGING IV TUBING ON A CENTRAL VENOUS CATHETER

1. Prepare the environment by washing your hands and cleansing the bedside table with alcohol.
2. Prime the new IV tubing, maintaining sterility of distal end of tubing.
3. Open package of sterile gloves. Using the package as a sterile barrier, add 4 × 3 inch gauze to the sterile barrier, Betadine swab, and alcohol swab stick.
4. Don sterile gloves.
5. Pick up catheter with sterile 4 × 3 inch gauze.
6. Scrub catheter junction with Betadine for 1 minute.
7. Allow junction to air-dry for 1 minute.
8. Scrub catheter junction with alcohol for 1 minute.
9. Using 4 × 3 inch gauze as a sterile protector, clamp catheter and disconnect old IV tubing.
10. Turn on new IV solution, using 4 × 3 inch gauze as sterile protector.
11. Pick up new IV tubing with 4 × 3 inch gauze and let fluid drip into hub of catheter until completely filled.
12. Connect IV tubing to catheter.
13. Unclamp catheter.

14. Assure the solution is being infused.

15. Tape catheter/tubing connection and secure to client's dressing.

The procedure for the reconnection of an infusion to a capped central venous catheter is the same as that just described with the following difference. Before connecting the IV tubing, flush the catheter with 3 to 5 ml of normal saline to assure patency of the catheter. Sterile technique should be maintained while drawing up and injecting the saline.

HEPARINIZATION OF A CENTRAL VENOUS CATHETER

The purpose of CVC heparinization is to prevent catheter clot formation when the catheter is not in use. The strength of heparin to be infused is based on the client's body size:

- For clients of less than 5 kg, infuse 1 ml of 10 units/ml every 12 hours
- For pediatric clients weighing more than 5 kg, infuse 1 ml of 100 units/ml every 12 hours
- For adult clients, infuse 1 1/2 ml of 100 units/ml every 12 hours.

The procedure is as follows:

1. Prepare the environment by washing your hands and cleansing the bedside table with alcohol.
2. Using a small-gauge needle and 3-ml syringe, draw up the appropriate amount of heparin. Assure that all air is removed from the syringe and needle.
3. Scrub the end of the heparin cap for 1 minute with a povidone-iodine swab stick.
4. Allow the povidone-iodine to dry for 1 minute.
5. Scrub the end of the heparin cap for 1 minute with an alcohol swab stick.
6. Insert syringe into heparin cap and gently flush catheter. Stop the infusion if resistance is met.
7. Withdraw the needle as the last 0.25 ml of the heparinized solution is injected.
8. Tape and secure the catheter junction to the patient's CVC dressing.

CHANGING AN INJECTION CAP ON A CENTRAL VENOUS CATHETER

The injection cap on a central venous catheter should be changed every 48 hours or after blood has been drawn.

1. Prepare the environment by washing your hands and cleansing the bedside table with alcohol.
2. Open package of sterile gloves. Using the package as a sterile barrier, add 4 × 3 inch gauze, sterile injection port, 3-ml syringe, small-gauge needle, Betadine swab, and alcohol swab stick.
3. Don one sterile glove. Using aseptic technique, draw up appropriate amount of heparin solution.
4. Don second glove. Flush air out of heparin syringe and insert into heparin cap. Fill injection cap with heparin. Leave the needle in the rubber cap.
5. Pick up catheter with sterile 4 × 3 inch gauze.
6. Scrub catheter junction with Betadine for 1 minute.
7. Allow junction to air-dry for 1 minute.
8. Scrub catheter junction with alcohol for 1 minute.
9. Using 4 × 3 inch gauze as sterile protector, clamp catheter and disconnect old injection cap.
10. Pick up heparin syringe attached to new injection cap.
11. Fill hub of catheter with drops of heparin.
12. Twist new injection cap onto catheter.
13. Unclamp catheter.
14. Flush catheter with ordered amount of heparin solution.
15. Withdraw needle from injection cap while flushing last 0.25 ml of solution.
16. Tape junction and secure catheter to client's dressing.

DRAWING BLOOD FROM A CENTRAL VENOUS CATHETER

Before performing this procedure, an order should be obtained for the maximum amount of blood that may be drawn at one time.

1. Prepare the environment by washing your hands and cleansing the bedside table with alcohol.
2. Open package of sterile gloves. Using the package as a sterile barrier, add a 4 × 3 inch gauze, sterile injection port, a 3-, 5-, and 10-ml syringe; small-gauge needle, Betadine swab, alcohol swab stick, and the appropriate syringes and needles for blood collection.
3. Place the vials of heparin solution and normal saline and appropriate blood tubes next to sterile field.
4. Don one sterile glove. Using aseptic technique, draw up appropriate amount of heparin solution and 5 to 10 ml of normal saline.
5. Don second glove. Flush air out of heparin syringe and insert into heparin cap. Fill injection cap with heparin. Leave the needle in the rubber cap.

6. Pick up catheter with sterile 4 × 3 inch gauze.
7. Scrub catheter junction with Betadine for 1 minute.
8. Allow junction to air-dry for 1 minute.
9. Scrub catheter junction with alcohol for 1 minute.
10. Using 4 × 3 inch gauze as a sterile protector, clamp catheter and disconnect old injection cap.
11. Attach 5-ml syringe and withdraw appropriate amount of blood discard. (The amount of discard is determined by the size of the catheter lumen, approximately 5 ml.)
12. Clamp the catheter lumen.
13. Attach syringe for blood collection.
14. Withdraw appropriate amount of blood for ordered blood tests.
15. Clamp the catheter lumen.
16. Attach syringe with normal saline; unclamp catheter and gently flush.
17. Clamp catheter.
18. Pick up heparin syringe attached to new injection cap.
19. Fill hub of catheter with drops of heparin.
20. Twist new injection cap onto catheter.
21. Unclamp catheter.
22. Flush catheter with ordered amount of heparin solution.
23. Withdraw needle from injection cap while flushing last 0.25 ml of solution.
24. Tape junction and secure catheter to client's dressing.
25. Inject blood into appropriate specimen tubes.

CHAPTER 7

Central Venous Catheter Complications

Phyllis Fichtelman Nentwich, RN, MS

Complications During Insertion
> Inadvertent Arterial Puncture
> Pneumothorax, Hydrothorax, and Hemothorax
> Catheter Embolism
> Subclavian Vein Thrombosis
> Hemorrhage/Hematoma
> Improper Catheter Tip Location
> Brachial Plexus Injury
> Extravasation

Infusion-related Complications
> Catheter Occlusion
> Air Embolism
> Catheter-related Sepsis

Though the advantages of central venous catheter placement outweigh the disadvantages, significant risks are associated with the insertion and maintenance of a central venous catheter. This chapter will identify the clinical manifestations, nursing implications and preventive measures for each complication.

COMPLICATIONS DURING INSERTION

Inadvertent Arterial Puncture

Inadvertent arterial puncture is the cannulation of an artery rather than a vein during catheter insertion. The clinical manifestations of this complication include bright red blood return with a high back pressure. The nursing implications are those of any arterial cannulation: remove the cannula immediately and apply a sterile pressure dressing to the insertion site for approximately 10 minutes. Proper site assessment and client immobilization during insertion will assist in the prevention of this complication.

Pneumothorax, Hydrothorax, and Hemothorax

Sharp chest pain, cough, decrease in breath sounds, dyspnea, cyanosis, and shock are the clinical manifestations of a pneumothorax, hydrothorax, or hemothorax.

A pneumothorax occurs when the pleura is punctured by the catheter. As the prefix indicates, a hydrothorax results when fluid is infused directly into the chest. A hemothorax occurs as a result of traumatization of the subclavian vein or vessels around the insertion site that allows blood to leak slowly into the thorax.

Preventive measures include proper assessment of venous placement and client immobilization during insertion. Upon assessment of the complication, the nurse should monitor vital signs, notify the physician, prepare the client for chest X rays, and prepare for the insertion of a chest tube if ordered.

Catheter Embolism

Manipulation of the catheter and needle during insertion can shear off the tip of the catheter causing a catheter embolism. Signs and symptoms of this complication vary, depending on where the segment lodges, but include irregular pulse, chest pain, dyspnea, and increased temperature. Nursing implications include monitoring vital signs, notifying the physician, and preparing the client for a chest X ray. Upon verification of the embolism, the segment must be surgically removed by the physician.

Subclavian Vein Thrombosis

Clot formation in the vessel containing the catheter is identified as a subclavian vein thrombosis. The clot may dislodge and become an emboli. Acute pleuritic chest pain, shortness of breath, and unilateral edema of the arm, neck, or face on the side of the catheter are the clinical manifestations of a subclavian vein thrombosis. The nurse should notify the physician and prepare the client for an upper extremity venogram and the removal of the catheter if ordered. Administering the appropriate amount of heparin at the ordered times will prevent clot formation.

Hemorrhage/Hematoma

A bloodstained dressing, frank blood at the insertion site, or bruising indicates hemorrhage or a hematoma. This complication can be prevented by maintaining a pressure dressing over the insertion site for 1 hour after a Broviac or Hickman catheter placement. Nursing implications include applying a sterile pressure dressing over the site, notifying the physician, monitoring vital signs, and elevating the head of the bed to a 30-degree angle unless contraindicated.

Improper Catheter Tip Location

When the tip of the catheter lies in a branch vessel, the right atrium, or the right ventricle but not in the vena cava, it is improperly placed. This complication is identified when an X ray is taken to verify placement of the catheter. Arrhythmias and pain and/or edema of the head, neck, or arm on the catheter side are clinical manifestations of improper catheter tip location. Upon assessment of these signs and symptoms, notify the physician and prepare the client for a chest X ray. The physician will move the catheter to its proper location and x-ray the site again for confirmation of placement. Immediate X ray confirmation will prevent the signs and symptoms of this complication.

Brachial Plexus Injury

Brachial plexus injury occurs when the network of spinal nerves that supplies the arm, forearm, and hand is injured. Clinical manifestations include tingling of the fingers, pain in the arm, and sensory-motor deficit or paralysis in the arm or hand. Immobilizing the client during catheter insertion will assist in preventing this complication. Long-term physical therapy may assist in returning function to the affected limb.

Extravasation

Extravasation is the infusion of fluid into tissues outside the vein. The clinical manifestations are similar to those of a peripheral infiltration: pain; edema of the neck, chest, or arm on the catheter side; sluggish IV rate; and inability to aspirate blood from the catheter. Prevention measures include confirmation of catheter placement via X ray, assuring that the catheter sutures are intact to prevent slippage, and securing the catheter and tubing to prevent tension on the catheter. Upon assessment of this complication, the nurse should notify the physician, decrease the IV rate, prepare the client for neck/chest X rays, and monitor vital signs.

INFUSION-RELATED COMPLICATIONS

Catheter Occlusion

The catheter may become occluded because of positional kinking of the tubing or catheter. Prolonged occlusion prevents the solution from infusing and can lead to clot formation in the catheter. Signs of a possible occlusion include lack of blood return when aspirated, an infusion that will not run at a set rate, the infusion pump alarming of *occlusion*, the IV tubing popping apart as a result of back pressure, the client's neck or arm becoming edematous on the catheter side, and resistance when the catheter is irrigated.

A catheter occlusion requires immediate attention by the nurse. The infusion rate should not be increased, and if resistance is met when irrigating the catheter, the nurse should stop irrigating. If the tubing has become disconnected, clamp the catheter and cleanse the catheter end with povidone-iodine and alcohol prior to aspirating any air that may have entered the catheter. Prepare a new IV setup while irrigating the catheter with 3 to 5 ml of normal saline. If resistance is met, stop the irrigation and notify the physician.

A catheter occlusion can be prevented by assuring that the tubing is not kinked before leaving the client. The IV line should be assessed hourly thereafter.

Air Embolism

An air embolism is defined as air entering a vein and traveling to the right ventricle via the superior or inferior vena cava. This is a medical emergency, because the air bubble impedes the pumping ability of the ventricle, reducing cardiac output to the pulmonary system.

Clinical symptoms depend on the amount of air entering the system. They include chest pain, dyspnea, apprehension, cyanosis, tachycardia, increased venous pressure, decreased arterial blood pressure, syncope, *Mill-house* murmur over the pericardium, bradycardia, and coma.

Upon assessment of these symptoms, the nurse should place the client in a left-lateral decubitus position in Trendelenburg, administer oxygen by mask, notify the physician, assess vital signs, prepare for a thoracotomy or needle aspiration of the right ventricle by the physician, and stay with the patient to provide reassurance.

The following steps will prevent an air embolism from occurring. Clamp the central venous catheter whenever it is open to air. If the catheter cannot be clamped with a padded alligator clamp or hemostat, place the client in the Trendelenburg position and have the client perform Valsalva's maneuver during tubing changes. All IV tubing connections should be taped in a spiral fashion and the catheter taped to the dressing to prevent tension. Assess the catheter for cracks or leaks. During catheter removal the client should perform Valsalva's maneuver and an occlusive dressing should be applied.

Catheter-related Sepsis

Catheter-related sepsis occurs when bacteria enter the bloodstream via the catheter or when the catheter becomes the source of infection from another entry site, producing a systemic septic reaction. The clinical manifestations are those of any systemic septic reaction—increased temperature, glycosuria, chills, lethargy, tachycardia, hyperglycemia, and hypotension. A septic workup will be ordered by the physician if these symptoms are identified.

The nurse should notify the physician of the client's symptoms, obtain peripheral and central blood cultures, send the infusing IV solution and tubing to the laboratory for culture, assess the insertion site and culture any exudate that may be present, assist the physician with catheter removal if indicated, and administer antibiotics as ordered.

A septic reaction can be prevented by using strict aseptic technique during catheter insertion and maintenance as outlined in Chapters 5 and 6.

UNIT IV

PRINCIPLES OF IV MEDICATION ADMINISTRATION

CHAPTER 8

Pharmacokinetics

Marcia Miller, RN

Phases of Drug Action in the Body
Techniques of Pharmacokinetics
Factors Affecting Drug Function
Special Factors Affecting Younger Populations

Clinical pharmacology is the study of the disposition, actions, and effects of drugs when given to or taken by patients. Clinical pharmacology includes pharmacodynamics and, more specifically, pharmacokinetics, the study and evaluation of how a drug is absorbed, its distribution within the body, the changes in the drug after administration, the concentration of the drug at varying times, the site and mechanism of action, and the elimination of the drug.

Pharmacokinetic study not only increases the base of knowledge related to drug therapy, it also aids individualization of therapy. The knowledge gained through years of study and research is applied in light of information acquired about the particular patient and the goals of drug therapy to provide workable guidelines for safe, effective drug treatment.

Pharmacologists are becoming increasingly involved in assisting physicians with drug therapy. It is no longer sufficient merely to order the correct drug for any given condition or monitor the patient clinically for a response. Pharmacokinetics can assist in determining the correct dosage and dosing intervals to allow for the most appropriate effect of the drug while limiting or eradicating its potential adverse effects.

Nurses have little direct connection with the field of pharmacokinetics but are hearing more of its terminology and, through physicians' orders, are complying with recommendations made by a pharmacologist who is exercising judgment based on pharmacokinetic information.

PHASES OF DRUG ACTION IN THE BODY

A review of what occurs in the body after drug administration will increase understanding of pharmacokinetics and its implications for patient care.

With the exception of drugs administered topically or to a localized area for "on-site" effect, drugs must enter the circulation before achieving their desired effect. *Absorption* is the term used to indicate drug movement from the site of administration to the bloodstream. This phase is absent in IV administration, since these drugs are injected directly into the circulation.

The next phase consists of the drug's arrival at the site where it is to act. To accomplish this it must pass through the microcirculatory system heading toward the cells it must attack, support, or alter. This is the *distribution* phase.

Some drugs, depending on their structure, have an affinity for protein molecules and bind to them. Streaming through the circulation bound to a protein molecule, they will eventually reach their intended site of action, but until they are released they are not free to exert their desired effect. Protein-binding has the tendency to delay the distribution of the drug and its onset of action.

When a drug remains primarily in the bloodstream or within organs with a high blood flow, it is said to be a single- or one-compartment drug. However, if a portion of the drug enters tissue or another fluid system where its rate is slower than its distribution through the circulation, it is said to be a multiple- or two-compartment drug.

As the molecules of the injected drug reach their site of action, they begin the process for which they were intended. At the same time, however, the body's enzyme system initiates its complex function of altering the injected chemical. This metabolic process of, in essence, detoxification is termed *biotransformation* or metabolism.

At this point the processes of absorption and distribution are almost complete and the drug is returned to the general circulation. From there the kidney or liver, primary organs of filtration, will process the free or altered drug for removal from the body. This phase is called *excretion.*

TECHNIQUES OF PHARMACOKINETICS

Evaluation of this entire process—absorption, distribution, biotransformation, and excretion—is the essence of pharmacokinetics. To follow this sequence of events, multiple blood samples are obtained during the interval from just before injection of a drug until the next dose is due. Because activity is greatest near the time of drug administration, samples are taken more frequently during the first 2 hours. Remaining samples, drawn at less frequent intervals, define the slower processes of biotransformation and excretion. Serum or plasma is then separated from the blood and assayed for the amount of the drug present or, at times, the products formed by biotransformation. Plotting the levels obtained versus time after dose produces curves similar to the ones shown in Figure 8.1.

To the pharmacologist these curves indicate not only the peak (maximum) and trough (minimum) concentration of the drug during the dosing interval, but also the volume into which the drug is distributed and the rate of elimination.

Once the normal process of a drug has been determined, usually during the investigational phase of that drug, levels can be adjusted to provide just the trough and peak levels for therapeutic monitoring. From these determinations, recommendations can be made as to the advisability of changing the dose or dosing interval or maintaining present therapy.

FACTORS AFFECTING DRUG FUNCTION

Each drug has a half-life, the usual amount of time it takes for a serum concentration to decrease by 50 percent. It will take approximately four to five half-lives for the body to reach a point where the amount of drug given equals the amount of drug excreted. This is defined as *steady state*. For example, if the half-life of a drug is listed as 12 hours, it will take about 48 hours of repeated dosing for the patient to be considered at steady state. Impairment of renal or hepatic function, significant changes in circulation, interference with the

Figure 8.1   Drug levels versus time after dose.

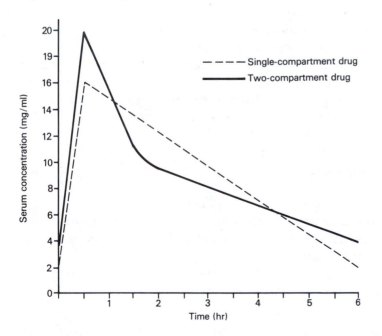

accurate or timely administration of the drug, or alteration in the metabolic process can change the time required to achieve steady state.

Steady state is important in therapeutic drug monitoring because the serum levels used to determine the accuracy of the drug dose and interval of administration are reliable only when the body achieves this state.

Nothing can be done to change the time it takes to achieve steady state, but when a drug with a long half-life is needed rapidly, a loading dose of that drug can be given, which will provide the body with enough of the chemical to initiate therapy and more quickly *approach* steady state.

In general, all IV drugs follow the pattern previously described—administration, distribution, biotransformation, and excretion. This implied simplicity belies the actual individuality and complexity of drug therapy. With hundreds of different drugs that can be given intravenously, there are a variety of factors that can influence their function within the patient.

- Some drugs remain free (unbound) in circulation and speed to their site of action, while others are bound to protein or other circulating components and are not able to function until released.
- Many drugs are given in a form in which they can immediately begin action, while others must first be chemically changed within the body to release the free (active) drug.
- While one drug will satisfy its objective within the circulatory compartment, another must diffuse through another compartment before its activity can begin.
- The site where the drug is required to exert its effect (organ, tissue, cell) varies from drug to drug.
- Drugs act to create normalization of function, alter function, accomplish planned destruction, or protect existing function. To achieve the desired effect, the drug must act in a specifically planned method either inside or outside the cell.
- The body's metabolic processes for biotransformation utilize potentially multiple enzyme systems or alternate processes that vary with each drug given.
- Drugs can be excreted through saliva, tears, mucus, sweat, and cerebrospinal fluid, although the primary organs of elimination are the kidneys and liver.

Add to all of this the uniqueness of the patient receiving the drug—the state of health or disease, possible alteration in metabolic or enzyme processes, and any existing deficiencies—and the potential for combination with additional drugs (IV or otherwise) and the factors influencing the action of a single drug magnify the complications of an already complex system.

SPECIAL FACTORS AFFECTING YOUNGER POPULATIONS

Pharmacokinetic studies in pediatric patients are not routinely required by the FDA before a drug is marketed. Of all the drugs presently administered intravenously to these patients, only a small portion have been studied to determine their actual processes in this young population. From work already completed, it is known that neonates and premature infants do not always handle drugs in the manner predicted by studies of adults. These infants have underdeveloped enzyme systems, many of which are needed for metabolic conversion and biotransformation. In addition, their renal excretion of many chemicals is depressed, often leading to a delay in ridding the body of the drug. Extending the dosing interval, with a possible change in the dose itself, allows therapy with the desired drug while taking into account the physical immaturity of the individual client.

Throughout infancy and childhood the body grows and matures. It is assumed that major systems responsible for handling injected chemicals rapidly mature to the point of acceptably utilizing, degrading, and eliminating drugs given.

BIBLIOGRAPHY

Levine, R. 1978. *Pharmacology Drug Actions and Reactions.* Boston: Little, Brown & Co.
Russell, H. 1980. *Pediatric Drugs and Nursing Intervention.* New York: McGraw-Hill Book Co.
Wang, R. 1979. *Practical Drug Therapy.* Philadelphia: J. P. Lippincott Co.
Wiriter, M. E. 1980. *Basic Clinical Pharmacokinetics.* San Francisco: Allied Therapeutics, Inc.

CHAPTER 9

Medication Administration and Site Selection

Marcia Miller, RN

ADVANTAGES AND DISADVANTAGES OF IV DRUG ADMINISTRATION

There are five golden rules of drug administration:

- Give the correct drug
- In the correct dose
- By the correct route
- At the correct time
- To the correct patient

No one has ever argued these rules. They are watchwords for whoever undertakes the responsibility of giving a medication to a patient.

Much has been written about drug delivery. Nurses are admonished to keep informed about the drugs their patients are to receive, including dosages, actions, desired effects, potential adverse effects, length of treatment, and responsibilities of care as it specifically relates to use of the drug. Our ability to meet these requirements has led to the addition of the intravenous route to our drug administration methods. It is a responsibility not to be taken lightly.

IV drug administration is not simply another technical skill to be acquired, but a more advanced and effective form of drug therapy.

IV administration of medications provides certain advantages over administration by other methods:

1. Delivery of the drug can be guaranteed.
2. The rate of delivery of the drug can be controlled.
3. There is a more rapid onset of action by the drug.
4. The stage of absorption is virtually eliminated, since the drug enters the bloodstream directly.

While these advantages are unquestionable, there are also disadvantages:

1. The drug must be in solution. For some drugs, particularly when given to small infants, the minimum dilutional volume may create problems in fluid management of the patient.
2. Many drugs can be irritating to the vein, particularly at the site of injection, leading to discomfort for the patient, phlebitis, and eventual loss of that particular IV site. Especially sensitive are the small vessels encountered in pediatric patients. Attempts to solve this problem by adding a buffer, lidocaine, or increasing the dilution *may* change the chemical structure of the drug or increase the fluid volume the patient is getting.
3. Extravasation of the drug into surrounding tissue as the result of infiltration may lead to discomfort, improper effect of the drug, or possible local tissue injury.
4. An error in drug, dose, or timing cannot readily be corrected. Assuming the drug enters the body in its free (active) form, it will begin its prescribed function almost immediately.
5. IV drug therapy requiring administration of two or more medications at the same time increases the potential for drug interaction before infusion is complete if they are not given correctly. Incompatibilities of drugs are not always visible, and failing to take into account interactions between drugs may lead to their chemical alteration and potential ineffectiveness.
6. Some drugs adhere to the IV tubing permanently or temporarily, thus preventing or delaying delivery of the drug.
7. Microorganisms at or near the IV injection site may be introduced into the IV system, putting the patient at risk for bloodstream or disseminated tissue infection.
8. Injection of microemboli in the form of air or particulate matter can lead to complications, including respiratory distress or seizures.
9. Cardiovascular problems *may* ensue after rapid IV injection of a drug, since it arrives in the heart in a concentrated form.

Nevertheless, if attention is paid to details in this critical form of therapy, the patient will more than likely benefit from its advantages rather than suffer from its potential disadvantages.

METHODS OF PROVIDING IV DRUGS

IV drugs can be provided to the patient in one of two ways, continuous infusion and intermittent dosing.

Continuous Infusion

This method is most commonly used for short-acting drugs or in situations where maintaining a steady level of drug in the circulation is most beneficial. The most common drugs given by continuous infusion are:

- Cardiotonic medications, pressor agents, or drugs given to directly influence cardiac or vascular function
- Bronchodilators given for acute pulmonary problems
- Glucose
- Electrolytes
- Vitamins, minerals, and trace elements
- Blood and blood products

Drugs given by continuous infusion are generally mixed into the primary container of IV solution or into a chamber designed to hold several hours of the prescribed admixture. Identification of additives with warnings for high-concentration solutions is vital.

Gravity flow

This is the simplest form of continuous infusion. It requires only the container of solution and appropriate tubing. It does have disadvantages, however, particularly in pediatric patients:

- A change in the distance between the drip chamber and the IV itself can alter the flow rate.
- Activity of the patient, especially as it influences the IV site, can speed up or slow down a previously regulated rate.
- A change in pressure affecting blood flow through the vessel can also affect the IV flow rate.
- Exceptionally slow IV rates cannot be accurately maintained.
- The potential for an unobserved rate increase is great and may compromise the patient, not only with a more rapid infusion of medication

than desired but with a fluid overload, unless measures are taken to restrict the amount of solution available to the patient at any given time.

Gravity flow with an added in-line rate controller

This device can be set to prevent delivery of the solution at a rate above that which is desired. Since it cannot prevent a lower rate, it is most advantageous with higher flow rates. Care must be taken to prevent patients from playing with the settings.

Controller

This machine has the ability to sense the drip rate and create constriction or allow expansion of the IV tubing to adjust the flow to the preset rate. It is more accurate than unattended gravity flow but, again, may be less accurate with slower rates.

Infusion pump

Many models of this type of equipment are now marketed. Their purpose is to provide a controlled, accurate, and constant rate of fluid delivery with built-in alarms to warn of problems or task completion. Use of an infusion pump is considered a *must* in continuous infusion of a drug whenever there is a physical risk if the rate varies from that prescribed. Drugs that affect the cardiovascular or pulmonary systems are safest when infused under the control of such a pump. Slow IV rates can also be assured without risk of fluid overload or insufficient volume, which may increase the potential for clotting of the IV line.

Intermittent Dosing

This method is commonly used for drugs with intermediate or long action or those needed quickly for prompt action. At evenly spaced intervals for prolonged therapy or as a one-time dose, they are injected into the IV system or directly into the patient. Drugs most commonly given by intermittent dosing are:

- Antibiotics
- Anticonvulsants
- Diuretics
- Steroids

- Sedatives
- Emergency drugs

Intermittent doses of IV medications need not, and should not, be limited to injection via the IV bag. Although this may afford a measure of safety, it may also compromise accurate drug delivery.

There are a number of possible methods for injecting drugs, either as part of or in addition to the existing IV system.

Fluid chamber (Buretrol)

Drugs injected into a fluid chamber receive the benefit of additional dilution, which in some cases may limit the discomfort experienced by the patient. It must be noted, however, that drugs given by this method are delayed in reaching the patient, and the interval of infusion is usually prolonged. It is important to remember that the medication must complete a journey through the IV tubing before it even reaches the patient. Emptying of the fluid chamber does not indicate completion of infusion—the tubing must also be cleared of the drug before the delivery is completed. This is crucial for patients whose IV rates are increased for the purpose of drug delivery, then decreased to an IV maintenance rate.

The extended time of delivery is of particular importance for drugs such as aminoglycosides and chloramphenicol, which do not clear IV tubing in a predictable time, especially at low flow rates. If drug therapy utilizes a combination of medications, a second drug given before the first has cleared the tubing may alter or negate the action of both. Unfortunately, not all such reactions are visible within the tubing. An understanding of the infusion method and the drugs being given is important.

Y-sites, flashballs stopcocks, and T-pieces

These injection sites, which are part of the IV tubing or added to the IV system, allow access for injection at points nearer to the patient. For drugs with recommended times over which they are to be delivered, and particularly with slow IV rates, one of these sites offers the potential for more accurate administration. To determine the most appropriate point of injection, it is necessary to know the tubing volumes from each site to the patient, as well as the rate at which the IV is running. A decision can then be made as to where to give the drug so that it will be infused in the recommended time.

With drugs known to have potentially serious side effects, the tendency has been to play it safe and give the drug through a fluid chamber. Unfortunately, this may compromise the accuracy of delivery. The goal should be not merely safety but also accuracy and effectiveness.

Piggyback

In the piggyback method, a container of prepared, diluted drug is connected by shorter tubing to a site in the existing IV tubing. This system can be run by gravity, with a controller or infusion pump. Its primary disadvantage in pediatrics is the volume of the diluted drug to be infused. There will also be some drug remaining in the secondary tubing, which will either be discarded or remain until the next dose is hung unless the container and tubing are flushed. Using new tubing each time is an expense to the patient. Keeping the previously used tubing hanging but closed off may be sufficient if the drug remaining in the tubing is stable and if only compatible drugs are run through that system.

Retrograde

A fairly new addition to the methods of drug delivery is the retrograde system. In this method a coil of tubing is added to the usual IV setup. On each end of the coil is a stopcock. Taking into account the IV rate, the drug is diluted so as to allow its infusion over the desired time. Once prepared, the diluted drug is injected in a retrograde fashion through the stopcock closest to the patient, displacing IV fluid out into a syringe at the distal stopcock. The IV solution then pushes the drug steadily forward into the patient. There are presently two sizes of coils—10 ml and 60 ml—each capable of handling half its volume in medication. The bulk of the coil may be a bit cumbersome, and an infusion pump is recommended when the retrograde coil is used, but drug delivery may be smoother and better defined by use of this system than with antegrade methods.

Syringe pumps

Syringe pumps are small infusion pumps designed to hold a syringe of prepared medication, which is attached to a stopcock or existing port in the IV line. The pump is programmed to deliver the syringe volume over a set time. It can be operated with the maintenance IV solution running or stopped, as long as the drug is compatible with the IV solution. Although expensive, it is probably the most accurate method of drug delivery. In most cases it is reserved for use with medications requiring precise delivery times or when very low rates make drug infusion more difficult.

FACTORS IN SITE SELECTION

Pharmacologic studies over the past several years have indicated that safe and accurate delivery of drugs to a patient must be based on knowledge of the drug, the IV system, the potential problems of delivery, and the total IV drug therapy ordered for the patient. Some drugs have a wide margin of efficacy regardless of how they are administered. Other drugs, those usually included in therapeutic drug monitoring, such as aminoglycosides, require more precise infusion to be effective. Problems with drug delivery are compounded by low IV rates and fluid restrictions, as well as sensitive blood vessels, problems that occur with the greatest frequency in pediatric patients.

Careful consideration should go into the plans for giving an IV medication. When an order is given for a drug to be administered intravenously, the following information is needed to help make the most appropriate site selection:

1. Is the patient presently running a continuous IV infusion, or is a heparin lock available for drug administration?
2. What IV solution is running, including additives?
3. What is the IV rate?
4. Can or should the IV rate be changed for drug delivery? If so, what rate has been recommended?
5. What is the recommended rate of infusion of the drug?
6. Are any other IV drugs scheduled to be given at the same time?
7. Are there any listed incompatibilities with the IV solution, additives, or other IV medications the patient is scheduled to receive?
8. Is there any record of drug instability once in solution?

If the drug to be given is compatible with the IV solution, the decision as to the site of injection is based primarily on the IV rate and the recommended rate for infusion of the drug. Should an incompatibility exist, the question is whether a second setup of a compatible solution should be utilized or whether the drug could be injected into the IV system near the patient, preceded and followed by a saline flush.

A number of sites exist for injection of the drug. The possibilities vary depending on the IV system used. If hospital policy allows in-line antegrade injection of medications, it is advisable to post a list of tubing volumes for each potential injection site. This list should also include extension sites and/or stopcocks that may be added to the standard tubing. Particular injection sites in the IV system and methods of adding to an existing system should be used *only* when approved by your institution and supported by written guidelines.

Once the most appropriate site of injection has been selected, a notation should be made on the medication sheet so that all subsequent doses will be given in a consistent manner. A change in the IV rate may necessitate a change in the site of injection. If this occurs, a notation should be made.

ADMINISTERING THE DRUG

When the drug is ready for injection, the IV should be checked for patency and the site for any evidence of infiltration or inflammation. If there is any question about the IV or the condition of the blood vessel, a new IV route should be established.

Strict aseptic technique should be followed when injecting a drug into the IV system. Cleansing of the site with an iodine-based swab followed by a 30-second drying time, then clearing with an alcohol swab, is ideal for any rubber-stoppered ports. Entry into these ports should be with a small-gauge (25-gauge) needle to prevent compromise of the port's integrity. Luer-Lok sites should be kept covered with a sterile protective cap when not actually being used.

If there is any question of the drug's incompatibility with the IV solution or with a drug that may have been previously injected into the IV system, a normal saline flush should be used both before and after the drug is given.

The rate of antegrade injection at a site within the tubing should be slow enough to avoid undue pressure within the blood vessel. In other words, the smaller the IV, the slower the injection rate. During the injection, the tubing immediately distal to the injection site should be occluded to prevent retrograde flow. If an infusion pump is being used to maintain the IV rate, it should be turned off temporarily during the time of the injection. At the completion of the injection, be sure the IV is running at the desired rate.

It has been estimated that up to 36 percent of IV drugs given is discarded when the IV tubing is changed. While there is evidence to support the advisability of routine tubing changes, it is also important to take into consideration the timing of drug administration. If dosing schedules and the characteristics of drug clearance are kept in mind when the tubing is to be changed, the aims of both infection control and assured drug delivery will be met.

No matter how a drug is given, it remains crucial to observe the patient for response to drug therapy. This means watching for both adverse effects and evidence of a therapeutic response.

Documentation of administration, including the site of injection, condition of the IV site, and patient response, is helpful in therapeutic drug monitoring as well as being a vital nursing responsibility.

There is presently no one perfect solution to IV drug administration. As long as there is a diversity of drugs, and the conditions they treat, a variety of IVs and IV systems, and an extremely wide range of patients, there will be challenges to ideal drug delivery.

UNIT V

PRINCIPLES OF HOME INTRAVENOUS THERAPY

CHAPTER 10

Home IV Antibiotic Administration

Phyllis Fichtelman Nentwich, RN, MS

The Interdisciplinary Team
Mutual Participation
Agreement for Participation in the Home IV Antibiotic Program
Home IV Antibiotic Teaching Plan
Follow-up

The administration of intravenous antibiotics in the home is now a widespread practice for diseases requiring extensive IV therapy. Clients with illnesses such as osteomyelitis, endocarditis, or cystic fibrosis with an underlying infection find confinement in the hospital for 4 to 6 weeks costly. Such clients, with proper supervision and education, can and should be discharged to continue parenteral therapy at home. This provides two benefits: the chance to recover surrounded by family and reduced expenses for both family and third-party payor. This chapter will describe the health team's responsibilities when a client administers antibiotics at home and will explain the mechanics of a home IV antibiotic program. A patient education guide for home IV antibiotic administration is included.

THE INTERDISCIPLINARY TEAM

An interdisciplinary team, consisting of a physician, registered nurse, and pharmacist, should provide the client with the needed equipment and instruction to administer the medications at home. The physician is responsible for assessing the client medically, for designating the potential candidate for home administration, and for prescribing the specifics of administration, including the antibiotic, diluent, rate of infusion, length of therapy, insertion of the heparin lock, and heparin solution. Follow-up medical assessment, including the ordering of serum, drug monitoring, and discharge from the program, are also the responsibilities of the physician. The pharmacist dispenses the antibiotics and equipment and is responsible for monitoring serum drug levels throughout therapy.

The nurse is responsible for assessing the potential client for the ability to understand the instructions provided and for evaluating the home environment. Figure 10.1 provides an example of a form that documents the nurse's assessment. The nurse is also responsible for patient and family education, follow-up assessment, documentation, insertion of the heparin lock, and continuity of care referral.

The client should meet the following criteria:

1. The client could be discharged home or would not need to be admitted if not for the need of ongoing IV antibiotic therapy.
2. The client has demonstrated previous compliance with medical regimes.
3. The client takes an active part in care.
4. The client's home environment is adequate for storage of the supplies.
5. The client demonstrates a readiness to participate in home IV therapy and a willingness to demonstrate competency.

Figure 10.1   Nursing assessment of home IV antibiotic client.

Client Name _____   Date of Birth _____

Address _____   Age _____

_____   Phone Number _____

Primary Physician _____

Primary Person to Administer IV Medications _____

Support Person to Administer IV Medications _____

Medication Profile

Weight _____   Allergies _____

Brief Medical History _____

_____

_____

Current Medication Profile _____

_____

Prescribed IV Antibiotic _____

Duration of Therapy _____

Home Environment

Available Facilities for Administration

a. Electrical supply   _____ Yes   _____ No
b. Plumbing   _____ Yes   _____ No
c. Adequate and safe storage space   _____ Yes   _____ No
d. Working refrigerator and freezer   _____ Yes   _____ No

Resources

Proximity of local health facility (time and miles)_____

_____

Transportation resources_____
Are work and/or school arrangements necessary?   Tutor?
Notification of school/occupational nurse?_____

   Contact Person _____

   Phone Number _____

Response to Illness

Does client have an understanding of disease process and necessity for IV antibiotic
therapy? _____

Does client comply with medical regime?_____

   If no, explain: _____

Does client take an active part in care? _____

   If no, explain: _____
Does client demonstrate readiness to participate in home IV therapy and willingness
to demonstrate competency? _____

RN Signature _____

Adapted from Nursing Assessment of Home IV Antibiotic Client Children's Hospital,
Columbus, Ohio 1983.

MUTUAL PARTICIPATION

Home IV antibiotic administration is a treatment plan of mutual participation. Once the client is assessed by the physician and nurse as appropriate
for the program, the client should weigh the advantages and disadvantages of
administering IV antibiotics at home. The nurse or physician can assist the
client in making the decision by outlining the following.

Advantages of Home Therapy

- The client will be in the comfort of his or her own home rather than
  in the hospital environment and will be able to maintain a normal
  eating and sleeping pattern.

- The client, with the physician's permission, may continue work or school.
- The client will receive training in IV therapy and will be able to practice until he or she can demonstrate competence.
- Health personnel are available 24 hours a day for assistance by phone.

Disadvantages of Home Therapy

- In the hospital there are health professionals to care for the client and handle emergencies.
- There are several precautions that must be taken even in the home environment, such as not getting the IV wet.
- Two responsible individuals must learn the techniques required to administer the IV medication safely.
- The daily routine of the client and support person will have to be altered to accommodate the medication schedule.
- If the IV becomes dislodged, the client must return to a health facility or notify a home health nurse to have it replaced.

AGREEMENT FOR PARTICIPATION IN THE HOME IV ANTIBIOTIC PROGRAM

To continue the philosophy of mutual participation in home administration of IV medications, an agreement form should be signed by the client and the nurse educator. The form should outline the responsibilities of both parties. By signing, the client is agreeing to administer medications in the prescribed manner at the appointed times and to keep all follow-up appointments. The client is also agreeing to notify the health professionals if any problems occur.

The nurse represents the health care team and, by signing, is agreeing that education and 24-hour emergency care will be provided, that the treatment plan will be mutually determined, and that the necessary supplies will be provided.

Figure 10.2 outlines such an agreement.

HOME IV ANTIBIOTIC TEACHING PLAN

Once the participants have mutually agreed upon the program, the educational process begins. As previously stated, two people must learn the procedure. If the client is capable of learning, the client may self-administer the antibiotics. A back-up person should be available to reinforce the procedure and to administer medications in the event the client cannot.

Figure 10.3 outlines the teaching plan for a client receiving IV antibiotics at home. As each objective is met, the nurse initials and dates the column next

Figure 10.2   Home IV antibiotic client agreement.

Consent for IV Therapy at Home
Medical Record Copy

I, _____, hereby make request for
                        parent or guardian
_____ to participate in the home IV program.
              patient
I am aware that there are risks and responsibilities involved. I have been instructed
in the theory and technique necessary for the administration of _____
                                                                  drug
to _____ and I understand the instructions given.
              patient
To continue my participation in this program I will:

- Keep all follow-up appointments
- Administer the medication in the prescribed manner at the appointed times
- Inform the IV therapy nurse clinician, pulmonary clinical nurse specialist, and/
  or my physician of any problems

I expect the professional staff to:

- Provide necessary education
- Provide 24-hour coverage for problems
- Include me in developing the treatment plan and keep me informed of any
  necessary changes
- Arrange for provision of all necessary supplies

I understand that as long as these conditions are met to the satisfaction of both
parties, the home IV therapy program can continue. Either party has the option of
discontinuing this agreement if not satisfied with the performance of the other party
or if the therapy becomes too difficult to handle at home.

_____   _____
Parent or Legal Guardian   Date

_____   _____
Signature of Witness   Date
(must be over 18 years of age)

Figure 10.3 Home IV antibiotic teaching plan.

OBJECTIVE	OBJECTIVE MET DATE/ INITIAL
1. To state that the patient education materials on home IV therapy have been read	_____
2. To state the purpose of the heparin lock	_____
3. To identify the purpose of heparinization	_____
4. To describe the care of a heparin lock	_____
5. To identify restrictions on activity due to a heparin lock	_____
6. To demonstrate proper hand-washing technique	_____
7. To list the supplies needed for administration of each antibiotic	_____
8. To demonstrate aseptic technique with the equipment	_____
9. To describe appropriate storage of the equipment and medications	_____
10. To state the name, purpose, dosage, length of therapy, and side effects of all medications to be administered intravenously	_____
11. To demonstrate the individualized procedure for administering the IV antibiotics	_____
12. To identify specific signs and symptoms of the complications that can occur during an infusion	_____
13. To describe the appropriate actions to take if a complication occurs	_____
14. To describe the procedure for removal of the heparin lock	_____

I understand all instructions given and can administer the IV antibiotics safely at home.

Client signature _____

RN signature _____

to it. Upon completion of the teaching, the client signs the form. The teaching plan then serves as documentation of the client's ability to administer the medications and becomes a permanent medical record. Table 10.1 outlines the appropriate content for each behavioral objective of the teaching plan. Table 10.2 lists the equipment needed.

Figure 10.4 is an example of a comprehensive patient education guide. The client should use this to learn the procedure initially and then refer to it often in the home setting to reinforce and confirm the steps of the procedure.

Table 10.1 BEHAVIORAL CONTENT AND RATIONALE

Behavioral Objective	Content
To state that the patient education materials have been read	Provide the client with all materials prior to the teaching/learning session.
To state the purpose of the heparin lock	The purpose of the heparin lock is to provide a means for intermittent administration of medications through an IV.
To identify the purpose of heparinization	Heparin is a medication that prevents blood from clotting in the catheter when an intermittent infusion is indicated.
To describe the care of a heparin lock	The dressing over the IV site must be kept clean and dry. For bathing, wrap the IV site with plastic wrap to prevent water from entering the dressing. Avoid strenuous use of the arm with the heparin lock. Cover the heparin lock with clothing when engaging in activities such as sports.
To identify restrictions on activity due to a heparin lock	Very few restrictions are necessary due to the heparin lock. Swimming should be avoided as well as strenuous activities with the IV arm. For example, carry books with the opposite arm.
To demonstrate proper hand-washing technique	Always wash and rise your hands thoroughly with soap and water before touching any part of the IV equipment. Wash your hands using a rubbing motion for 1 to 2 minutes. Dry hands thoroughly with a paper towel. Do not handle anything other than the IV supplies during the procedure or wash and dry hands again prior to handling equipment.
To list the supplies needed for administration of each antibiotic	IV antibiotics can be administered by IV push or IV piggyback. IV push is a method of administering antibiotics directly into the bloodstream. IV piggyback is a method of administering antibiotics in a diluted form by dripping the medication directly from the bag of IV solution and medication. The major factor determining the method of administration is the irritation of the drug to the vein. Equipment needs are based on the type of method chosen (see Table 10.2).
To demonstrate aseptic technique with the equipment	To keep the equipment sterile, the following points should be demonstrated: 1. Do not touch any part of the equipment that will come in contact with the IV medication or the bloodstream. (continued)

Table 10.1   continued

Behavioral Objective	Content
	2. Keep IV medication in the freezer or the refrigerator to prevent bacterial growth.
	3. When using the IV piggyback method, change the tubing every 24 hours.
	4. Do not cough or sneeze on the IV equipment.
	5. Do not allow pets around the equipment.
To describe appropriate storage of the equipment and medications	Always keep the equipment out of the reach of small children. Store equipment in a clean dry cabinet. Medication should be stored in a clean, dry cabinent, refrigerator, or freezer. See "Home Stability" under each drug profile.
To state the name, purpose, dosage, length of therapy, and side effects of all medications to be administered intravenously	See drug profiles.
To demonstrate the individualized procedure for administering the IV antibiotics	See Figure 10.4
To identify specific signs and symptoms of the complications that can occur during an infusion	See Figure 10.4
To describe the appropriate actions to take if a complication occurs	See Figure 10.4
To describe the procedure for removal of the heparin lock	Loosen the stabilizing tape and dressing. Then while applying pressure over the IV site with a cotton ball, remove the catheter at the same angle it was inserted. Maintain pressure over the site until the bleeding has stopped. Apply a bandage over the site. The IV can be discontinued if a complication occurs or if treatment is complete. Contact the physician prior to removal of the heparin lock.

Table 10.2   EQUIPMENT NEEDS

IV Push Method

- One syringe of normal saline and heparin
- Medication record
- Pen
- Heavy box or coffee can for needle disposal
- 23-gauge needle
- Syringe of medication
- Povidone-iodine swab

IV Piggyback

- One syringe of normal saline and heparin
- Medication record
- Pen
- Heavy box or coffee can for needle disposal
- 23-gauge needle
- IV solution with antibiotic
- IV tubing and hanger
- Povidone-iodine swab

Successful learning takes place in a quiet, private environment with audio-visuals available for demonstration. The nurse should demonstrate the procedure on a mannequin or doll and then allow the client to practice on the mannequin until proficiency is obtained. The nurse should then evaluate the client's learning through return demonstration. The client should administer at least one dose of the medication under the supervision of the nurse. Once the client demonstrates proficiency, the client can be discharged to the home setting with the needed supplies and instructions for follow-up.

Supplies may be dispensed by either the participating hospital or a pharmaceutical supply company. Materials supplied by the participating hospital tend to cost less and are easily available for the hospital nurse or pharmacist to collect for the client. Smaller hospitals may find this dispensing difficult to organize when few patients may benefit, however. Pharmaceutical supply companies are prepared to produce large quantities of specified IV products. Additionally, many such companies employ nurses to assess the home environment and support the client's needs on an ongoing basis.

(Text continues on p. 109)

Figure 10.4 Home IV antibiotic patient education guide. (From *Helping Hand,* Homegoing Education and Literature Program. Copyright 1983, Children's Hospital Inc., Columbus, OH. Reprinted with permission.)

Helping Hand

Children's
HOSPITAL

Homegoing Education and Literature Program

Children's Hospital
Columbus, Ohio 43205   614/461·2000

I. V. ANTIBIOTIC THERAPY AT HOME

HH-II-73
6/83 Rev. 12/86

Intravenous (I.V.) antibiotic therapy is a method of giving antibiotics directly into the blood stream. Before the child goes home from the hospital, two responsible people must be able to demonstrate that they know how to give the medication through a heparin lock.

WHAT IS HEPARIN LOCK?

A heparin lock (also called a heparin well) is a needle or plastic catheter that is inserted into a vein and left in place. The lock is kept filled with a solution containing heparin. Heparin is a medicine that keeps blood from clotting in the catheter when I.V. fluid is not running through it. A rubber seal on the end of a short length of tubing keeps the heparin in the lock. The purpose of a heparin lock is to permit the I.V. tubing to be disconnected between doses of antibiotics.

SPECIAL TIPS ABOUT THE HEPARIN LOCK:

● Keep the dressing over the I.V. site clean and dry.
● Before bathing, wrap the I.V. site with plastic wrap. Do not wrap the arm too tightly but try to seal the edges. Do not put the arm with the I.V. into water.
● Avoid strenuous use of the arm with the I.V. Carry books, open doors, etc. with your other arm.
● If you are outside or engaging in activities around dirt or dust, cover the I.V. site with clothing or a light cloth dressing.
● Put the arm with the I.V. through sleeves of clothing first. Do this carefully so that the I.V. does not catch on clothes and become dislodged.
● Hold the I.V. when inserting or removing needles from rubber seal by grasping the hub of the t-connector and the male adapter with your thumb and index finger.

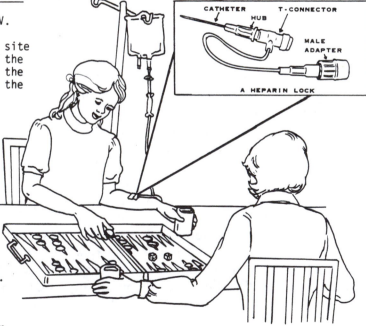

Picture 1   A heparin lock allows you to receive I.V. therapy at home.

METHODS OF ADMINISTERING I.V. ANTIBIOTICS:

I.V. antibiotics can be given by either a "drip" or "push" method. The method you will
be using is prescribed by your doctor.
● I.V. push is done by injecting the medicine from the syringe into the vein (through the
heparin lock) in the amount of time ordered by the doctor.
● I.V. drip is done by allowing a bag of diluted medication to drip through I.V. tubing
into the vein over 20 to 60 minutes. This method is used to prevent complications caused
by giving the medicine too fast. This method must be used if the medicine is very
irritating to the vein.

USE AND CARE OF EQUIPMENT:

Since the medication will be given directly into the blood stream, it is important to
keep all equipment clean. Certain pieces of the equipment and all the medication must be
kept sterile (free of bacteria). The first rule to follow is: WASH AND RINSE YOUR HANDS
BEFORE HANDLING ANY EQUIPMENT (Picture 2). The second rule is: USE ASEPTIC (WITHOUT
BACTERIA) TECHNIQUE. Aseptic (a-SEP-tic) technique means not touching those parts of the
equipment that must remain sterile. Below is a list of equipment you will be using at
home. Included is a short description and a notation of whether it is to be kept clean
or sterile. Picture 3 shows equipment used to administer medication by the push method.
Picture 4 shows equipment used to administer medication by drip method. Refer to
Picture 3 or 4 to learn the names of the equipment you will be using.

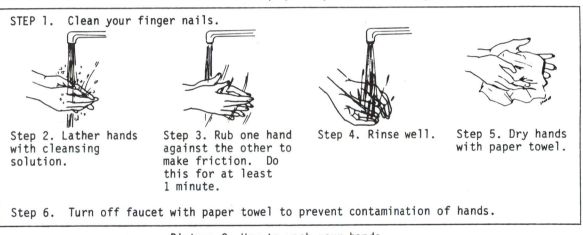

STEP 1. Clean your finger nails.

Step 2. Lather hands with cleansing solution.

Step 3. Rub one hand against the other to make friction. Do this for at least 1 minute.

Step 4. Rinse well.

Step 5. Dry hands with paper towel.

Step 6. Turn off faucet with paper towel to prevent contamination of hands.

Picture 2   How to wash your hands.

EQUIPMENT FOR PUSH METHOD:

1. <u>23-gauge needle</u> - comes packaged with needle in protective cover. Keep rim and inside of hub sterile. Keep cover clean. Keep needle STERILE.
2. <u>Syringe</u> - glass. Keep clean.
   a. <u>Adapter for needle</u> - comes with protective cover. Keep clean. When cover is removed keep STERILE.
   b. <u>Plunger</u> - plastic rod inside syringe. Keep STERILE.
   c. <u>Inside of syringe</u> - keep STERILE.

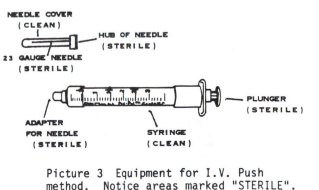

Picture 3 Equipment for I.V. Push method. Notice areas marked "STERILE".

(continued)

Figure 10.4 continued

EQUIPMENT FOR DRIP METHOD:

1. Medication bag - clear plastic bag
   containing medication and fluid.
   Outside the bag should be kept clean.
   a. Spike entrance - plastic tubing
      covered with protective material.
      Keep clean until protective
      material is removed. The rim
      and inside of tubing must be
      kept STERILE.
2. I.V. TUBING - length of tubing should
   be kept clean.
   a. Spike - hard plastic with pointed
      end with protective cover. Keep
      clean until protective cover is
      removed--then keep STERILE.
   b. Drip chamber - clear plastic with
      metal needle inside. Keep clean.
   c. I.V. tubing holder - prongs at top
      of roller clamp. Use to hang I.V.
      tubing when not in use. Keep clean.
   d. Clamp - roller clamp used to regulate
      I.V. drip rate. Keep clean.
   e. Arm end of tubing - hard plastic
      with tapered end to hold needle.
      Comes with protective cover.
      Keep clean until protective cover
      is removed. Then keep STERILE.
   f. 23-gauge needle - comes packaged
      with needle in protective cover.
      Keep rim and inside of hub STERILE.
      Keep cover clean. Keep needle STERILE.

HOW TO KEEP EQUIPMENT CLEAN:

1. Wash and rinse hands thoroughly with
   soap and warm water for at least one
   (1) minute (Picture 2, page 2).
   The friction caused by rubbing hands
   together is more important than using
   extremely hot water.
2. Dry hands thoroughly, preferably with
   paper towels. (Cloth towels can
   retain bacteria.)
3. Turn off water taps using paper towels.
4. Do not handle anything other than the
   I.V. supplies until after medication is
   started. If you do, wash and dry hands
   again before handling equipment.
5. Do not let any equipment touch the
   floor or an obviously dirty area.
6. Store I.V. supplies (except medication)
   in a clean area and away from children
   and pets.

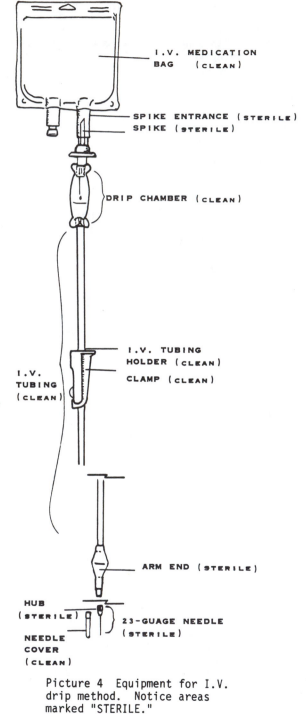

Picture 4 Equipment for I.V.
drip method. Notice areas
marked "STERILE."

HOW TO KEEP EQUIPMENT STERILE:

1. Do not touch any part that is listed on Picture 3 and 4 as STERILE.
2. Discard sterile parts that accidentally touch anything (fingers, clothes, nonsterile equipment). Use a new, sterile supply.
3. Keep I.V. medications in a clean area in the freezer until the evening before they are given. Store them in a plastic container with a lid.
4. Remove only the number of doses of medication that will be used in the next 24-hour period. Store these in a clean area in the refrigerator.
5. Remove the medication from the refrigerator 1/2 hour before it is to be administered.
6. Use a new set of I.V. tubing every 24 hours.

PREPARING TO ADMINISTER THE ANTIBIOTIC:

1. Wash, rinse and dry your hands (see Picture 2, page 2).

2. Locate a dry, clean work area. The kitchen counter or table is usually the most convenient. Wash the table or counter top, rinse and dry it.

3. Assemble necessary equipment:

PUSH METHOD	DRIP METHOD
□ I.V. medication syringe(s)	□ I.V. medication bag
□ 1 package of normal saline and and heparin cartridges	□ 2 needles (23-gauge)
□ 1 23-gauge needle for each syringe of medication	□ 1 package of normal saline and heparin cartridges
□ cartridge holder	□ cartridge holder
□ 1 betadine swab	□ I.V. tubing
□ medication record	□ 2 betadine swabs
□ pen	□ tape
□ puncture resistant container such as used bleach bottle or coffee can for syringe disposal	□ I.V. pole
	□ medication record
	□ pen
	□ puncture resistant container such as used bleach bottle or coffee can for syringe disposal

4. Read the label on the medication bag or syringe for name of drug, dosage and expiration date. The label should read:

PATIENT NAME: _____

I.V. SOLUTION: _____

DRUG: _____

DOSAGE: _____

EXPIRATION DATE: _____

5. Check the bag or syringe to make sure I.V. solution is clear. If it is not clear, use another bag or syringe and return the cloudy solution to the supply company.

(continued)

Figure 10.4   continued

HOW TO PREPARE THE NORMAL SALINE (SODIUM CHLORIDE) AND HEPARIN:

1. Wash, rinse and dry your hands (see Picture 2, page 2).
2. Open the package of sodium chloride and heparin.
3. Remove one cartridge of sodium chloride. (Be sure to read the label.)

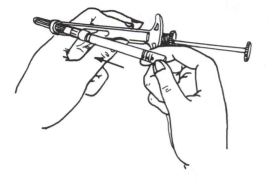
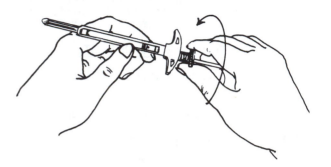

4. Place cartridge of sodium chloride in cartridge holder.

5. Push the white plunger down to meet the screw inside the syringe. Then turn the plunger clockwise until resistance is felt. Turn blue screw until it stops.

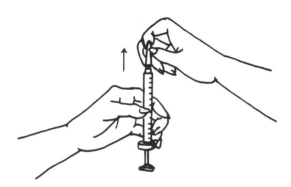
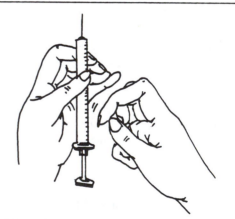

6. Remove protective covering from end of needle being careful not to touch the needle.

7. Hold syringe up. Tap the syringe gently to make air bubble rise to top. Gently push plunger up to force air bubbles out. Check syringe to make sure it contains 2 cc of sodium chloride solution.

8. Carefully put cover over needle to prevent sticking your finger.
9. Repeat steps 3 through 8 to prepare the second syringe of sodium chloride and the 1 cc syringe of heparin.
10. To remove used syringes from cartridge holder, reverse the instructions to steps 3 through 5.

PUSH METHOD

HOW TO ADMINISTER THE MEDICATION BY THE PUSH METHOD:

1. Wash, rinse and dry your hands (see Picture 2, page 2).

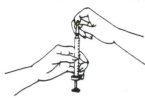
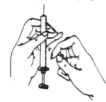
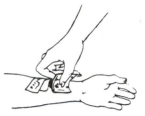

2. Remove protective cover from syringe containing medication. Attach a 23-gauge needle. To lock in place, push and and twist at the same time.

3. Remove protective cover from needle. Hold syringe with needle pointed up. Tap the syringe gently to make air bubbles rise to the top. Gently push plunger up to force air bubble out. Check syringe to make sure it contains the correct dosage.

4. Wipe the end of the heparin lock with a betadine swab and let it dry for 30 seconds.

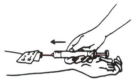

Sodium Chloride

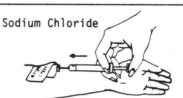
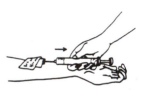

5. Insert the sodium chloride syringe into the heparin lock.

6. Gently push the plunger of the syringe forward flushing the sodium chloride into the heparin lock. IF ANY RESISTANCE IS MET, or any swelling is noted at the I.V. site STOP and call the hospital.

7. Remove syringe and needle from heparin lock.

Antibiotic

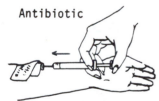

Sodium Chloride

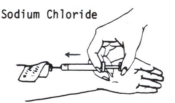

Heparin

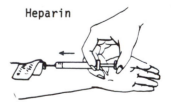

8. Repeat steps 5, 6 and 7 to administer the antibiotic. Administer the antibiotic over _____ minutes.

9. Repeat steps 5, 6 and 7 using the second syringe of sodium chloride.

10. Repeat steps 5, 6 and 7 using the syringe of heparin. Heparin should always be the last syringe you use.

11. Record administration of medications on chart (see page 13).
12. CAUTION: If you accidentally puncture your skin after the medication has been given, wash your hands and apply Hydrogen Peroxide to the puncture site. Call your doctor.

(continued)

Figure 10.4   continued

<u>HOW TO DISPOSE OF USED NEEDLE AND SYRINGE:</u>

CAUTION: The law states that the syringe must be "rendered inoperable". This means the needle must be broken. This will keep anyone from reusing a disposable syringe.

1. Carefully put cover over needle to keep from accidentally sticking yourself with the used needle..
2. Bend covered needle back and forth slowly and carefully until it snaps off inside the cover. Firmly push cover onto syringe.
3. Put syringe and needle into a puncture resistant container with cover such as a used bleach bottle or a coffee can. If a can is used, seal the lid with adhesive tape before disposal.
4. Do not let the container get too full. When the container is almost full, dispose of it in a closed plastic bag.

> CAUTION: Be sure to keep syringes and supplies out of the reach of children and others who might misuse them.

DRIP METHOD

<u>SETTING UP EQUIPMENT FOR THE DRIP METHOD:</u>

1. Remove I.V. tubing from box and place it on clean table or hang over I.V. pole. Take care never to let the end of the I.V. tubing touch the floor or other unsterile surface.
2. Close the clamp on I.V. tubing.
3. Remove protective coverings from medication bag and spike of I.V. tubing being sure not to touch expose ends. Insert spike of I.V. tubing into entrance of medication bag, being careful not to puncture sides of medication bag. Discard any punctured bags and use a new one.
4. Hang medication bag on I.V. pole or hook.
5. Squeeze the drip chamber 2-3 times to fill it 2/3 full.
6. Open the clamp.
7. Hold the end of the I.V. tubing below the bag and let the I.V. solution flow through the tubing to flush all air out of the tubing.
8. Close the clamp when all air is removed from tubing.
9. Hang tubing on I.V. pole until ready to use.

<u>HOW TO ADMINISTER THE ANTIBIOTIC BY THE DRIP METHOD:</u>

1. Wash and dry your hands (see Picture 2, page 2).

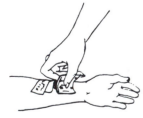

Sodium Chloride

2. Wipe the end of the heparin lock with a betadine swab and and let it dry for 30 seconds.

3. Insert the sodium chloride syringe into the heparin lock.

4. Gently push the plunger of the syringe forward flushing the sodium chloride into the heparin lock. IF ANY RESISTANCE IS MET, or any swelling is noted at the I.V. site, STOP and call the hospital.

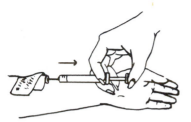

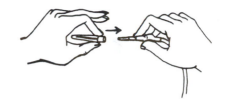

5. Withdraw the needle and syringe.

6. Remove protective covering from end of
    I.V. tubing. Place a 23-guage needle
    with protective cover on the end of the
    tubing. Do not touch end of tubing or hub
    of needle with your fingers. (For a secure
    connection between needle and I.V. tubing
    push and twist at the same time.)

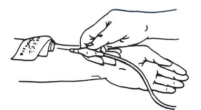

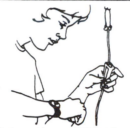

7. Remove protective covering from
    needle and insert needle into
    heparin lock. Tape the I.V
    tubing securely.

8. Administer the antibiotic over
    _____ minutes. Count _____ drops
    per minute. Use the roller clamp to
    adjust the rate of the drops. Observe
    for any signs of redness, swelling or
    pain at the I.V. site during the
    infusion (refer to page 10).

AFTER THE ANTIBIOTIC ADMINISTRATION:

1. Wash, rinse and dry your hands (see Picture 2, page 2).

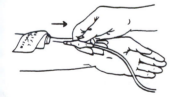

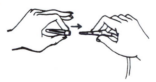

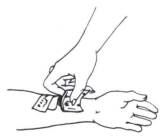

2. Remove needle and
    tubing from heparin
    lock.

3. Disconnect the tubing
    from the needle without
    touching the end of the
    tubing. Place a new
    needle with protective
    cover on the end of the
    tubing to keep it clean.
    Hang tubing on I.V. pole.

4. Wipe the end of the
    heparin lock with a
    betadine swab and let
    it dry for 30 seconds.

(continued)

Figure 10.4 continued

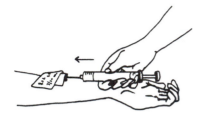

Sodium Chloride

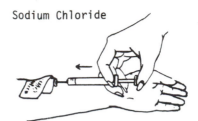

5. Prepare second syringe of sodium chloride. (This can be done ahead of time while medication is infusing.) Insert the syringe of sodium chloride into the heparin lock.

6. Gently push the plunger forward flushing the sodium chloride into the heparin lock. IF ANY RESISTANCE IS MET, or any swelling is noted at the site, STOP and call the hospital.

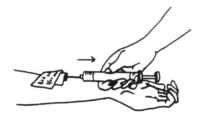

Heparin

7. Remove syringe of sodium chloride.

8. Repeat steps 5,6, and 7 with the syringe of heparin.

9. For subsequent medication doses:
   • Use new medication bag for each dose. (Carefully remove spike of I.V. tubing from old bag and insert into new bag.)
   • Use same I.V. tubing for only 24 hours.
   • Use new needles for each dose.
10. Record administration of medication on chart (see page 13).
11. CAUTION: If you accidentally puncture your skin after the medication has been given, wash your hands and apply Hydrogen Peroxide to the puncture site. Call the doctor.

HOW TO DISPOSE OF USED NEEDLE AND SYRINGE:

CAUTION: The law states that the syringe must be "rendered inoperable". This means the needle must be broken. This will keep anyone from reusing a disposable syringe.
1. Carefully put cover over needle to keep from accidentally sticking yourself with the used needle.
2. Bend covered needle back and forth slowly and carefully until it snaps off inside the cover. Firmly push cover onto syringe.
3. Put syringe and needle into a puncture resistant container with cover such as a used bleach bottle or a coffee can. If a can is used, seal the lid with adhesive tape before disposal.
4. Do not let the container get too full. When the container is almost full, dispose of it in a closed plastic bag.

> CAUTION: Be sure to keep syringes and supplies out of the reach of children and others who might misuse them.

OTHER INFORMATION AND SAFETY:

When administering antibiotics by I.V. there can be problems that may occur, so you need to know what to look for and what to do. Below is a list of things to look for before, during and after each antibiotic administration. Also included are possible causes of the problems and what you should do about it. If you have any questions or concerns, do not hesitate to call the nurse or your local emergency room.

PROBLEM	POSSIBLE CAUSE	WHAT TO DO
1. Swelling, redness, or hardness at I.V. site	a. End of catheter has come out of vein. b. Medication is irritating vein.	a. Contact nurse at Children's Hospital Home I.V. Antibiotic Program or local emergency room. b. Contact nurse or local emergency room.
2. Leakage of fluid at I.V. site	a. Needle on I.V. tubing or syringe is not tight enough. b. Needle is not inserted far enough into heparin lock. c. T-connector/male adapter is not connected tightly. d. I.V. catheter has become dislodged.	a. Tighten connection between needle and I.V. tubing. b. Insert needle farther into heparin lock. c. Tighten connection between t-connector/male adapter. Stabilize catheter by grasping the hub of the catheter with thumb and index finger of one hand. Gently push and twist the t-connector/male adapter clockwise with the other hand. d. If the I.V. continues to leak call the nurse or local emergency room.
3. Air in I.V. tubing	a. Drip chamber or tubing not filled before beginning infusion.	a. Disconnect tubing from heparin lock. Without touching the needle, flush tubing with I.V. solution until air is gone. Clean heparin lock again with betadine. Replace needle and continue infusion.
4. Resistance met when flushing the heparin lock with sodium chloride	a. Syringe of sodium chloride, heparin or medication not assembled correctly. b. Catheter has come out of vein. OR Blood clot has formed in catheter.	a. Withdraw syringe from heparin lock and recheck assembly. Be sure medication comes out of needle when plunger is pushed. b. If even slight resistance is met in heparin lock STOP. Do not force medication heparin or sodium chloride into vein. Call the nurse or your local emergency room.

(continued)

Figure 10.4 continued

PROBLEM	POSSIBLE CAUSE	WHAT TO DO
5. Medication running too fast	a. Clamp on tubing has moved.	a. Readjust clamp until proper drip rate is reestablished.
	b. Distance between arm with I.V. and medication bag has increased.	b. To prevent this problem, keep medication bag at the same height above the arm with I.V. during the infusion.
6. Medication running too slow or not at all	a. Clamp on tubing has moved.	a. Readjust clamp until proper drip rate is reestablished.
	b. Distance between arm with I.V. and Medication bag has decreased.	b. Hang I.V. medication bag higher above I.V. arm.
	c. End of catheter is against wall of vein.	c. Remove I.V. tubing from heparin lock. Put needle cover back over needle. Attempt to flush heparin lock with sodium chloride. If resistance is felt STOP and call nurse or local emergency room. If heparin lock flushes easily, reconnect I.V. tubing.
	d. Catheter is displaced or clotted off.	d. If I.V. continues to infuse slowly or not at all, call nurse or local emergency room.
7. Pain at I.V. site	a. Medication is irritating vein or catheter has come out of vein.	a. STOP infusion. Inspect I.V. site for swelling, hardness or redness. If any of these signs are present call your nurse or local emergency room. If no signs are noted restart infusion at slower rate. If pain continues STOP infusion and call nurse or local emergency room.
8. Bleeding at I.V. site	a. Heparin lock has been dislodged.	a. Call nurse or local emergency room.
9. Heparin lock comes out of skin	a. Heparin lock has been dislodged.	a. Put pressure on the bleeding site for 3 to 5 minutes or until bleeding stops. Use a clean piece of gauze or cotton then call your nurse or local emergency room.

HELPFUL HINTS:

• Since you probably do not have an I.V. pole at home, here are some other items you may have that you could use to hold the I.V. bag and tubing:

   - use a clothes hanger - hang on drapery rod, lamp with heavy base, coat rack, or anything above the level of the arm with the I.V. (medication bags can also be hung on any of the items listed above without using the clothes hanger.)
   - use a secure nail or picture hanger already in wall. (Remove picture during medication administrations.)

• I.V. tubing in use can be attached to the clamp on the tubing by slipping it between the prongs. This keeps tubing from touching anything unsterile.
• If your heparin lock comes out in the middle of the night, hold bleeding site for 3 to 5 minutes or until bleeding stops. You may wait until morning to have it restarted unless you are specifically told otherwise.
• When coming in to have your I.V. restarted bring an extra t-connector, male adapter, convenience pack, and cartridge holder with you.
• Always call your doctor or nurse before coming to the hospital to have your I.V. restarted.
• Keep all I.V. supplies out of reach of small children and pets.
• Keep this Helping Hand with your I.V. supplies for easy access.

HOW TO REMOVE THE HEPARIN LOCK:

DO NOT remove the heparin lock unless:
• You are told to do so by your doctor, nurse or emergency room personnel.
• You have completed your ENTIRE course of antibiotics.

1. Gently loosen tape around catheter and male adapter.
2. Hold heparin lock with one hand. Have a clean gauze or cotton ball in the other hand.
3. Carefully pull heparin lock out of the vein with one smooth, continuous motion. Pull the heparin lock out parallel to the skin.
4. Apply pressure to the bleeding site with gauze or cotton as soon as catheter is out. Continue applying pressure for 3 to 5 minutes or until bleeding stops.
5. Apply a clean bandaide over the I.V. site.
6. Look at the catheter and make sure all of the catheter came out of the vein. If you think any of the catheter is left in the vein, proceed with the following emergency measures:
   • Apply pressure on the vein with your fingers slightly above the I.V. site.
   • Have the child lie as still as possible and not move the arm or leg that the I.V. was in.
   • Call the emergency squad and take the child to the nearest hospital emergency room.
   • Take the catheter with you.

IMPORTANT PHONE NUMBERS:

Fill in the phone numbers, copy it and tape by your phone.

Children's Hospital Emergency Room: 614-461-2500 _____

Doctor: _____

I.V. Therapy Nurse Clinician: _____

Pulmonary Clinical Nurse Specialist: _____

Local Emergency Room: _____

Equipment Supply Company: _____

Local Emergency Squad: _____

(continued)

Figure 10.4 continued

MEDICATION RECORD:

PATIENT NAME: _____

MEDICATION: _____

DOSE: _____

EXAMPLE:

FIRST WEEK:

Date → Time ↓	11/15	11/16
8 Am	PF	PF
2 Pm	PF	2:30 PM
8 Pm	PF	PF
2 Am	1:30 PF	PF

DIRECTIONS: Put your initials in the appropriate square after medication is given. If time of administration differs from assigned time, please record time in appropriate square.

FIRST WEEK:

Date: → Time: ↓							

SECOND WEEK:

Date: → Time: ↓							

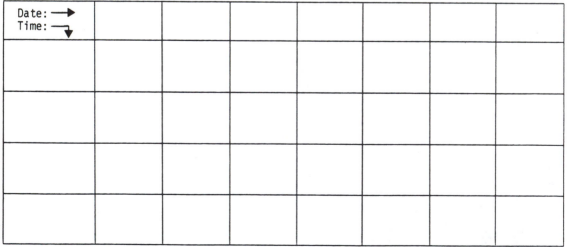

FOLLOW-UP

Continuity of care for the home IV antibiotic client includes provision for additional supplies, assurance of venous access, and 24-hour emergency coverage. Foresight should be used when initially ordering the supplies. Additional supplies should be sent home in case of accidental contamination. Further supplies should be ordered from either the hospital or pharmaceutical company in advance of the expected time of use. Clients should be told where and by whom their IV will be reinserted if needed. If the IV becomes dislodged or infiltrates during the night, the client should be instructed to remove the catheter and notify the home care agency or hospital in the morning for reinsertion. The physician or nurse should make provisions for medical follow-up during the day or night. Notifying the local emergency room ahead of time that the client is on antibiotics at home can facilitate emergency treatment if needed.

If the client will be returning to school or work, the school or occupational nurse should be notified of the client's health status, restrictions due to venous access, and what to do in case of an emergency.

Upon completion of the prescribed antibiotic regime, the client should notify the physician. The client may be instructed on the procedure for discontinuing the IV. Follow-up then is based on the physician's recommendations.

BIBLIOGRAPHY

Children's Hospital. 1983. *Nursing Assessment of Home IV Antibiotic Client.* Columbus, Ohio: Children's Hospital.
Children's Hospital Homegoing Education and Literature Program. 1985. *IV Antibiotic Therapy at Home.* Columbus, Ohio: Children's Hospital.

CHAPTER 11

Home Total Parenteral Nutrition

A Nurse's Guide to Home Total
Parenteral Nutrition
Patient Education Care Guides

Carla Powell, RN

Edited by Paul L. Cerrato, BS, MA

INTRODUCTION

Total parenteral nutrition (TPN) was first used in the mid-1960s at the University of Pennsylvania. There it was shown that normal growth and a positive nitrogen balance could be maintained with TPN in animals and humans having inadequate intestinal absorption (Dudrick 1968). The causes for such malabsorption include radiation enteritis, bowel infarction, multiple bowel resections resulting from Crohn's disease, and intestinal fistula. In children, causes can include severe trauma to the intestines, allergies, and congenital short bowel (when the bowel is too short, the remaining intestinal tract cannot absorb the nutrients necessary to sustain life). For such patients, TPN can ward off starvation when administered over a short- or long-term period. Those requiring long-term care frequently require special training to enable them to administer the regimen at home. Home parenteral nutrition (HPN) was first described by Scribner, Cole, and Christopher (1970) and is being used by a steadily increasing number of patients each year. The Shils registry reports 552 patients on HPN prior to 1981.

For patients to successfully adjust to HPN, they and their families must learn to do everything that the nurse and pharmacist do while administering TPN in the hospital setting. To help them accomplish that feat, we will describe the mechanics of instructing and discharging a patient on HPN.

The goals of this chapter are:

- To provide the nurse with the instructional materials needed to assist the patient and family in acquiring the knowledge and skills necessary to infuse HPN
- To minimize the emotional strain associated with HPN
- To provide instruction for the patient and family in the assessment, prevention, and treatment of complications of HPN and motivate the patient to seek assistance when problems occur
- To provide the patient and family with information concerning community resources

The responsibilities of each member of the HPN team are outlined in Table 11.1. While each has his or her own duties, some duties are shared across disciplines. The physician informs the patient and family of the prognosis, the chances of adapting, the cost of HPN, potential complications, mortality, and benefits (Ament 1984). The nurse reinforces and clarifies the information, allowing the patient to give a truly informed consent. The social worker provides more details on cost and then helps the patient and family determine how they can pay for the therapy. The nurse and social worker evaluate the support system the patient and family can utilize in performing HPN. If the patient will be mixing TPN solutions at home, a pharmacist will help the nurse evaluate the patient's dexterity and ability to comprehend instructions. The phar-

Table 11.1 ROLES AND RESPONSIBILITIES OF THE HPN TEAM

Physician
- Selects patients
- Obtains informed consent information
- Makes prognosis
- Estimates cost
- Treats complications
- Prescribes HPN formula and medications
- Monitors patient

Nurse
- Obtains pre-HPN information
- Assesses support system
- Obtains precatheter placement information
- Determines catheter exit site
- Conveys patient information to home supply company
- Instructs patient concerning catheter care, infusion techniques, and complications of IM and IV medication administration
- Records fluid intake and output (I&O) and sugar and ketones (S&K)
- Coordinates home supply needs and discharge date with home supply company
- Provides instructions to all agencies following patient at home

Pharmacist
- Monitors patient
- Selects parenteral solution
- Instructs patient concerning preparation of parenteral solutions

Dietitian
- Performs pre- and postdischarge nutritional assessment
- Takes diet history
- Provides diet consultation

Social Worker
- Assists in placing patient in extended care facility or foster home
- Coordinates financial reimbursement for HPN
- Evaluates emotional and psychosocial support

Home Referral Agency
- Evaluates HPN technique
- Organizes and assures arrival of all supplies
- Evaluates environmental conditions of home (e.g., cleanliness, presence of screens on windows)
- Draws blood samples and provides HPN physician with lab results
- Reevaluates HPN technique every 6 months
- Reports information obtained during evaluation to nutrition support service

Nutrition Support Service or Home Care Physician
- Follows up on patient
- Evaluates weight, intake and output (I&O), sugar and ketones (S&K), and laboratory values
- Reformulates solution when needed
- Provides diet consultation during weaning from HPN

macist and nurse will also stay in communication with the agencies charged with following the patient in the home. The home supply company may also play a role in HPN upon the advice of the nutrition support team.

If the patient is a child, two adults in the home should be given instruction. If the patient is an adult, the patient and a significant other person should be given instruction in HPN procedures and possible complications. The amount of time devoted to instruction—approximately 20 to 40 hours over 7 to 14 days—should be confirmed with the physician, patient, and family.

The cost of HPN depends on whether the HPN solution is premixed or mixed by the patient and varies from $140 to $250 a day. The method of paying for HPN must be discussed, since many patients have limited financial resources. A situational assessment form (Figure 11.1) evaluates the patient's understanding of the illness, perception of support from family and friends, and financial situation (see also Parrish, Mirtallo, and Fabri 1982). The nurse or social worker reviews the form, contacts the home supply company, and informs the patient of how much he or she will have to pay and how much will be covered by either major medical insurance or Medicare/Medicaid. Some home supply companies will continue to supply the patient even after insurance has been depleted (Steiger et al. 1986, 659). Many patients on Medicare and Medicaid are unable to return to work. Even if they are able to work, most are unable to meet the cost of HPN. When this is so, the social worker and home supply company may seek alternative means of payment.

The motor skills, vision, and ability of the patient to comprehend instructions are evaluated as instruction proceeds.

If the patient is unable to perform the procedures and a family member cannot be instructed, an extended care facility must be considered. About 15 percent of patients discharged on HPN require admission to extended care facilities.

Patients need to know that they can reach someone on the nutrition support team, at the home supply company, or at the home health nursing agency 24 hours a day. Knowing about resources, newsletters, and the existence of other people with similar situations is also a form of support for the HPN patient. The *Life Liner** newsletter, for instance, is available to anyone requesting to be put on the mailing list. The home supply company may also have newsletters for the patient.

PSYCHOSOCIAL ISSUES

Patients on HPN face more than just financial burdens. The short bowel syndrome, one common indication for IV nutritional therapy, presents many psychosocial problems as well. The problems described in the subsections be-

*Address: Oley Foundation, 214 Ham Memorial, Albany Medical Center, Albany, New York 12208.

Figure 11.1 HPN patient education program.

Situational Assessment

Please complete this form so we can get to know you better. Knowing something about you will help us give you information that is meaningful.

If you are unsure about any questions, please seek your nurse's assistance.

1. What is your main health problem? _____

   _____

2. Other health problems: _____

   _____

3. Care when home:

   a. Who will help care for you at home? _____

   b. How is the health of the caregiver? _____

   c. Is the caregiver employed? _____ Yes _____ No

      If employed, work phone number: _____

   d. What is the best time for your caregiver to come to the hospital for instruction?_____

      _____

   e. Do you feel your family understands your condition and therapy?

      _____ Yes _____ No _____ Somewhat

      If yes, in what way? _____

      If no, why not? _____

4. Finances:

   a. How much do you spend per month on medications, clinic visits, blood work, etc.?

      _____

   b. What hospital insurance do you have? _____

   c. Do you currently receive: _____ Medicare _____ Medicaid

      _____ Pension _____ Social Security Disability _____ State or county assistance

   d. What financial assistance do you have? _____

   e. Do you think you might need financial assistance in the future?

      _____ Yes _____ No

   f. Have you tried to obtain financial help from any agencies?

      _____ Yes _____ No

      If yes, what agency? _____

Psychological Assessment

Q1

1	2	3	4	5

I have not been satisfied with prior treatment for any medical condition; it was too costly: they did not listen to me

I have been satisfied with prior treatment; it was worth the expense; they cared about me and treated me promptly.

Q2

1	2	3	4	5

My faith is an important part of my daily life; I pray and attend church regularly.

I have little faith in a supreme being or God; I do not pray or attend church.

Q3

1	2	3	4	5

I don't like a lot of change all at once; I like continuity and stability in my life.

I enjoy change and variety in my life; I accept it as a part of living.

Q4

1	2	3	4	5

I am the only one at home who can do the necessary steps correctly for my hyperalimentation.

Hyperalimentation is bothersome; someone else should be responsible for my care.

Q5

1	2	3	4	5

My health is poor; I do not feel well.

I am in good health and feel well.

Q6

1	2	3	4	5

I do what I can and what I am told to keep my health.

I have lost all interest in keeping myself in good health.

Q7

1	2	3	4	5

I don't know what I would do if a problem arose: I am confused about who to contact; I would feel bad if I called the wrong person on the team.

I feel capable in my abilities to manage problems: I know who to contact if I have problems that I can't manage; I wouldn't hesitate to call anyone on the team.

Q8

1	2	3	4	5

I realize that I can't eat the way I used to, but I still enjoy being with my family at mealtime.

At mealtime, I feel left out and awkward; I don't like to sit at the table while others are eating.

Q9

1	2	3	4	5

Since I am medically stabilized, symptoms will not occur.

I realize that symptoms may develop during my therapy even though I am medically stable.

Q10

1	2	3	4	5

If I feel the need to change my therapy, I will contact a team member first, and then follow their instructions.

If I feel the need to change my therapy, I will change it and then contact a team member.

Q11

1	2	3	4	5

I distrust the team; they are closed and guarded; they listen to me superficially; they inwardly reject what I say; I question their judgement; I do not feel I am a part of this team.

I trust the team: they respect what I say and use the information that I provide for them; I have faith in their judgment; I feel I belong to the team.

(continued)

Figure 11.1 continued

Q12				
1	2	3	4	5

My family has not supported my decision to start home hyperalimentation.			My family has been supportive in my decision to start and continue home hyperalimentation.	

Q13				
1	2	3	4	5

My occupation was important to me; I want to work again if possible; I plan my daily activities around my therapy.			I'm glad I don't have to work; I didn't like my occupation; therapy stops or keeps me from doing my daily activities; I do as little as possible.	

low may result from machine dependency, fluid and food restrictions, compliance problems, poor self-care, drug use, and hospitalization.

Organic Brain Syndrome

Presenting as either an acute or chronic condition, this syndrome can be caused by drug abuse, metabolic disorders, and sepsis. It can result in inadequate attention span, inability to remember information, and poor judgment. It must be dealt with before a home training program can begin. Informing the institution's staff of the condition can help prevent patients being placed in situations where they are incapable of comprehending verbal or written instructions (Gulledge and Gipson 1979).

Distorted Body Image

It is important that patients have an opportunity to discuss the disfigurement or alterations in body appearance or function that result from being attached to a central IV line. Their feelings and concerns need to be understood and handled appropriately. If there are no cognitive problems or major causes of anxiety, most patients will learn aseptic care and heparinization within a week (Gulledge and Gipson 1979).

The initial reactions of patients with short bowel syndrome are worth noting. If the syndrome is a result of a chronic illness, such as Crohn's disease, HPN is usually viewed as a new lease on life and the patient focuses attention on learning the procedures. If the short bowel syndrome is a sudden loss, such as that resulting from bowel infarction, then the patient may suffer anxiety due to loss of bowel function. In that case the patient will have to work through a grieving process as well as learn to care for the catheter (Price and Levine 1979; Steiger et al. 1986, 658).

Depression

Patients on HPN may become depressed as a result of chronic illness, intensive hospitalization, pain, dependency on drugs or family, malnutrition, or depletion of finances. These burdens may necessitate intensive supportive psychotherapy.

In working with the depressed patient, both the clinician and the family must focus their efforts on helping the patient move from a sick role to a more active life-style. The family may also need help in adjusting, especially if the HPN patient was once the family breadwinner (Gulledge 1982; Johnslos 1981; Gulledge and Gipson 1979).

Drug Problems

Patients who are drug abusers must go through a drug withdrawal program before having a permanent catheter inserted. Good communication between staff and patient, however, may decrease the craving for drugs (Gulledge and Gipson 1979).

Equipment Dependency

Patients may be grateful to be alive, but the quality of life remains an issue. Independent people resent losing control of their lives. Daily routines and social contacts must be planned around catheter care and machine function. Equipment malfunction, frequent nocturnal voiding, and noise are common patient worries. Expense, maintenance, and equipment supply are concerns if a reliable home health care agency is not following the patient.

Strained Interrelationships

The stress of HPN is very significant for patients and for those who live with them. HPN may accentuate problems between couples if their relationship is not strong.

Couples who have successfully worked through problems together in the past adapt better to HPN than those with stormy relationships. The home care nurse may have to spend extra time in an unstable home environment to help the patient, spouse, and children adjust to HPN (Steiger et al. 1986, 658; Johnslos 1981; Gulledge and Gipson 1979).

Some patients have sexual concerns as well. They may be concerned about getting tangled in the lines or dislodging the catheter during sexual activity. Single people worry about finding a mate. Chronically ill patients may use sickness as an excuse to avoid sexual activity. As patients begin to feel and look better, they may become concerned about what their partner expects of them sexually. These concerns can usually be resolved quickly if the spouse and patient are brought together, the issues discussed, and the patient reassured that too much too soon will not be forced on him or her (Gilbert 1986; Gulledge and Gipson 1979).

A backup person must be trained so the HPN patient does not feel solely responsible. On the other hand, when another person is totally responsible for backup support, he or she may become resentful. Resentment may develop because of the time required for HPN or the constant reminder that the patient is not normal. The patient may be angry because the procedures are not being done correctly or feel guilty because HPN demands so much of the spouse (Gulledge and Gipson 1979).

Overprotectiveness by family members is another potential problem. As the medical staff tries to increase the patient's activity and independence, some family members may become unduly concerned about the patient's welfare. In a situation like this, the patient's quest for independence should be reinforced. The nursing staff will also need to spend time with the family to help them overcome their unrealistic fears. This will allow the family to vent their anger and anxiety as they redefine their relationship with the patient (Gulledge and Gipson 1979).

Food is another issue to be explored. Is mealtime when the family gets together? If so, alternatives may need to be discussed. Is eating a way of handling emotional problems? Again, alternatives need to be explored to help the patient learn new ways to cope (Gulledge and Gipson 1979). If the patient who is supposed to be NPO eats, this may cause diarrhea, increase ostomy and fistula drainage, and result in dehydration and rehospitalization. Patients who eat despite orders not to become aware very quickly of the damaging effect that eating has on their fluid and electrolyte balance.

The physician may order the patient not to eat, but the decision to eat or not can only be made by the patient. Dehydration occurs less often if the nurse assumes the patient will eat and then observes the losses over several days. The additional losses can then be replaced each day in the TPN solution or infused after TPN is discontinued.

It is important to explore potential family and individual problems prior to beginning HPN. The physician can then determine whether HPN will complicate an already stressful situation or restore quality to the patient's life.

PEDIATRIC CONSIDERATIONS

The normal growth and development of children is a prime concern of home parenteral nutrition. The recommendations of Colley, Wilson, and Wilhen (1977) are summarized below.

Neonates and Infants

Neonates and infants gain more weight and develop more rapidly when they receive auditory, visual, kinesthetic, and tactile stimulation.

Stimulation should be scheduled every 3 to 4 hours when an infant is on HPN. Pacifiers can be used to teach the sucking reflex and satisfy sucking needs. Rocking, holding, and touching—preferably by the parent—are necessary to promote parent-infant bonding.

Toddlers

Ages 1 to 3 constitute a time of increasing autonomy when the toddler needs as much freedom as possible. However, parenteral nutrition prohibits oral intake and tends to restrict mobility. Restraints may be necessary to prevent the IV feeding apparatus from becoming dislodged. Safe age-appropriate activities are necessary to let the child expend energy, such as splashing water, throwing a ball, and putting objects into containers.

Food intended for other family members should not be prepared or eaten in the child's presence. If oral intake is allowed, give patients their favorite food at intervals. For children who cannot take foods orally, lollipops are a good pacifier.

Preschoolers

Problems encountered in the 3 to 5 age group result from immobility, fears, fantasies, and a rudimentary understanding of bodily function. Because the child is restricted by parenteral nutrition, an outlet for energy and aggression is needed, such as racing cars across the bed or knocking down blocks. With guidance by parents, the use of a tricycle and other playroom activities may be allowable.

Physiology is a mystery and a source of fear for preschoolers. Discussion and reassurance can calm their fears. Mealtimes are frustrating, since children may not be able to eat. Allowing the child to talk of favorite foods may help. Most important of all is to make the child aware that parenteral nutrition is not a punishment. To provide children with some control over the situation, encourage them to bathe, dress, and brush their teeth.

Older Children and Adolescents

Patients in this age group face problems with self-esteem, a sense of identity, values, maturation, and control over their lives. They need rational explanations for their problems. Self-esteem and body image are of special concern. Nutritional deficiencies may have resulted in poor growth, delayed puberty, and an unattractive appearance. Helping patients improve their appearance will promote self-esteem. Proper body hygiene, the use of moisturizing lotions, makeup, and wearing their own clothes rather than pajamas can all give the adolescent a mental lift.

Adolescents need independence and control over their environment. To help them gain these, include them in arranging the daily care plan. Friends should also be encouraged to visit. Lastly, patients need to be given information about parenteral nutrition and allowed to discuss their concerns as often as needed.

INFUSION TECHNIQUE

The number of hours the patient is to infuse and the infusion device to be used in the home must be determined. The patient can infuse at a continuous rate or over a shorter period to permit some time off the infusion. A 24-hour portable infusion system is now available (Englert and Dudrick 1978). It allows the patient to wear a vest that contains a small infusion pump and two IV bags of TPN solution. This method allows patients who do not have the flexible schedule necessary for cyclic TPN—12 hours on TPN and 12 hours off—to receive treatment. The portable system is also appropriate for patients whose blood glucose cannot be controlled with cyclic TPN.

Adults and children who can fit cyclic TPN into their schedule adjust well to the rapid infusion rates required by this procedure (Ament 1984). To adjust the child to cyclic TPN, Ament recommends decreasing the time it takes to administer the infusion by 1 hour each day and increasing the rate proportionately to infuse the required volume. To discontinue the infusion, Ament recommends decreasing the infusion rate by 50 percent for 15 minutes and 50 percent again for 15 minutes and then discontinuing TPN as outlined in his protocol. A rapid infusion rate should be tapered to prevent rebound hypoglycemic reactions.

Cyclic TPN in adults can begin with 4 hours off and 20 hours on, if tolerated, and then progress to 8 hours off and 16 hours on. The patient may be left on this schedule for 2 to 3 days to allow for continuity during home instruction. The nurse instructor will then be able to observe the patient beginning TPN at 4 PM and discontinuing it at 8 AM the following day. To taper off the solution, it is recommended that the infusion rate be decreased to 50 ml for the last 2 hours of infusion.

To improve communication and coordination, an instruction checklist should be attached to the nursing Kardex (Figure 11.2). The clinician doing patient teaching should record the information taught in the nursing notes and on the instruction checklist. Then anyone who wants quick information concerning what the patient has been taught or whether the patient is able to perform the procedure adequately can refer to this checklist.

CHARTING HPN

Charting of each instruction session is necessary for legal documentation. The charting should include:

- *The content taught.* There is no need to document each session's instruction in detail. Only the procedure title should be charted (e.g., "Discontinuing TPN" or "Heparinizing the catheter demonstrated and practiced").

Figure 11.2 Home parenteral nutrition instruction checklist.

	Staff Nurse	Dates of Teaching (use codes)	Performs Adequately	Unable to Perform Adequately
I. *CVC* Description				
Purpose				
Insertion				
II. *Care of Catheter* Dressing change				
Line maintenance				
III. *Preparation of Solution* Measuring drugs in syringe				
IV. *Administration of Solution* Infusion pump				
Parenteral nutrition solution Formula _____ Flow rate _____				
Parenteral fluid solution Formula _____ Flow rate _____				
V. *Administration of IM, IV Meds* Injection site selection/ cleaning				
Insertion of needle				
Injection of drug				
VI. *Drawing Blood from Hickman*				
VII. *Complications* Clotting				
Infection				
Air embolism				
Inadvertent displace- ment				
Severed catheter				
Thrombosed vein				
Metabolic imbalance (hypoglycemia/ hyperglycemia)				
Equipment malfunction (alarms)				

(continued)

Figure 11.2 continued

	Staff Nurse	Dates of Teaching (use codes)				Performs Adequately	Unable to Perform Adequately
VIII. *Monitoring Techniques* I&O							
Daily weights							
Sugar and Ketones							
24-hour urines							

CODES: ✔ Knowledge/skill adequate   Preplacement assessment
     ® Reinforcement needed   Given _____
     F Family included   Reviewed _____

Adapted from the Ohio State University Hospitals Home Parenteral Nutrition Manual 1983.

- *The patient or family response to instruction.* Include answers to the following questions in your charting: Did the family and patient comprehend the information? Were appropriate questions asked during and after instruction? Are there any skill deficits that need to be evaluated?
- *Plans for continued instruction.* Document when the next instruction session will take place and whether there is a need to reinforce any of the information just taught.

EVALUATION

The patient's ability to perform HPN procedures should be evaluated as instruction progresses. Further evaluation is made every 6 months by the home health supply company or the public health agency following the patient. The patient readmitted for septic complications should be reevaluated.

Patients' verbal feedback will help to determine whether they know what community resources are available, what needs to be done when equipment malfunctions, and how to recognize and handle specific complications.

The home care nurse should demonstrate each procedure in the instruction manual supplied to the patient. After the patient has been shown the procedures, he or she should be able to give a demonstration correctly at least twice. The instructor should observe the demonstration to insure proper technique and to confirm the patient's ability to follow instructions.

Instruction booklets, cassette tapes, pictures, or videotapes are invaluable in reinforcing information. The patient and significant other should be made responsible for assembling all supplies for all procedures from the first or second day to the last teaching session.

DISCHARGE PLANS

Discharge plans begin at the time the patient is identified as an HPN candidate. Once the home supply company is notified, arrangements are made for a nurse to see the patient in the home on the day of discharge.

The HPN instruction manual supplied by the nutrition support nurse includes a continuity of care instruction sheet (Figure 11.3). This form tells the patient what the solution consists of, the infusion rate, vitamins to be administered, when each procedure is to be performed, when the monitoring procedures are to be performed, and when laboratory results are needed. This form serves two purposes. It gives patients concise information concerning what is expected of them in the home setting, and a duplicate in the patient's permanent chart provides legal documentation that the patient received basic education.

The nurse reviews the instruction sheet with the patient and family at the beginning of the instruction session as each procedure is taught and before discharge to confirm all information. The patient is also given telephone numbers that he or she can call 24 hours a day, including the home and hospital numbers of the nurse, pharmacist, resident, and physician, and the number of the home supply company. All numbers can be listed in the HPN manual.

The patient should be seen in the clinic 2 and 4 weeks after discharge and then once a month until stable. After that, the patient will return only as needed.

For children, follow-up is ongoing. To promote normal growth, caloric requirements must be reevaluated every month for the first year of life. After that, patients should be seen every 3 months.

Ament (1984) recommends that children have anthropometric measurements taken along with those for serum potassium, sodium, calcium, magnesium, total protein, and albumin.

Blood samples should be drawn for liver function studies and a complete blood count at each home visit. Trace metals should be monitored quarterly or every 6 months (Ament 1984, 343). The child's growth and development are monitored and caloric adjustments are made as needed.

A NURSE'S GUIDE TO HOME TOTAL PARENTERAL NUTRITION*

I. *Central Venous Catheter Description and Purpose*
   A. Describe the entrance and exit sites of a central venous catheter.
      1. The catheter (a thin tube with a small cuff) enters the body through a vein in the upper chest area near the clavicle.
      2. The catheter exits the body midway down the front of the

*Adapted from the Ohio State University Hospitals Education and Training Program.

Figure 11.3   Continuity of care instruction sheet.

**Referral for Continuity
of Patient Care
Supplement Sheet**

To:

Instructions Enclosed   ☐ Yes   ☐ No

☐ Nursing services   ☐ Social services

☐ Physical therapy   ☐ Nutrition services

☐ Occupational therapy   ☐ Respiratory Therapy

☐ Speech Therapy

Formula   Rate

1. Dextrose   _____gm   Start _____ an hour × _____
   Travasol with electrolytes   _____gm   Infuse _____ an hour × _____
                                            Wean _____ an hour × 2°

   Sodium chloride   _____meg
   Potassium chloride   _____meg
   Calcium gluconate   _____gm
   Magnesium sulfate   _____gm
   Trace elements   _____ml

   _____ replacement fluids _____ ml
   Other
   Other
   Total volume
   See procedure for starting TPN infusion.

2. MVI 12 _____ 5ml vials added to each TPN solution before infusion.

3. Vitamin K _____ ml (10 mg/ml) added to TPN solution once a week.

4. Lipids 500 cc 2 × a week. See procedure for lipid infusion.

5. Heparinize permanent central venous catheter once a day after all IV infusions are complete. See procedure for discontinuing TPN infusion.

6. Permanent central venous catheter dressing change _____ × a week with _____ dressing. See dressing change procedure. Notify nutrition support service (NSS) of tenderness, redness, or fever greater than 100°F.

7. Urine checks for sugar and ketones to be done once a day with first voided specimen after TPN discontinued. S&K to be recorded on I&O sheet. Notify NSS of 4 + urine checks.

8. Intake and outputs to be recorded on I&O sheets provided by NSS.
   a. Notify NSS of 500-cc difference in I&O over 2 to 3-day period.
   b. I&O sheets are to be brought to clinic on return visits.

9. 24° urine to be brought with patient on return clinic visit. They should be done on monthly intervals if clinic visits are not scheduled.

10. Laboratory work request form included with continuity form.

    Laboratory results are to be mailed to: physician or nutrition support service name and address

11. Resource telephone numbers are included in patient's Home Parenteral Nutrition Manual. These are 24-hour numbers. Please do not hesitate to call.

Information included:
_____ Home Parenteral Nutrition Manual
_____ Laboratory work request prescription
_____ Blood-drawing procedure
_____ List of home supplies
_____ Patient Home Parenteral Nutrition Manual
    _____ a. Going on TPN
    _____ b. Discontinuing TPN and heparinizing catheter
    _____ c. Complication list for Hickman and home parenteral nutrition
    _____ d. Lipid infusion
    _____ e. Medication additive instructions
    _____ f. Resource telephone numbers
    _____ g. TPN formulation and rate information
    _____ h. I&O sheets
    _____ i. TPN dressing change clean/sterile
    _____ j. Alarm and trouble-shooting information sheet
    _____ k. Other
    _____ l. Other

Signature	Phone	Date

Adapted from the Ohio State University Hospitals Home Parenteral Nutrition Manual 1983.

    chest wall (usually above the nipple area), or it exits from the abdomen.
  B. Explain where the catheter tip is placed within the body.
    1. The tip of the catheter lies in a large vein at the entrance to the right atrium, the upper chamber of the heart, or it is placed within the atrium.
    Note: Point out the sites and tip placement on a diagram or show an actual catheter.

  C. Explain the purpose(s) for which the central venous catheter will be used.

   1. To administer intravenous fluids

    a. Total parenteral nutrition (TPN) (also called hyperalimentation) is used to provide adequate long-term nutrition for patients who cannot eat in the usual manner. The high concentration of nutrients found in the TPN solution requires rapid, high-volume blood flow. This is best obtained by administering the solution through a large central vein.

    b. Electrolyte solutions (e.g., lactated Ringer's) may be given via a central venous catheter.

    c. Lipids are supplied by means of an intravenous fat emulsion, which supplies calories and essential fatty acids.

   2. To withdraw blood for lab tests.

  D. Identify and demonstrate use of the home care equipment needed to perform the following HPN procedures:

   1. Preparation of solutions

   2. Administration of IM/IV solutions

   3. Line maintenance including heparinization and changing injection cap

   4. Care of the exit site

  E. Demonstrate at least twice, the correct aseptic method for performing the above procedures.

  F. Describe how to obtain equipment from home supply company. The nurse or pharmacist must make a list of patient supplies, which can be given to the home supply company.

 II. *Insertion of Central Venous Catheter*

  A. Describe the patient's participation in preoperative care.

   1. Informed consent is required.

  B. Describe the nurse's role in catheter insertion.

   1. The nurse marks the catheter's exit site with indelible ink before the catheter is inserted.

    a. The nurse consults the physician and the patient for exit site preferences. The exit site may be on the abdomen, between the breasts, or on the chest. The patient needs to be aware of the benefits and burdens of the different sites.

     i. When the exit site is between the breasts the catheter can be tucked into the bra. This area may be more moist than other sites, however.

ii. Using the abdominal site provides a large area on which to tape the catheter. This area is also out of the way of constrictions, including the waistband, bra, and belt. If the patient's clothing is tight, however, the catheter may cause an unsightly bulge.

iii. If the chest area is used, the catheter should be low enough for the site to be viewed for cleaning.

b. If possible, the catheter should be placed on the patient's nondominant side. Some complain of a pulling sensation in the chest if the catheter is on dominant side.

2. Physical care

    a. Patient should be prepared as if going for a general anesthetic.

    b. Antiseptic soap showers may be ordered prior to surgery.

    c. Patient should be NPO after midnight prior to surgery.

3. Preoperative medication may be given to relax the patient.

C. Describe intraoperative care of the patient.

1. Intravenous fluids are given.

2. Skin is washed with povidone-iodine solution from neck to armpit, upper arm, chest below the nipple line, and abdomen.

3. Patient is placed in supine or slightly elevated position for comfort.

4. Anesthesia

    a. *Local*—The catheter insertion site is numb. Patient may complain of a stinging sensation. Patient is awake and able to answer questions and follow instructions. Patient may be asked to hold breath, move arm, or comment about degree of numbness. The local anesthetic may be supplemented with a sedative or a mild inhalation anesthetic.

    b. *General*—Patient is asleep during the procedure.

5. Catheter placement technique

    a. To create an entrance site, a 2 to 3" incision is made in the area of the vein to be used (the cephalic vein in Figure 11.4).

    b. A tunnel under the skin and into the fat tissue is then made from the entrance site to the exit site.

    c. The catheter is threaded through this tunnel and out the exit site, where it is anchored with a stitch. The tip of the catheter is then introduced into the large vessel

Figure 11.4 Placement of the catheter.

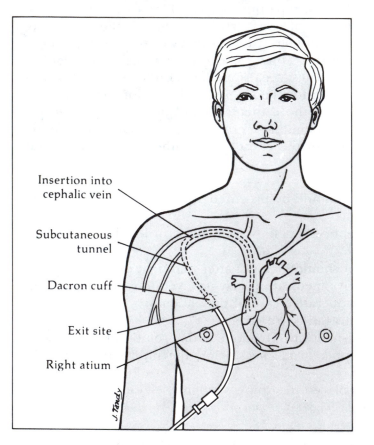

Insertion into cephalic vein

Subcutaneous tunnel

Dacron cuff

Exit site

Right atium

J. Tandy

entering the upper right chamber of the heart. This is done under fluoroscopy (X ray) so that the doctor can see where the tip of the catheter is being placed.

    d. A small cuff on the catheter is situated within the tunnel near the exit site. This cuff helps stabilize the catheter and is a barrier against infection.

    e. A dressing is placed at the entrance site under the clavicle and at the exit site.

    f. The catheter is either immediately hooked up to an IV or flushed with a heparin solution and capped.

D. Describe postoperative care of the patient.

    1. Patient under local anesthesia returns directly to room from operating room.

    2. Patient under general anesthesia goes to recovery room first.

        a. Frequent check on blood pressure, pulse, and respirations.

      b. Routine pulmonary care to clear secretions, including coughing, deep breathing, and turning.

      c. Dressing is checked for bleeding.

      d. Relief for any nausea or vomiting is provided.

   3. Pain medication is given to relieve incision site discomfort, which can last for 4 to 5 days after the procedure.

   4. Patient may experience slight burning at the exit site when it is cleansed during dressing change.

III. *Catheter Care*

  A. Describe the purpose and principles of aseptic technique.

    1. Purpose: To prevent infection

    2. Principles

      a. Microorganisms cause infection.

      b. Microorganisms exist on everything that is not properly sterilized.

      c. Microorganisms multiply rapidly, increasing the risk of infection.

      d. Microorganisms multiply more rapidly in a wet environment.

      e. Microorganisms are more virulent in cancer patients because they are on immunosuppressive drugs.

IV. *Preparation of Patient-Mixed TPN Solution*

  A. Some institutions send the patient home on a three-in-one parenteral mixture. The patient or pharmaceutical company must then mix all three components (fat, carbohydrates, and amino acids) into one bag. All ingredients come packaged separately. This procedure significantly lowers the cost of HPN, and since the patient has to mix the solution, he or she is aware of its exact composition.

  B. The solutions have to be mixed in a specific order (fat, carbohydrates, and amino acids) in a ratio of 1/2:1:1.

  C. To prevent precipitate formation, $\leq$ 15 meq of calcium, $\leq$ 30 meq of phosphorus, and $\leq$ 10 meq of magnesium should also be mixed into the three-in-one solution.

  D. In the home setting, only one day's supply of TPN solution should be mixed each day. There are two reasons for this.

    1. Bacteria will grow in a solution that is inadvertently contaminated. This growth may not be detected with the eye. If a contaminated bag is used the day it is mixed, bacteria have less of a chance to grow.

    2. Mixing one solution a day will also cut down on medication errors.

E. If the three-in-one solution is mixed by the pharmaceutical company, it should remain stable for 7 days.

F. If an IV filter is to be used for the solutions, a 4.4-micro filter is required. This allows passage of lipid particles.

G. Preparation of work area

1. Review aseptic technique and how to prevent and recognize contamination during the procedure. Include:
   a. Cleaning work area
   b. Washing hands
   c. Cleaning connection
   d. Not touching sterile parts, plunger of syringe, needle, rubber seal of TPN bag, or spike tubing.
   e. If there is a possibility that an item has been contaminated, *do not use.*

2. Discuss with patient which area of the home can be used solely for HPN procedures (e.g., an area of dining room or bedroom).
   a. Choose an area away from the mainstream of traffic that is easy to clean and that has a good light source.
   b. To prevent draft—which could carry bacteria—close all windows, doors, and air vents.
   c. Put away anything that might carry bacteria, including food, plants, and other organic matter.

3. Find a large, flat surface to work on (e.g., card table, top of chest of drawers, countertop or table covered with formica). Clean the surface with alcohol and let it dry.

4. Give an idea of amount of supplies the company will send during a 1- or 2-month period.
   a. Supplies for mixing solutions may fill a 2′ × 6′ closet. Syringes, needles, swabs, dressing supplies, and medications require additional space.
   b. A jar with lid for disposing of needles will be needed.
   c. Instruct patient to rotate supplies by putting new supplies behind older ones.
   d. Supplies should be stored under constant temperature, preferably in the home rather than the garage.

5. Place the equipment needed to prepare the TPN solution on the clean work surface.
   a. Check the sterile bottles for cracks or loss of vacuum. If you suspect the solution is contaminated, do not use the product.

H. Preparation of TPN

1. Instruct patient to wash hands as follows.

    a. Wash for 2 minutes with an antiseptic soap, cleaning between fingers. Use fingernails or orange stick to clean under nails with soapy solution.

    b. Rinse from fingertip down to wrist.

    c. Dry hands with towel.

    d. Turn water off with towel.

    e. Use towel to move IV pole if it is still hooked up to TPN.

2. Review with the patient the supplies needed to prepare the solution:

    a. Amino acid solution

    b. Dextrose solution

    c. Lipid emulsion for three-in-one mix

    d. Multivitamin solution

    e. Electrolyte solution

    f. Trace element solution

    g. Syringes (1 per additive)

    h. Needles (1 per syringe)

    i. Filter needles for ampules

    j. Final container with attached transfer tubing

    k. Alcohol swabs

    l. Povidone-iodine swabs

    m. IV pole

    n. Scissors

    o. Trash can

3. Before patient performs actual procedure, conduct mock sessions. Patient should practice with needle and syringe until comfortable.

    a. Attach needle to syringe. Do not touch hub of needle or tip of syringe. Turn needle clockwise to secure to syringe.

    b. When drawing air up into the syringe, touch only the syringe barrel and the end of the plunger.

    c. It is especially important for the patient to be adept at removing the needle cover.

4. Determine if patient knows dosage, volume, concentration, and purpose of all medications being added to TPN formula.

5. Transfer of drugs from a vial

    a. Clean amino acid or dextrose bottle seals with povidone-iodine swab.

    b. Remove plastic cap from medicine vial. Clean rubber seal with povidone-iodine and alcohol swabs.

    c. Draw amount of air into syringe equal to amount of medicine to be drawn up.

    d. Insert the needle—bevel up to prevent coring of vial—into medication vial.

    e. Invert vial, syringe and needle straight up to ceiling. Inject air into vial. (Sometimes it is difficult to push all the air into the vial. If so, allow syringe to fill with medicine, and push remainder of air in to draw out the rest of medicine.)

    f. Draw medication into syringe. Always keep needle below medication fluid level to obtain all medicine from vial.

    g. Remove the vial and tap syringe so air rises to top. Push all air out of syringe. Remember that the needle has to be straight up to expel air.

    h. Clean amino acid or dextrose bottle seal with alcohol swab.

    i. Inject medicine into TPN bag. Now repeat procedure for all medicines.

6. Transfer of drugs from an ampule

    a. Hold the ampule upright and lightly tap the top in order to free any solution adhering to the walls.

    b. Swab the neck with a povidone-iodine and alcohol swab.

    c. Wrap the same swab around the neck and grasp the ampule on each side of the neck with the thumb and forefinger. Snap the ampule so that the glass particles will be moving away from you.

7. Transfer of solution to 3-liter viaflex bag

    a. Place an empty 3-liter viaflex bag on the work surface and close both clamps on the bag's tubing.

    b. Remove metal caps from all bottles.

    c. Remove the latex cover from one of the bottles, grasping it with an alcohol swab to avoid contamination of the underlying bottle stopper.

    d. Remove the protective cover from one of the spikes on the viaflex bag's tubing. Insert the spike into the large part of the dextrose bottle, being sure not to touch the spike with your fingers.

    e. Invert and hang the bottle to be transferred onto the IV pole. Place the empty viaflex bag flat on the counter.

    f. Open the clamps on the tubing to allow the solution to flow into the viaflex bag.

g. When the transfer is complete, close the clamp on the tubing, pull the spike from the bottle, and repeat with the other bottles. Then close the clamps on the tubing and cut off the excess tubing.

    8. Invert the final solution to assure complete mixing of the ingredients.

    9. Store the final solution in the refrigerator until ready to use.

  I. Patient will need to perform this procedure two times in presence of instructor.

V. *Additives for Premixed TPN Solution*

  A. A premixed solution contains amino acids, dextrose, electrolytes, and trace elements in a ready-to-be-infused form. Because multivitamins and vitamin K do not remain stable in solution over long periods, the patient will have to add these on the day the solution is infused.

  B. Steps in procedure

    1. Clean work area with alcohol and wash hands. Clean connections with povidone-iodine, letting air-dry for 2 minutes. Then cleanse with alcohol.

    2. Review supplies needed for premixed adult TPN.

      a. 3-liter viaflex bag

      b. 2- to 5-ml vials of multivitamin solution to be added every day and 10 mg of vitamin K, added *only* once a week. (Pediatric multivitamins are dosed per age and weight. Vitamin K is included in pediatric multivitamin preparations.)

      c. 10-ml syringe with needle

      d. 3-ml syringe with needle for adding vitamin K

      e. Povidone-iodine and alcohol swabs

    3. Discard any packages that are not completely sealed. This includes any TPN bags that do not contain a plastic cover over the end where the spike is inserted.

    4. Make sure the patient knows the frequency, volume, and dosage of each drug to be added to TPN bag.

    5. Attach needle to the syringe, being careful not to touch the hub or tip of syringe. (Make sure the patient knows what part of the syringe is sterile and cannot be touched.)

    6. Pull the plunger back to draw up air equal to the number of ml of medication to be drawn up, touching only the barrel of the syringe and the end of the plunger.

    7. Have patient practice removing the needle cap from the syringe and drawing up fluids from vial. Have patient do a mock demonstration before performing with TPN bag.

8. Repeat procedure for all medicines.

   Note: If foreign particles are found floating in solution, or if solution is cloudy, or even if the patient only suspects this is the case, the solution should not be used.

VI. *Parenteral Fluid Flow Rate*

  A. Make sure the patient knows the volume, number of hours, infusion rate, and taper time.

   Over _____ hours

   Start _____ ml/hr × _____ hour

   Taper _____ ml/hr × _____ hours

  B. Tell the patient how to use the infusion pump as an alarm clock when it's time for the taper.

  C. Review signs and symptoms of hyperglycemia and hypoglycemia and the importance of not changing the TPN infusion rate without physician consent.

  D. Review how to prevent rebound hypoglycemia when TPN is stopped suddenly. The solution may have to be abruptly discontinued when a clot forms in a permanent catheter, when the low battery alarm goes off, or when the electricity goes off.

   1. In emergency situation try to taper at 50 ml/hour × 2 hours in order to prevent hypoglycemic reaction.

   2. Treatment for hypoglycemia includes protein or complex carbohydrates (milk and crackers) (Lodewick 1983).

   3. If the patient is unable to absorb the complex carbohydrates because of short bowel syndrome, an oral glucose gel or tablets, available in drug stores, may be the safest way to treat the problem. The patient should take 1 tube or tablet, letting it dissolve in the mouth. It's easy to take and can be kept at the bedside without refrigeration.

  E. If the patient is infusing at night, safety dictates that the IV be discontinued. If not, the patient will have to risk a bolus of hypertonic gravity-driven infusion.

  F. Make sure the patient knows how long the battery in the pump will last and how to recharge the battery.

  G. The instructions provided for the TPN infusion pump vary from brand to brand. Patients should follow the instructions each time they go on, no matter how well they know the procedure.

VII. *Preparing Patients to Administer TPN*

  A. Review equipment needed.

B. Review assessment, prevention, and treatment of complications.

C. Review touch contamination in patient instruction booklet, asking questions such as: Are all packages sealed? Which part of the equipment can't be touched? Tell patients to throw out anything they suspect is contaminated.

D. Review use of clamps. A padded clamp or one that has smooth edges prevents the catheter from being torn. If preferred, the patient may put tape on the catheter to prevent tearing. Vary position on the permanent catheter each time the catheter is clamped to prevent wear and tear on any one spot.

E. First day
   1. Demonstrate how to use infusion pump and review alarms.
   2. Have patient do a return demonstration.

F. Second day
   1. Have patient do mock demonstration of starting TPN and correcting alarm situation. Review all alarms with patient.
   2. If patient is comfortable with the procedure, have patient begin TPN infusion that night.

G. The physician, pharmacist, and nurse communicate during this time so that the cycle can begin at hour 20 of the first day and hour 16 of the second day, when the patient will go on the formula at 4 PM and come off at 8 AM the next morning. This allows the person giving instructions to be available when patient goes on and off.

H. The patient will stay on the 16-hour cycle for 2 to 3 days.

I. When the patient is changed to a 12-hour cycle (usually 8 PM to 8 AM), the nursing staff needs only to reinforce the information and should not need to spend excessive time instructing the patient.

J. After 4 to 5 days, the patient should be doing the procedure alone.

VIII. *Starting TPN Infusion*
   A. Review equipment needed:
      1. Alcohol
      2. Hibiclens
      3. Tape (optional if using Luer-Lok connection)
      4. TPN solution
      5. Travenol 8100 pump tubing
      6. Alcohol prep pads (1)
      7. Povidone-iodine prep pads (1)
      8. Clamp

B. Review complications that can occur with procedure and how they can be prevented:
  1. Air emboli
  2. Hyperglycemia
  3. Hypoglycemia
  4. Sepsis
  5. Machine malfunction

C. Steps in procedure
  1. Wash hands.
  2. Assemble supplies.
  3. Clean table with alcohol.
  4. Place tubing on table.
  5. Open alcohol and iodine swabs.
  6. Wash hands with antiseptic soap.
  7. Clean connection of central venous catheter and injection cap with povidone-iodine swab.
  8. Hang IV bag on pole.
  9. Remove plastic tab from bag.
  10. Clamp tubing with slide and flow-controller clamp.
  11. Remove protector cap from spike; insert spike into IV bag.
  12. Push white button on cassette down and forward. It should click in place.
  13. Fill drip chamber half full by squeezing chamber.
  14. Apply black drop detector to drip chamber.
  15. Open slide clamp.
  16. Invert cassette, white button towards floor.
  17. Open flow-control clamp.
  18. Close flow control.
  19. Insert cassette into machine cradle, white button up. (Round portion goes into cradle first.)
  20. Cleanse injection cap connection with alcohol swab.
  21. Clamp Hickman catheter with padded clamp.
  22. Remove injection cap.
  23. Remove plastic cap from tubing. Connect tubing to Hickman catheter.
  24. Raise cradle on infusion pump. All alarms should light up.
  25. Unclamp Hickman and IV tubing.
  26. Set infusion rate. Return cumulative volume to zero by pressing Clear Volume.
  27. Set dose volume. Press Up arrow until desired ml appear in dose view box.
      a. Remind patient to subtract taper volume when setting dose volume. The machine's alarm will go off when all but taper volume has infused.

        b. The patient must reset the dose volume to 100 ml and set rate to 50 ml per hour.

    28. Push Run button.

  D. Patient should perform this procedure two times with instructor watching.

IX. *Infusion of Fat Emulsion*

  A. The purpose of the solution is to prevent a fatty acid deficiency. Dosage is usually 3 to 4 percent of caloric requirements.

  B. Lipids can normally be run by gravity when piggybacked into the TPN tubing. Some HPN teams prefer an infusion pump, however. In that case, a second pump will be necessary, or the lipids can be infused with the first pump after the TPN has infused.

  C. Review equipment needed for procedure.

    1. Fat emulsion

    2. Air-vented tubing

    3. Needle

    4. Povidone-iodine swab (1)

    5. Alcohol swab (1)

    6. Tape

  D. Steps in procedure

    1. Remove tubing and fat emulsion from box.

    2. Assemble other supplies.

    3. Wash hands.

    4. Clean Y-injection port closest to catheter with povidone-iodine swab.

    5. Remove metal rim from fat emulsions.

    6. Clamp fat emulsion tubing and apply needle with plastic cover to end of tubing. Set aside.

    7. Remove cap from spike on tubing. Do not contaminate spike.

    8. Insert spike into fat emulsion through largest indentation in rubber seal.

    9. Hang bottle.

    10. Fill drip chamber half full by squeezing chamber.

    11. Open clamp and allow tubing to fill.

    12. Clean Y-injection port closest to catheter with alcohol.

    13. Insert needle into Y-injection site.

    14. Tape needle securely so it does not slip out.

    15. Run simultaneously with TPN over 4 hours. (Drip chamber 10 qtt/ml, 25–30 qtt/min for an adult.)

    16. After infusion is completed, remove tubing and needle and discard.

E. Frequency: usually 2 to 3 times a week.

F. Patient will need to perform this procedure on him- or herself at least once before discharge.

X. *Discontinuing TPN and Heparinizing the Catheter*

A. Clarify heparin dosage to be used. For example, in Seattle, Washington, 30 to 10 u/ml are used; the Cleveland Clinic uses 2000 to 1000 u/ml; the Ohio State University uses 250 to 100 u/ml for HPN patients.

B. Have patient practice working with needle and syringe, removing cap, removing needle with cap, and drawing up solution without contaminating plunger, needle, or hub.

C. Review dosage, volume, concentration, and purpose of heparin.

D. Review complications that may occur with this procedure:

   1. Air emboli

   2. Sepsis

   3. Bleeding, if wrong dose is given

E. Stress checking dose and concentration of heparin.

F. Review supplies necessary for procedure.

   1. Heparin

   2. 25-gauge needle and 3-ml syringe

   3. Injection cap

   4. Clamps

   5. Povidone-iodine swabs (3)

   6. Alcohol swabs (3)

   7. Tape

   8. Trash can

G. Steps in procedure

   1. Clean table with alcohol.

   2. Wash hands.

   3. Open all equipment and place in order of use.

   4. Turn off machine.

   5. Remove tape and clean permanent catheter and injection cap connection with povidone-iodine.

   6. Remove plastic cap from heparin cap and clean rubber disk in heparin vial with povidone-iodine.

   7. Tighten needle onto syringe by twisting in opposite direction.

   8. Cleanse rubber disk in vial with alcohol.

   9. Draw 2 ml of air into syringe.

   10. Inject air into heparin vial.

   11. Invert heparin vial and syringe; draw out required ml of heparin.

12. Hold syringe with needle straight up. Tap syringe to get air to the top of syringe. Push all air out.
13. Replace needle cap and set within reach.
14. Apply clamp to catheter.
15. Clean connection with alcohol.
16. Disconnect tubing and attach injection cap.
17. Remove clamp.
18. Inject heparin into catheter.
19. Tape connection of tubing and injection cap.
20. Tape catheter tubing to chest.
H. This protocol should be followed each time TPN is discontinued. If TPN is infused every other day, then heparinize every day. In this case, change injection cap when coming off TPN or once a week.

XI. *Dressing Change*
  A. Dressing changes may be done using sterile or clean technique. If sterile technique is used, the first day should be spent explaining to the patient how to don sterile gloves, set up a sterile field, and open a sterile package.
  B. Povidone-iodine ointment may or may not be used. There is no proven benefit from using ointment under a central venous catheter dressing (Maki and Band 1985; Powell et al. 1985).
  C. The dressing can be made of semipermeable membrane, which can stay on 7 days (Powell et al. 1985), or gauze and tape, which can be changed two to three times a week. Some HPN programs advocate no dressing.
  D. Approximate costs of each type of dressing
    1. Sterile technique with dressing kit—$5.50. The dressing kit contains transparent dressing, sterile gloves, and sterile drape.
    2. Sterile technique without dressing kit—$2.00. This requires sterile acetone alcohol swab sticks, povidone-iodine swab sticks, and transparent dressing.
    3. Clean technique—$1.60. This includes bottled alcohol and povidone-iodine, cotton swab sticks, and transparent dressing.
    4. No dressing—up to 50¢ depending on cleansing process: no charge for soap and water; 50¢ for povidone-iodine and acetone alcohol swabs.
  E. Review supplies necessary for procedure.
    1. Acetone alcohol swab sticks (2)
    2. Povidone-iodine swab sticks (1 package, 5 to package)

    3. 2" Scanpore tape

    4. Op-Site (5 × 7 cm or 10 × 14 cm)

    5. Alcohol

    6. Hibiclens soap solution to wash hands

F. Review principles of touch contamination.

    1. Wash hands per procedure described in mixing TPN solution.

    2. Hold all swab sticks so that cotton tip is above hand during cleansing.

G. Steps in procedure

    1. Assemble all equipment for dressing change.

    2. Clean table with alcohol.

    3. Open all swab stick packages. Leave swab in package with 1" to 2" of stick extending out of package. Do not touch swab stick with hand until you have washed hands. Place package so that the stick does not touch any surface.

    4. Open Op-Site.

    5. Remove old dressing and discard.

    6. Wash hands in Hibiclens soap for 2 minutes.

    7. Clean catheter exit site as follows:

        a. Start at the exit site and work outward in a circular motion, covering slightly more than the area to be dressed. Use 2 acetone alcohol swab sticks and 2 povidone-iodine swab sticks. One swab stick is to clean the catheter 2" to 3" out from exit site.

        b. Always clean from cleanest to dirtiest point. Never go back to exit site once the swab has moved away from it. Never touch exit site with fingers.

    8. Before applying Op-Site, dry the area. If you have sterile gauze, blot area dry.

    9. Apply Op-Site dressing in side to side manner. First pull paper backing half-way off, allowing sticky side to face the patient.

    10. Place dressing on skin with the halfway mark centered over catheter and the top portion of the dressing positioned 1" or more above the exit site of catheter.

        a. Never stretch Op-Site when applying to skin.

        b. Do not touch sticky side. If sticky side touches itself, it cannot be unstuck.

    11. Lift catheter 1/4" to 1/2" off chest. Pull remaining paper backing off. Pinch the dressing around the catheter and then apply to the skin in order to have a complete seal.

12. If patient will be swimming, the entire catheter and injection cap must be kept under Op-Site dressing.

13. Tape catheter to chest as desired.

XII. *Sterile Technique*

A. Review equipment necessary for procedure.
  1. TPN dressing kit
  2. Op-Site dressing (optional)

B. Review sterile technique. The patient has to master the following basic procedures before this procedure can be taught:
  1. Applying sterile gloves
  2. Opening a sterile package

C. Steps in procedure
  1. Clean off table with alcohol.
  2. Wash hands.
  3. Open TPN dressing kit.
  4. Remove old dressing. Clean area with Unisolve if needed.
  5. Put on sterile gloves.
  6. Open, remove from package, and place supplies in the order in which they will be used:
    a. Acetone alcohol swab sticks
    b. Povidone-iodine swab sticks
    c. Benzoin swab sticks
  7. Remove sterile barrier from kit and place it over catheter with the V opening directly below exit site.
  8. Cleanse around exit site, using circular motion, starting at the site and working outward. Use 2 acetone alcohol swab sticks (allow to air-dry for 2 minutes) and then 2 povidone-iodine swab sticks.
  9. Cleanse catheter with povidone-iodine swab, starting at exit site and moving outward.
  10. Using swab stick, draw a picture on the skin with benzoin 1" (one inch) from the catheter. (Optional)
  11. Apply povidone ointment to exit site. (Do not use ointment with Op-Site.)
  12. Remove sterile barrier.

Applying Op-Site

  13. Remove gloves.
  14. Apply Op-Site dressing, making sure to pinch it around and under catheter onto the skin.

15. Place strip of tape over bottom section of Op-Site.
16. Curl catheter neatly on top of this tape and securely tape to chest wall.

Applying regular gauze and tape

13. Cut gauze pad to desired size (1" × 1").
14. Tear tape to desired size. Stick on sterile plastic tray.
15. Apply gauze to exit site and hold in place.
16. Apply tape, making sure to pinch tape around and under catheter onto skin. Tape should completely seal gauze.
17. Remove sterile gloves.
18. Curl catheter neatly on top of tape and securely tape to chest wall.

   D. Two return demonstrations are necessary to certify patient in this procedure.

XIII. *Drawing Blood from a Permanent Central Venous Catheter*
   A. Review instructions and equipment necessary to perform procedure.
      1. Blue tube (1) (PT & PTT)
      2. Lavender tube (1) (CBC)
      3. Tubes for other lab work (4)
      4. Povidone-iodine prep pad
      5. Alcohol
      6. Padded clamp
      7. 10-ml syringe
      8. 30-ml syringe
      9. 5-ml syringe
      10. 20-ml syringe
      11. 2- to 10-ml vials of normal saline
      12. Injection cap
      13. Wythe heparin cartridge 100 u/ml, 2.5 ml
      14. Tubex
      15. 3- to 18-gauge needles
   B. Review possible complications.
      1. Air emboli
      2. Infection
      3. Inadvertently displaced or damaged catheter
   C. Explain need for discarded 30-ml syringe and separate 5-ml syringe when drawing from heparinized catheter.
      1. The first syringe is discarded to prevent prolonged and inaccurate PT & PTT results.

   2. If catheter is not heparinized, then 5- to 10-ml discard is appropriate.
 D. Steps in procedure
   1. Wash hands.
   2. Attach 18-gauge needle to 20-ml syringe and draw up 20 ml of saline. Insert Wythe heparin cartridge into Tubex.
   3. Cleanse injection cap and Hickman junction with povidone-iodine.
   4. Allow to dry 2 minutes and clean with alcohol swab.
   5. Clamp catheter.
   6. Remove injection cap.
   7. Attach 10-ml syringe.
   8. Unclamp catheter and draw up 10 ml of blood.
   9. Clamp catheter and *discard* syringe and blood.
   10. Attach 30-ml syringe, unclamp, and draw up 30 ml of blood.
   11. Clamp catheter, remove 30-ml syringe, and attach 5-ml syringe.
   12. Unclamp catheter and draw up 5 ml of blood. Clamp catheter.
   13. Remove 5-ml syringe, attach 20-ml syringe with saline, and irrigate catheter.
      Note: Have another person attach 18-gauge needle to 30-ml and 5-ml syringes and fill blood tubes. Fill PT & PTT and CBC tubes first so blood does not clot.
      a. Fill first: 1 blue—full
      b. Fill second: 1 lavender—full
      c. Fill third: 4 red and gray—half full
         Gently rotate tube to mix with anticoagulating solution.
   14. Unclamp catheter and slowly flush Hickman with saline.
   15. Clamp catheter, remove syringe, and attach new injection cap.
   16. Cleanse cap with povidone-iodine and alcohol.
   17. Inject 250 units of heparin into catheter.

XIV. *Complications of HPN*
 A. Clotting
   1. Definition: A blood clot forms inside the central catheter and prevents the flow of solutions through the catheter.
   2. Symptoms
      a. Occlusion alarm sounds.
      b. IV fluids will not infuse into catheter by gravity flow.
      c. Unable to aspirate (draw blood back) from the catheter.

      d. Resistance felt when injecting heparin into the inject-
ing cap. Do not force fluid in!

         Note: To develop the patient's assessment skills, have the
patient feel the normal pressure required to instill heparin. Then simulate excess resistance by temporarily
clamping the catheter and have the patient try to instill
heparin. (Make sure excess resistance is not caused by
a clamp or kinks in the line.)

  3. Prevention

      a. After TPN is discontinued, inject heparin into the cath-
eter daily as outlined above.

      b. Flush catheter with 10 ml of saline and follow with hep-
arin after blood withdrawal.

      c. Clamp catheter before opening to air to prevent back-
flash of blood into catheter.

  4. Treatment

      a. Call physician and prepare to make a visit.

      b. Physician may use medication to dissolve the clot. If this
does not work, the catheter will have to be replaced.

B. Infection

  1. Definition: Microorganisms growing around the catheter
exit site (local infection) or in the bloodstream

  2. Symptoms

      a. Local infection causes redness, swelling, warmth, ten-
derness, and/or drainage at exit site.

      b. Systemic infection causes fever, extreme fatigue, chills,
dizziness, and inability to function.

  3. Prevention (see XI. Dressing Change)

      a. Perform each procedure using proper technique as per
instructions.

         Note: If the patient is admitted to the hospital with a
catheter site infection or sepsis, request that the patient
or a family member demonstrate the dressing change
procedure to make sure there is no break in sterile technique.

  4. Treatment

      a. Call physician when temperature is greater than 101°F
and for any other signs and symptoms of infection, and
prepare to make a visit.

      b. Infection of catheter site and sepsis will both be treated
with systemic antibiotics. If neither resolves with antibiotics, the catheter may have to be replaced.

C. Air embolism

   1. Definition: Air is accidentally sucked into the bloodstream through a tear in the catheter or through the open end.

   2. Symptoms

      a. Anxiety

      b. Shortness of breath

      c. Lightheadedness

      d. Fast heartbeat

      e. Chest pain

      f. Bluish discoloration of skin

      g. Fainting

   3. Prevention

      a. Never allow catheter to become open to air unless it is clamped.

      b. Make sure injection cap is screwed on tightly or taped securely in place.

      c. Tape catheter to dressing so that it does not hang loose.

      d. Keep scissors away from catheter to prevent accidental cutting.

      e. Use a padded clamp to prevent the catheter from breaking.

   4. Treatment

      a. Call emergency squad.

      b. Immediately lie down and turn on left side.

D. Catheter displacement

   1. Definition: Accidental movement of catheter from its original position

   2. Symptoms

      a. Chest pain

      b. Burning

      c. Cuff of catheter may be showing.
Note: Show patient a permanent CVC and point out the cuff. Check with physician on actual position of catheter cuff.

      d. Length of catheter outside of chest is longer than normal.

      e. Swelling may occur between insertion area and exit site. (This rarely occurs unless large volumes of fluids are being given.)
Note: The catheter normally moves in and out slightly with breathing.

   3. Prevention

        a. For the first 2 months after placement, observe that the suture is attached to the catheter and exit site at each dressing change.

        b. Coil the excess catheter and tape to chest or dressing.

    4. Treatment

        a. Call physician and prepare to make a visit. Catheter may need to be replaced.

        b. Coil excess catheter and tape to chest or dressing.

E. Severed catheter

    1. Definition: A hole or tear in catheter

    2. Symptoms

        a. Bleeding from catheter

        b. Signs of air in bloodstream (see C. Air Embolism above)

    3. Prevention

        a. Be careful not to accidentally cut or tear the catheter.

        b. Do not use scissors to trim the dressing.

        c. Use only clamps that cannot tear (e.g., padded hemostat or plastic clamp without teeth).

        d. Always coil excess catheter and tape to chest or dressing so catheter is not pulled.

    4. Treatment

        a. Clamp catheter with fingers, and check to see if clamp was cause of tear.

        b. If clamp was not the cause, use clamp between the cut or tear and chest.

        c. The catheter can be repaired within 20 minutes with a repair kit. Make sure these are available.

        d. Call physician and prepare to make a visit.

F. Thrombosed vein

    1. Definition: Blood clots and/or impaired blood flow in the catheterized vein as a result of catheter irritation

    2. Symptoms

        a. Swelling or discomfort in upper arm or shoulder, at or near the catheter insertion site

        b. Tightness or pressure in middle of chest

        c. Appearance of small veins around insertion site

    3. Prevention

        a. None

    4. Treatment

        a. Call physician and prepare to make a visit.

G. Metabolic imbalances

Note: To prevent metabolic imbalances, monitor daily weights, intake and output (I&O), and sugar and ketones (S&K) as per routine schedule while patient is hospitalized. Instruct patient in obtaining daily weights, I&O, and S&K on first voided urine in the morning. Have patient practice.

1. Fluid/electrolyte imbalance
   a. Definition: An imbalance of various electrolytes (minerals) and/or volume of fluid in blood and body tissues
   b. Symptoms
      i. Weakness, easily fatigued
      ii. Tingling in arms, legs, hands, feet
      iii. Thirst
      iv. Weight loss or gain
      v. Swelling
      vi. Nausea, vomiting, diarrhea
      vii. A 500-ml difference between intake and output over a 2-day period
   c. Prevention
      i. Monitor electrolyte blood levels specified by physician.
      ii. Keep accurate measurements of weight and intake/output.
      iii. Contact health professional if nausea, vomiting, or diarrhea lasts longer than 24 hours.
   d. Treatment
      i. Physician will prescribe any necessary addition or deletion of electrolytes or fluids.
2. Hyperglycemia
   a. Definition: An increase in the blood glucose above normal.
   b. Symptoms: Can result when infusion rate is too fast. Include:
      i. Frequent urination
      ii. Thirst
      iii. Nausea
      iv. Weakness
      v. Headache
      vi. Positive glucose (sugar) in urine
   c. Prevention
      i. Start TPN at beginning rate for 1 hour, then set to higher rate as prescribed by nutrition support service.
      ii. Maintain constant flow rate.
   d. Treatment: Decrease slowly the rate of TPN infusion.
3. Hypoglycemia

      a. Definition: A decrease in the blood glucose above normal.

      b. Symptoms: can result from interruption in flow rate. If so, occlusion alarm sounds in 15 to 30 minutes. Include:

         i. Cold and clammy skin

         ii. Jittery feeling

         iii. Nervousness

         iv. Headache, nausea, and hunger

     c. Prevention

         i. Maintain constant flow rate.

         ii. Taper off HPN at end of infusion, as prescribed by nutrition support service.

     d. Treatment

         i. Glucose gel or tablet. Repeat dose in 20 minutes if symptoms persist.

         ii. Eat something sweet, such as hard candy or sugar-sweetened orange juice.

H. Malfunction of TPN equipment or supplies

  1. Definition: Any malfunction of pump, alarms, or cassette/tubing that prevents safe, proper administration of HPN or problems with dressing kit

  2. Symptoms

     a. Electric shock or tingling sensation when infusion pump is touched

     b. A nonfunctioning pump will cause an alarm signal.

     c. Dressing kit with plastic covering open or missing supplies or dry swab sticks.

  3. Prevention

     a. Have certified electrician check house for proper grounding.

     b. Use three-prong plug in room where HPN is administered (Jacobson, Boger, and Harrison 1981).

     c. Do not use other electrical appliances while pump is running. Run pump on battery if other appliances must be used.

     d. Keep machine plugged in at all times.

     e. Keep machine clean.

  4. Treatment

     a. Battery is recharged by plugging it in for 16 hours during use.

     b. Repeat the procedure for starting TPN, following the instruction booklet step by step.

     c. For infusion pump malfunction, call home supply

agency immediately to arrange for a replacement
pump.

   d. For alarms, refer to alarm trouble-shooting sheet.

   e. Replace cassette if not functioning. Repeat the procedure for starting TPN, following instruction booklet closely.

   f. Call home supply agency to arrange for cassette replacement.

      i. Be sure to save package in which cassette came.

      ii. Packaging and nonfunctioning cassette go back to NSS nurse with description of problem.

   g. Do not use defective dressing kit.

      i. The home supply company will provide reimbursement.

      ii. Keep the damaged kit's stock number for nurse.

XV. *24-Hour Urine Collection*

  A. Review equipment necessary for collection:

    1. Container to hold and transport collected specimens (washed-out 1/2-gallon plastic milk containers are excellent)

    2. Container for each voided specimen

  B. The 24-hour collection does not have to be repeated just because a patient misses one specimen. If the amount can be estimated, just note the mishap on the lab slip.

  C. Have patient start the collection with first voided morning specimen.

  D. Steps in procedure

    1. Upon awakening, void, discard this specimen, and note the time.

    2. Collect and save all urine for the next 24 hours.

    3. The last specimen collected should be taken approximately 24 hours after the first one.

  E. Frequency: once a month.

XVI. *Intake and Output Chart*

  A. A 30-day intake and output chart is shown in Figure 11.5.

  B. All output, including urine, emesis, drainage from fistula, and diarrhea, should be recorded in milliliters for each 24-hour period.

  C. All fluid taken in, including IV infusion and oral intake, should be recorded in milliliters for each 24-hour period.

    1. Intake and output for each 24-hour period should be recorded on a separate data sheet, then totaled and entered on the chart.

Figure 11.5 30-Day intake and output data sheet.

Date	Weight	IV Intake	Oral Intake	Total Intake	Total Output	Sugar and Ketone	Urine Output	Emesis	Other Output

2. The amount of all intake and output should then be totaled.

D. The patient will be required to record intake and output until his or her weight is stable and there are no fluid and electrolyte imbalances.

E. Dehydration resulting in weight loss and overhydration resulting in weight gain are two common complications to watch for.

F. Weight should be recorded once a week.

G. The patient should take the record to the clinic to be reviewed by the physician.

XVII. *Urinary Sugar and Ketone Testing*

A. The following information should be given to the patient:

    1. The urine should always be negative for sugar and ketones.

    2. For the HPN patient, sugar in the urine can indicate that the body is not tolerating the IV glucose load.

    3. Ketones in the urine mean the body is burning too much fat.

    4. Flu, systemic or CVC site infections, or any other stress may cause sugar to be released into the urine.

    5. Whenever sugar or ketones are found in the urine, notify the physician or nurse.

B. Steps in the procedure

    1. Gather materials:

        a. Keto-Diastix reagent strips

        b. Timer or watch with second hand

    2. Check expiration date on bottle. Do not use an expired bottle of reagent strips. Discard if bottle has been open longer than 4 months.

    3. Collect fresh urine specimen in a clean, dry container. (Be sure to do the test on the first voided morning specimen after coming off TPN.)

    4. Open the bottle, immediately remove one test strip, and replace cap on bottle. Hold the plastic end of the strip and do not touch the test areas.

    5. Dip test areas of strip into urine and immediately remove it. As an alternative, pass the test end of the strip through a stream of urine. Begin timing.

    6. Compare the ketone test area to the ketone color chart exactly 15 seconds after wetting.

    7. Compare the glucose test area to the glucose color chart exactly 30 seconds after wetting. (The total time for glucose and ketone tests together is 30 seconds.)

    8. Record results of both tests in the correct column of the intake and output chart.

PATIENT EDUCATION CARE GUIDE*

TRAVENOL 8100 ALARM TROUBLE-SHOOTING SHEET

Alarm	Cause	Effect on Pump	How to Correct Problem
Battery low	Battery weak Running IV infusion on battery	Pump will stop infusing in 15 minutes	Keep plugged into electrical outlet at least 16 out of 24 hours. Infusion pump will recharge while in use, giving an 80% charge. Always keep plugged in when not in use.
Cassette	Cassette not properly set in pump Defective infusion set; check for leaks	No flow	Seat cassette into cradle (large rounded end goes into cradle while button is up). Push cassette cradle up. Change infusion pump tubing.
Dose end alternating with KVO (keep vein open)	Infusion complete	KVO 5 ml/hr or less	Reset infusion rate and dose volume to be infused. Start machine to taper glucose or infusion. Discontinue IV infusion. Stop alarm and pump by lowering cassette cradle.
Drop sensor	Drop sensor not attached to drip chamber Run switch pressed; occurs when dose control not being used Drop sensor unplugged on back of pump	No flow	Plug in drop sensor at back of pump. Attach drop sensor to drip chamber. Push stop. Push run switch. Dose control has to be set if drop sensor not used.
Failure alternating all with code number	Malfunction in pump Holding a digit midway between two numbers	No flow	Take pump out of service. Call home supply for new pump.

Alarm	Cause	Effect on Pump	How to Correct Problem
High flow	Liquid sloshing in chamber Defective infusion set Over-primed drip chamber Squeezing drip chamber while pump running	No flow	Reduce level of fluid in IV drip chamber. Stop cause of sloshing chamber. Insert new infusion set. Resume infusion.
Low flow	Empty IV fluid container Clamped tubing Occluded or kinked catheter at cassette Flooded drip chamber Dirty drop sensor eye Air in cassette chamber Drop sensor not attached to drip chamber Misprimed IV set	Keep open rate	Hang new bag. Unclamp tubing. Notify physician. Fill chamber only half full. Clean drop sensor with Q-tip and water. Remove air from tubing and/or cassette. Attach drop sensor to drip chamber. Resume infusion.
Occluded	IV tubing catheter below cassette clamped or kinked Clogged filter Catheter clamped or clotted 18-gauge needle inserted into Y site at distal end of IV tubing may occlude infusion from pump.	No flow	Push stop. Unclamp tubing or change filter. Push run. Pull needle back and secure or change needle size. Push start to resume infusion.
Rate	Start button pushed without rate of infusion dialed	No flow	Set rate of infusion. Push stop. Push run to resume infusion.
Stopped	Infusion pump not turned back on when stopped	No flow— alarm will sound every 5 minutes.	Push stop. Push run. If infusion completed, lower cassette cradle and disconnect from infusion per procedure.

DRAWING BLOOD THROUGH HICKMAN CATHETER

Gather all supplies. Open packages and place in order of use as listed below.

Equipment

1 blue tube (PT & PTT)
1 lavender tube (CBC)
4 tubes for other lab work
Povidone-iodine prep pads
Alcohol prep pads
Padded clamp
10-ml syringe
30-ml syringe

5-ml syringe
20-ml syringe
2- to 10-ml vials of normal saline
Injection cap
Heparin
3-ml syringe with needle
3- to 8-gauge needles

Practice Session	Steps in Procedure	Final Demo
	1. Wash hands.	
	2. Attach 18-g needle to 20-ml syringe and draw up 20 ml of saline. Draw up prescribed heparin dose in syringe.	
	3. Cleanse injection cap and Hickman junction with povidone-iodine.	
	4. Allow to dry 2 minutes and clean with alcohol swab.	
	5. Clamp catheter.	
	6. Remove injection cap.	
	7. Attach 10-ml syringe.	
	8. Unclamp catheter and draw up 10 ml of blood.	
	9. Clamp catheter and *discard* this syringe and blood.	
	10. Attach 30-ml syringe, unclamp, and draw up 30 ml of blood.	
	11. Clamp catheter, remove 30-ml syringe, and attach 5-ml syringe.	
	12. Unclamp catheter and draw up 5 ml of blood. Clamp catheter.	
	13. Remove 5-ml syringe, attach 20-ml syringe with saline, and irrigate catheter. *Note*: Have another person attach 18-gauge needle to 30-ml and 5-ml syringes and fill blood tubes.	

Fill first: 1 blue—full
Fill second: 1 lavender—full
Fill third: 4 red and gray—half
    full

14. Unclamp catheter and slowly flush Hickman with saline.
15. Clamp catheter, remove syringe, and attach new injection cap.
16. Cleanse cap with povidone-iodine and alcohol.
17. Inject 250 units of heparin into catheter.

PERMANENT CENTRAL VENOUS CATHETER DRESSING CHANGE (STERILE TECHNIQUE)

Frequency (as determined).

Equipment

TPN dressing kit
Op-Site (optional)

Practice Session	Steps in Procedure	Final Demo

1. Clean table with alcohol.
2. Wash hands.
3. Open TPN kit.
4. Remove old dressing.
5. Put on sterile gloves.
6. Open, remove from package, and place in order of use:
   • Acetone alcohol swab sticks
   • Povidone-iodine swab sticks
   • Povidone-iodine swab
   • Benzoin swab sticks
7. Remove sterile barrier from kit and place over catheter with the "V" opening directly below exit site.
8. Cleanse around exit site using a circular motion, starting at the site and working outward without returning to the center. Clean an area larger than the dressing will cover.

Use:
- 1 acetone alcohol swab stick (allow to air-dry for 2 minutes)
- 2 povidone-iodine swab sticks

9. Cleanse catheter with povidone-iodine swab, starting at exit site and moving outward toward end.
10. Using swab stick, apply benzoin like a picture frame to the skin 1 inch from the catheter. (Optional)
11. Apply povidone ointment to exit site. Do not use ointment with Op-Site.
12. Remove sterile barrier.

Op-Site

13. Remove gloves.
14. Apply Op-Site, making sure to pinch it onto the skin around and under catheter.
15. Place strip of tape over bottom section of Op-Site.
16. Curl catheter neatly on top of this tape and securely tape to chest wall.

Regular Gauze and Tape

13. Cut gauze pad to desired size (1 × 1 inch).
14. Tear tape to desired size. Stick on sterile plastic tray.
15. Apply gauze to exit site and hold in place.
16. Apply tape, making sure to pinch tape onto skin around and under catheter. Tape should completely seal gauze.
17. Remove sterile gloves.
18. Curl catheter neatly on top of tape and securely tape to chest wall.

PERMANENT CENTRAL VENOUS CATHETER (CVC) DRESSING CHANGE (CLEAN TECHNIQUE)

Equipment

2 acetone alcohol swab sticks
1 package providone-iodine swab sticks (3 to package)
2″ scanpore tape
Op-Site (5 × 7 cm or 10 × 14 cm)
Alcohol
Antiseptic soap solution to wash hands

Practice Session	Steps in Procedure	Final Demo

1. Assemble all equipment for dressing change.
2. Clean table with alcohol.
3. Open all swab stick packages. Leave swab in package with 1 to 2 inches sticking out of package. Do not touch swab stick with hand until you have washed hands. Place package so that the stick does not touch any surface.
4. Open Op-site.
5. Remove old dressing and discard.
6. Wash hands in antiseptic soap for 2 minutes.
7. Clean catheter exit site as follows: Start at the exit site and work outward in a circular motion, covering an area larger than the dressing will cover. This makes the exit the cleanest area. Use:
   - 2 acetone alcohol swab sticks
   - 2 povidone-iodine swab sticks
   - 1 swab stick is to clean the catheter 2 to 3 inches out from exit site.
8. Holding green edge of Op-Site, remove half (2 to 3 inches) of protective backing and apply this half to skin.
9. Pinch Op-Site around catheter or around portion of permanent catheter emerging from exit site.
10. Peel away remainder of paper backing while gently smoothing Op-Site onto skin. Care must be taken not to stretch Op-Site while placing on skin.
11. Remove green tabs from Op-Site dressing.
12. Anchor remainder of exposed catheter or IV tubing:
    - Place a piece of tape along lower border of Op-Site, leaving emerging catheter exposed by making a tear in the tape. This provides a base upon which more tape can be placed.
    - Place a second piece of tape directly over first piece, covering exposed tubing or catheter.
    - Loop remainder of catheter or tubing upward and secure to base tape and/or skin, using additional tape as necessary.

- Place small piece of tape on corner of Op-Site dressing and label with date, time, and initials.

Pertinent Information

1. Before Op-Site can be applied, the area has to be dry. If you have sterile gauze the area can be blotted dry.
2. Never stretch Op-Site when applying to skin.
3. Do not touch sticky side.
4. If sticky side touches itself, it cannot be unstuck.
5. Always pinch Op-Site around the catheter and then apply to the skin in order to have a complete seal.
6. If you will be swimming, the whole catheter and injection cap must be under Op-Site.

PREPARATION OF WORK AREA FOR MIXING TPN

Practice Session	Steps in Procedure	Final Demo
	1. Choose an area away from the mainstream of traffic that is easy to clean and that has a good light source.	
	2. To prevent drafts, which could carry bacteria, close all windows, doors, and air vents.	
	3. Put away anything that might carry bacteria, such as food, plants, or other organic agents.	
	4. Use a large flat surface, such as a table or countertop, which can be cleansed with alcohol.	
	5. Obtain a jar with lid for disposing of needles.	
	6. Clean the countertop with alcohol. Let the surface air-dry.	
	7. Place the equipment needed to prepare the TPN solution on the clean work surface.	
	8. Check the sterile bottles for cracks or loss of vacuum. If contamination of the solution is suspected, do not use the product.	

PREPARATION OF TPN

Equipment

Multivitamin solution
Electrolyte solution
Trace element solution
Syringes (1 per additive)
Needles (1 per syringe)
Final container with attached trans-
   fer tubing

Alcohol swabs
Povidone-iodine swabs
IV pole
Scissors
Trash can

Practice Session	Steps in Procedure	Final Demo

1. Wash hands thoroughly.
2. Review solution formula. Select supplies and medication necessary for solution.
3. Attach needle to syringe. Do not touch hub of needle or tip of syringe. Turn needle clockwise to secure to syringe.
4. When drawing air into syringe, touch only the barrel of syringe and the end of plunger.

Transfer of Drugs from a Vial

1. Clean amino acid or dextrose bottle seal with povidone-iodine swab.
2. Remove plastic cap from medicine vial. Clean rubber seal with povidone-iodine swab and alcohol swab.
3. Draw amount of air into syringe equal to amount of medicine to be drawn up.
4. Insert the needle into medication vial, bevel up to prevent coring into vial.
5. Invert vial, syringe and needle straight up to ceiling. Inject air into vial.
6. Draw medication into syringe. Always keep needle below medication fluid level to obtain all medicine from vial.
7. Remove the vial and tap syringe so air rises to top. Push all air out of syringe.
8. Clean amino acid or dextrose bottle seal with alcohol swab.
9. Inject medicine into TPN bag.
10. Repeat procedure for all medicines.

Transfer of Drugs from an Ampule

1. Hold the ampule upright and tap the top lightly in order to remove any solution there.
2. Swab the neck with a povidone-iodine and alcohol swab.
3. Wrap the same swab around the neck and grasp the ampule on each side of the neck with the thumb and forefinger. Snap the ampule at the neck so that the parts of the ampule will be moving away from you.
4. When the stem of ampule is removed, draw up drug using filter needle. Do not allow needle to touch side of ampule.
5. Replace filter needle with new sterile needle and set aside until needed.
6. Transfer solution to 3-liter viaflex bag.
   - Place an empty 3-liter viaflex bag on the counter top and close both clamps on the bag's tubing.
   - Remove metal caps from all bottles.
   - Remove the latex cover from one of the bottles, grasping the latex with an alcohol swab to avoid contamination of the underlying bottle stopper.
   - Remove the protective cover from one of the spikes on the viaflex bag's tubing. Insert the spike into the large part of the dextrose bottle, being sure not to touch the spike with your fingers.
   - Invert and hang the bottle to be transferred onto the IV pole. Place the empty viaflex bag flat on the counter.
   - Open the clamps on the tubing, allowing the solution to flow into the viaflex bag.
   - When the transfer is complete, close the clamp on the tubing, pull the spike from the bottle, and repeat with the other bottles until transfer is complete.
   - Close the clamps on the tubing and cut off the excess tubing.
   - Invert the final solution to assure complete mixing of the ingredients.
   - Store the final solution in the refrigerator until ready to use.

ADDITIVES FOR PREMIXED TPN SOLUTION

Equipment

TPN bag
Multivitamins—2- to 5-ml vials
　(added every day)
Vitamin K—10 mg (added *only* once
　a week)
10-ml syringe with needle

3-ml syringe with needle for adding
　vitamin K
Povidone-iodine swabs
Alcohol swabs
Other additives (Optional)

Practice Session	Steps in Procedure	Final Demo
	1. Review solution formula. Select supplies and medication necessary for solution.	
	2. Discard any packages that are not completely sealed. This includes TPN bags without a plastic cover over the end where the spike is inserted.	
	3. Attach needle to the syringe, being careful not to touch the hub or tip of syringe.	
	4. Pull the plunger back to draw up air equal to the milliliters of medication to be drawn up. Touch only the barrel of syringe and the end of the plunger.	
	Transfer of Drugs from a Vial	
	1. Clean the injection port on the TPN bag with povidone-iodine swab.	
	2. Remove the plastic cap from medicine vial. Clean rubber seal with povidone-iodine swab and alcohol swab.	
	3. Draw amount of air into syringe equal to amount of medicine to be drawn up.	
	4. Insert the needle into medication vial, bevel up to prevent coring into vial.	
	5. Invert vial and syringe needle straight up to ceiling. Inject air into vial.	
	6. Draw medication into syringe. Always keep needle below medication fluid level to obtain all medicine from vial.	
	7. Remove the vial and tap syringe so air rises to top. Push all air out of syringe.	
	8. Wipe TPN bag injection port with alcohol.	
	9. Inject medicine into TPN bag.	
	10. Repeat procedure for all medicines.	

STARTING TPN INFUSION (TRAVENOL 8100 INFUSION PUMP)

Equipment

Alcohol
Antiseptic soap
Tape
TPN bag
Clamp

Travenol 8100 pump tubing
Alcohol prep pads (1)
Povidone-iodine prep pads (1)
Needle

Practice Session	Steps in Procedure	Final Demo
	1. Wash hands.	
	2. Assemble supplies.	
	3. Clean table with alcohol.	
	4. Place tubing on table. Open alcohol and iodine swabs.	
	5. Wash hands with antiseptic soap.	
	6. Clean connection of catheter and injection cap with povidone-iodine swab.	
	7. Hang IV bag on IV pole.	
	8. Remove plastic tab from bag.	
	9. Clamp tubing with slide and flow-controller clamp.	
	10. Remove protector cap from spike and insert spike into IV bag.	
	11. Push white button on cassette down and toward round part of cassette. It should click in place.	
	12. Fill drip chamber half full by squeezing chamber.	
	13. Apply black drop detector to drip chamber.	
	14. Open slide clamp.	
	15. Invert cassette by positioning white button toward floor.	
	16. Open flow-control clamp and fill tubing, thumping Y-sites to remove air.	
	17. Close flow control.	
	18. Insert cassette into machine cradle. White button should face up toward ceiling. (Round portion goes into cradle first.)	
	19. Cleanse injection cap connection with alcohol swab.	
	20. Clamp catheter with padded clamp or clamp without teeth.	

21. Remove injection cap.
22. Remove plastic cap from tubing and connect tubing to catheter.
23. Raise cradle on infusion pump. All alarms should light up.
24. Unclamp catheter and tubing.
25. Set infusion rate. Reduce cumulative volume to zero by pressing Clear Volume.
26. Set dose volume. Press On/Clear button until 0000 appears. Press Up arrow until desired ml appear in dose viewbox.
27. Push Run button.

FAT EMULSION INFUSION

Frequency

As determined.

Method of Administration

As determined. NOTE: Bottle must be disconnected as soon as it is infused.

Equipment

Fat emulsion
Air-vented tubing
Needle

Povidone-iodine swabs (1)
Alcohol swab (1)
Tape

Practice Session	Steps in Procedure	Final Demo

1. Remove tubing and fat emulsion from box.
2. Assemble other supplies.
3. Wash hands.
4. Clean Y-injection port closest to catheter with povidone-iodine swab.
5. Remove metal rim from fat emulsion.
6. Clamp fat emulsion tubing and apply needle with plastic cover to end of tubing. Set aside.
7. Remove cap from spike on tubing. Do not contaminate spike.
8. Insert spike into fat emulsion through largest indentation in rubber seal.

9. Hang bottle.
10. Fill drip chamber half full by squeezing chamber.
11. Open clamp and allow tubing to fill.
12. Clean Y-injection port closest to catheter with alcohol.
13. Insert needle into Y-injection site.
14. Tape needle securely so it cannot slip out.
15. Run simultaneously with TPN over ____ hours ____ qtt/min.
16. When infusion is complete, remove tubing and needle and discard.

DISCONTINUING TPN AND HEPARINIZING CATHETER

Equipment

Heparin ____ u/ml ____ ml
25-gauge needle and 3-ml syringe
Injection cap
Clamps

Povidone-iodine swabs (3)
Alcohol swabs (3)
Tape
Trash can

Practice Session	Steps in Procedure	Final Demo

1. Clean table with alcohol.
2. Wash hands.
3. Open all equipment and place in order of use.
4. Turn off machine.
5. Remove tape and clean permanent catheter and injection cap connection with povidone-iodine.
6. Remove plastic cap from heparin and clean rubber disk in heparin vial with povidone-iodine.
7. Tighten needle onto syringe by twisting in opposite direction.
8. Cleanse rubber disk in vial with alcohol.
9. Draw 2 ml of air into syringe.
10. Inject air into heparin vial.
11. Invert heparin vial and syringe; draw out ____ ml of heparin.
12. Hold syringe with needle straight up. Tap sy-

ringe to get air to the top of syringe. Push
all air out.

13. Replace needle cap and set within reach.
14. Apply clamp to catheter.
15. Clean connection with alcohol.
16. Disconnect tubing and attach injection cap.
17. Clean connection cap with povidone-iodine
    and alcohol.
18. Remove clamp.
19. Inject heparin into catheter.
20. Tape connection of tubing and injection cap.
21. Tape catheter tubing to chest.

HPN COMPLICATIONS

Complication	Definition	Assessment	Prevention	Treatment
Clotting	A blood clot forms inside the permanent central catheter and prevents the flow of solutions thru the catheter.	Occlusion alarm sounds. IV fluid will not infuse into catheter by gravity flow. Unable to aspirate (draw blood back) from catheter. Resistance felt when injecting heparin into the injection cap. Do not force fluid in!	Inject heparin into the catheter daily as per procedure after TPN is discontinued. Flush catheter with 10 ml of saline and follow with heparin after blood withdrawal. Clamp catheter before opening to air to prevent back-flash of blood into catheter.	Call physician and prepare to make a visit. Physician may use medication to dissolve the clot. If this does not work, the catheter will have to be replaced.
Infection	Microorganisms growing around the catheter exit site (local infection) or in the bloodstream	Local infection: redness, swelling, warmth, tenderness, an/or drainage at exit site. Systemic infection: fever, extreme fatigue, chills, dizziness, inability to function	Perform each procedure using proper technique as per instruction.	Call physician when temperature is greater than 101°F and for any of the other signs and symptoms of infection, and prepare to make a visit. Infection of catheter site and sepsis will both be treated with systemic antibiotics. If neither resolves with

Complication	Cause	Signs and Symptoms	Prevention	What to do
Air Embolism	Air is accidentally sucked into the bloodstream through a tear in the catheter or through the open end.	Anxiety Shortness of breath Lightheadedness Fast heartbeat Chest pain Bluish discoloration of skin Fainting	Never allow catheter to become open to air unless it is clamped. Make sure injection cap is screwed on tightly or taped securely in place. Tape catheter to dressing so it does not hang loose. Keep scissors away from catheter to prevent accidental cutting. Use padded clamp to prevent breaking catheter.	Immediately lie down and turn on left side. Call emergency squad.
Catheter Displacement	Accidental movement of catheter from its original position *Note:* Catheter normally moves in and out slightly with breathing.	Chest pain Burning Cuff of catheter may be showing. Catheter length outside of chest is longer than normal. Swelling between insertion area and exit site (rarely occurs unless large volumes of fluid are being given)	For the first 2 months after placement, observe that the suture is attached to the catheter and exit site at each dressing change. Coil the excess catheter and tape to chest or dressing.	Call physician and prepare to make a visit. Catheter may need to be replaced. Coil excess catheter and tape to chest or dressing.
Severed Catheter	A hole or tear in catheter	Bleeding from catheter Signs of air in bloodstream (see Air Embolism above)	Be careful not to accidentally cut or tear the catheter. Do not use scissors to trim the dressing. Use only clamps that cannot	Clamp catheter with fingers, and check to see if clamp was cause of tear.

HPN COMPLICATIONS continued

Complication	Definition	Assessment	Prevention	Treatment
			tear (e.g., padded hemostat or plastic clamp without teeth). Always coil excess catheter and tape to chest or dressing so catheter is not pulled.	the cause, use clamp between the cut or tear and chest. Call physician and prepare to make a visit.
Thrombosed Vein	Blood clots and/or impaired blood flow in catheterized vein as a result of catheter irritation	Swelling or discomfort in upper arm or shoulder, at or near catheter insertion site Tightness or pressure in middle of chest Appearance of small veins around the insertion site	None	Call physician and prepare to make a visit.
Metabolic Imbalances	Imbalance in blood/body of various electrolytes (minerals) and/or volume of fluid	Weakness, easily fatigued Tingling in arms, legs, hands, feet Thirst Weight loss/or gain Swelling Nausea, vomiting, diarrhea A 500-ml difference between intake and output over a 2-day period	Monitor electrolyte blood levels as specified by physician Keep accurate measurements of weight and intake/output. Contact health professional if nausea, vomiting, or diarrhea lasts longer than 24 hours.	Physician will prescribe any necessary addition or deletion of electrolyte or fluids.
Hyperglycemia		Can result when infusion rate is too fast.	Start TPN at beginning rate for 1 hour, then set to	

Problem	Signs and Symptoms	Action
	Include: Frequent urination Thirst Nausea Weakness Headache Positive glucose (sugar) in urine	higher rate as prescribed by nutrition support service (NSS) Do not increase infusion rate above what NSS has set for you. Maintain constant flow rate.
Hypoglycemia	Can result from sudden interruption in flow rate. In so, occlusion alarm sounds in 15–30 minutes. Include: Cold and clammy skin Jittery feeling Nervousness Headache, nausea, hunger	Maintain constant flow rate. Taper off HPN at end of infusion as prescribed by NSS Glucose gel or tablet Eating something sweet such as hard candy or orange juice with sugar
Malfunction of TPN Equipment or Supplies	Any malfunction of pump, alarms, cassette/tubing that prevents safe, proper administration of HPN or problem with dressing kit. Dressing kits with open plastic covering, missing supplies, or dry swab sticks Electric shock or tingling sensation when infusion pump is touched A nonfunctioning pump will cause an alarm signal.	Have certified electrician check house for proper grounding. Use three-prong plug in room where HPN is administered. Do not use other electrical appliances while pump is running. Run pump on battery if use of other appliances is necessary. Keep machine plugged in at all times. Repeat procedure for starting TPN, following instruction booklet step by step.

HPN COMPLICATIONS   continued

Complication	Definition	Assessment	Prevention	Treatment
			For infusion pump malfunction, call home supply agency immediately to arrange for a replacement pump. Keep machine clean. For alarms, refer to alarm trouble-shooting sheet. For cassette and tubing, see alarm trouble-shooting sheet. Replace cassette if not functioning. Repeat the procedure for starting TPN, following instruction booklet closely. Call home supply agency with problem. Save package cassette came in and cassette. Home supply agency will replace cassette. Packaging and nonfunctioning cassette go back to NSS nurse with description of problem. Use new kit. Home supply company will reimburse you if made aware of problem. Keep stock number on kit for NSS nurse.	

TOUCH CONTAMINATION

Touch contamination means transmission of germs (i.e., bacteria and fungi) to a sterile object from a nonsterile source by physical contact. The most common source of touch contamination is your hands. In order to minimize the chance that you will contaminate your solutions while starting TPN, precautions such as good handwashing and aseptic technique should be followed.

Handwashing is important because your skin normally supports the growth of many germs. Your hands should be washed with warm water and soap and a brush used to free your skin and fingernails of as many bacteria as possible. You should not touch sterile components used to compound your solutions, since even the best handwashing will not kill all the germs present on your skin. Examples of sterile components are needles, solution, administration set spikes, bottle stoppers, and IV administration set tips.

Maintaining aseptic technique means always manipulating your equipment and solutions in a manner that will avoid contamination of a sterile area. Eliminating touch contamination is part of aseptic technique.

BIBLIOGRAPHY

Ament, M. E. 1984. "Home Total Parenteral Nutrition in Infants and Children." In *Nutrition and Feeding of Infants and Toddlers.* Boston: Little, Brown & Co.

American Society of Hospital Pharmacists, ed. 1986. Caloric agents. In *Drug Information 86.* Bethesda, Md.: American Hospital Formulary Service, p. 1248.

Colley, R., J. M. Wilson, and M. D. Wilhen. 1977. Intravenous nutrition: nursing considerations. *Issues in Comprehensive Pediatric Nursing* 1:5.

Dudrick, S. J., et al. 1968. Long-term parenteral nutrition with growth and development and positive nitrogen balance. *Surgery* 64:134–142.

Englert, D. M., and S. J. Dudrick. 1978. Principles of ambulatory home hyperalimentation. *American Journal of Intravenous Therapy* 5:11–28.

Gilbert, K. A. 1986. Needs theory and health education: a psychological approach to teaching home nutritional therapy. *Nutritional Support Service* 6:23–25.

Gulledge, A. D. 1982. Home parenteral nutrition and the family. *Nutritional Support Service* 2:44–46.

Gulledge, A. D., and W. T. Gipson. "Short bowel syndrome, and psychological issues for home parenteral nutrition." Paper presented at the McGaw Home TPN Team Concept Seminar, Las Vegas, Nevada, December 1979.

Jacobson, N., L. Boger, and S. Harrison. 1981. An electrical safety regimen for parenteral hyperalimentation patients. *Nutritional Support Services* 1 (Dec.): 17–19.

Johnslos, J. E. 1981. Home parenteral nutrition: the "cost" of patient and family participation. *Social Work Health Care* 7:49–66.

Lodewick, P. A. 1983. Think fast. *Diabetes Forecast* (May/June): 29–33.

Maki, D., and J. Band. 1985. A comparative study of polyantibiotic and iodophor ointments in prevention of vascular catheter related infection. *The American Journal of Medicine* (March): 739–44.

Ohio State University Hospitals Education and Training Department. 1983. *Home Parenteral Nutrition Manual.* Columbus, Ohio: Ohio State University Hospitals.

Parrish, R., J. Mirtallo, and P. J. Fabri. 1982. Behavioral management concepts with application for home parenteral nutrition patients. *Drug Intelligence and Clinical Pharmacy.* (July/Aug.): 581–86.

Powell, C., et al. 1985. Op-site dressing study: a prospective randomized study evaluating povidone-iodine ointment and extension set changes with 7-day op-site dressings applied to subclavian sites. *JPEN* (July): 443–46.

Price, B. S., and E. L. Levine. 1979. Permanent total parenteral nutrition: psychology and social responses of the early stages. *JPEN* 3:48–52.

Schribner, B. H., J. J. Cole, and T. G. Christopher. 1970. Long-term total parenteral nutrition. *Journal of the American Medical Association* 212:457.

Steiger, E. et al. 1986. "Home Parenteral Nutrition." In *Parenteral Nutrition.* Philadelphia: W. B. Saunders.

CHAPTER 12

Home IV Chemotherapy

Nurse's Guide to Home IV Chemotherapy
Patient Education Care Guides

Elaine Glass, RN, MS, CNA

NURSE'S GUIDE TO HOME IV CHEMOTHERAPY

DEVELOPING A HOME IV CHEMOTHERAPY PROGRAM

Introduction

An essential part of starting and maintaining a home IV chemotherapy program is to develop a philosophy and mission statement. If you are not starting this program alone, all the partners in your business or colleagues in your department should participate in writing the philosophy and mission statement. The philosophy should include what you believe is important to your program. Issues that you may want to address include cancer, health, home care, patients and families, home chemotherapy, the nursing staff, the interdisciplinary team, the company's or department's management style, and excellence. The following example illustrates what such a philosophy might express.

Home IV Chemotherapy Philosophy

Cancer

Cancer is a chronic illness that can affect anyone at any age. Cancer is not an automatic death sentence; many types of cancer can be cured or controlled for many years. Physical, psychoemotional, spiritual, and social well-being are all important to consider in living with cancer.

Health

Health exists on a continuum and is a unique state for every individual. It occurs when any human being, regardless of the presence of cancer, reaches an optimal state of physical, psychoemotional, spiritual, and social well-being.

All human beings have the inherent right to achieve and maintain optimal health. However, individuals vary in their interest and motivation in exercising this right.

Home care

Every person with cancer should have the opportunity to obtain high-quality, up-to-date, cost-effective, and individualized health care. If the client's condition and treatment are conducive to home care, the client should be offered the choice of receiving IV chemotherapy at home. We believe that the client's well-being can be improved by receiving chemotherapy in familiar surroundings, with family and perhaps pets nearby. We believe it is the nurse's role to:

- Assist the client and family in clarifying their situation, so they can make the decision that will best meet their needs
- Attempt not to impose values on the client and family when facilitating their decision-making

Finally, we believe that home administration of IV chemotherapy offers a safe and cost-effective alternative method of treatment that can help reduce health care costs. As a service to the community, 5 percent of the program's profits will be allocated to assist the indigent.

Clients and families

We believe that all human beings have intrinsic value and are equal regardless of race, ethnic background, sex, religion, or creed.

Clients, families, and significant others who are coping with cancer may have to deal with numerous changes in life-style and activities of daily living. The entire family is under stress and must be supported by:

- Providing adequate amounts of information, as it is requested, in terms that can be understood
- Including both the client and family members in decision-making regarding the original treatment program and any changes in this program
- Arranging flexible visiting times
- Facilitating family communication and social activity
- Encouraging clients and families to participate in support groups like I Can Cope and Make Today Count

Home chemotherapy

We believe that many IV chemotherapy drugs can be administered safely in the home. Side effects associated with chemotherapy may be reduced when chemotherapy is given in the home because the client may be more relaxed in familiar surroundings, more rested from not traveling and waiting in the physician's office or clinic, and less influenced by medical sights and sounds, especially other ill patients.

Nursing staff

All members of the nursing staff are unique individuals who must be confident in the technical and personal skills that they possess in caring for people with cancer. We believe that registered nurses in our home IV chemotherapy program must:

- Assume responsibility for assessing, planning, implementing, and evaluating the nursing care of their primary caseload of clients
- Be accountable for effective nursing care of their clients by performing and documenting the nursing process
- Assume responsibility for their ongoing education by reading current literature, attending in-service training, taking initiative to attend workshops and other educational programs, participating constructively in peer review, and eventually achieving national certification in oncology nursing
- Communicate and share openly their thoughts and feelings about caring for clients and families with cancer, so they can provide support for others as well as gain support from them
- Develop a balanced life-style with a variety of physical and mental coping mechanisms to deal with the stress involved in working with cancer clients and families
- Contribute to cost containment and reduce stress among peers by being prompt at work, maintaining good health habits to prevent illness, and organizing work schedules efficiently to reduce overtime
- Be assertive with peers, including physicians, in advocating client-centered care
- Demonstrate pride in the home IV chemotherapy program
- Behave in a mature and ethical manner

Interdisciplinary team

We believe that a number of health care professionals may need to share the responsibility of meeting the needs of cancer clients and their families. The home care chemotherapy nurse is responsible for initiating collaboration with and referral to other health care disciplines to insure that comprehensive care is provided.

Management style

The home IV chemotherapy program is managed by an oncology clinical nurse specialist who believes in participative management. However, democratic, autocratic, and laissez-faire leadership styles may be used on occasion. The manager strives to be open and responsive to the concerns and suggestions of staff members. Decisions are made primarily by consensus, and once made, are supported by everyone. Position in the program is not the basis for quality of ideas. All input is valued and encouraged and should be conveyed to the manager in a constructive and tactful manner.

The manager attempts to treat all members of the nursing staff fairly. Expectations are clearly defined. Numerous resources are available in the office and in several area hospitals. Concurrent record audits, on-the-spot feedback, and performance appraisals are carried out in a constructive manner to enhance the professional development of each nurse. The manager strives to create a work environment in which the nursing staff feel stimulated to grow and motivated to participate in problem-solving and decision-making. Each nurse is encouraged to develop a critical and inquisitive mind. Involvement in nursing research is encouraged and valued.

Excellence

We believe that all members of the home IV chemotherapy program are committed to excellence. Excellence begins with a positive attitude. Excellence is evidenced in actions that convey skill and caring. Excellence is demonstrated in communication that is honest and respectful of others. Excellence must be a part of all that is said and done.

Mission Statement

Although the philosophical statement may be rather lengthy, the mission statement should be very brief, a maximum of one or two sentences. It should explain succinctly the purpose of your program. For example:

Our mission is to administer IV chemotherapy in the home in a safe, skilled, and caring manner so that clients and families can achieve optimal well-being in familiar surroundings at a cost-effective price.

Goals of Home IV Chemotherapy

When setting up a program for home IV chemotherapy, you must decide which of the goals of chemotherapy to include in the program. Basically, there are three goals in IV chemotherapy administration: (1) cure, (2) control, and (3) palliation. These goals are based on both the type of cancer and the extent to which it has metastasized in each particular client.

Some professionals believe that only palliative chemotherapy should be given in the home. This belief is based on the rationale that the client has little chance of long-term survival so that the main effort is to keep the client comfortable. Since increasing the client's comfort by reducing the symptoms of the disease is the reason for administering palliative chemotherapy, home chemotherapy is appropriate.

Some professionals believe that when the goal of chemotherapy is control, the client should not receive chemotherapy at home. The rationale is that since the client has a chance for long-term survival, the client should be followed and examined closely by a physician. This necessitates visiting the physician in an office, clinic, or hospital each time the chemotherapy is scheduled for administration.

Other professionals believe that a consideration in long-term survival is quality of life, which can be improved by decreasing the amount of time the client and family spend in health care facilities. Additionally, with scarce health care resources and the expense of long-term cancer therapies, home care therapy is more cost effective (Rees 1985, 1407). Thus, the client should be given the option of home IV chemotherapy with periodic visits to the office, clinic, or hospital for examination by a physician. Between these visits, a nurse can assess the client for signs of dose-limiting toxicities and symptoms of disease progression that would necessitate immediate physician attention.

If the goal of chemotherapy is curative, some professionals believe that the client should be followed and examined closely by the physician with each chemotherapy administration (Rees 1985, 1407). When cure is possible or probable, they believe the client's health would be risked with only periodic visits to the physician. Furthermore, as a rule, curative chemotherapy is more aggressive and the client is subjected to potentially more life-threatening toxicities than with other chemotherapies. Therefore, there is a need for frequent follow-up requiring the skills of a physician. However, some types of curative therapy may be considered for home administration if low toxicities are expected. This would generally be true of adjuvant or maintenance chemotherapy.

Regardless of whether the goal of chemotherapy is palliation, control, or cure, if the chemotherapy includes continuous 24-hour infusions, it may be considered for home administration. With these types of therapies, the physician sees the client on the first day of therapy and determines the appropriateness of administering the therapy. The patient is then started on a continuous infusion portable pump in the physician's office or clinic. Follow-up maintenance care of this continuous chemotherapy infusion pump is done at home by the home IV chemotherapy nurse.

The goals of chemotherapy that will be included in the home IV chemotherapy program must be made explicit so that they can be written into the program's admission criteria. Based upon the physician's initial assessment of the feasibility of home IV chemotherapy, the client and family should be allowed to make the decision for or against it after the risks have been adequately explained.

CLIENT REFERRAL TO THE PROGRAM

Admission Criteria

Six issues need to be addressed in the admission criteria: (1) the goal of the chemotherapy, (2) the specific antineoplastic and supportive agents to be used, (3) physician availabilty, (4) objective follow-up measures, (5) family support, and (6) reimbursement. The first issue, the goal of chemotherapy, has been discussed.

The second issue is the specific agents that can be administered in the home. Drugs that have an appreciable risk of hypersensitivity reactions should not be administered in the home. These drugs are listed in Table 12.1. Antineoplastic agents with an infrequent or low risk of hypersensitivity should be used with caution in the home, and some programs may choose to exclude some of these drugs as well. Drugs included in these two categories are listed in Tables 12.2 and 12.3.

Table 12.4 lists antineoplastic agents that are generally not known to produce hypersensitivity reactions and are, therefore, relatively safe to administer in the home.

Investigational drugs that are in Phase II and III testing and intravenous antiemetics must also be considered. Ifosfamide is an example of a Phase III drug that has been studied and used for a number of years but has not yet become commercially available. As indicated in Table 12.4, ifosfamide has not been associated with any hypersensitivity reactions. Therefore, depending on the nature of the investigational drug and how long it has been in use, some programs may decide to include Phase II and III drugs in their policies if they are being administered by physicians in their communities.

Because many of the antineoplastic agents cause moderate to severe nausea and vomiting, some of the antiemetics are most effective when administered intravenously. However, several antiemetics, including Compazine, Reglan, Inapsine, and Haldol, are associated with extrapyramidal reactions. Therefore, if these drugs are given IV in the home, IV Benadryl (and IV Cogentin for Haldol and Reglan) must be a part of the standing physician's orders for treating these reactions. Other drug reactions must also be anticipated and addressed in the program's policy, which should give specific guidelines for

Table 12.1   DRUGS WITH APPRECIABLE RISK OF REACTIONS

Asparaginase
Cisplatin
Etopside

Adapted from Brager 1984, 140

Table 12.2   DRUGS WITH INFREQUENT RISK OF REACTIONS

Adriamycin	Cytoxan	Methotrexate
Bleomycin	Daunorubicin	

Adapted from Brager 1984, 140–41

nursing actions. These policies should also include routes, doses, or methods of administration that the home IV chemotherapy program will not use.

A third issue to be addressed in the admission criteria is that of physician availability. Either the admission or referral form should have a section for the physician's signature, indicating the physician's availability by phone at the time of chemotherapy administration. This is highly recommended in the event of an unusual circumstance or unexpected reaction while the client is receiving treatment in the home. If the client's primary physician is not readily available, the home IV chemotherapy physician should be available as a backup. Of course a severe anaphylactic reaction would require an immediate call to the closest emergency squad for life-saving assistance if the client is a full code.

A fourth area for consideration in the admission criteria is what objective tests will be performed, how they will be done, and who will monitor them. For example, plicamycin may be administered in the home to maintain a reasonably low serum calcium level when the calcium level increases due to boney metastasis. Clotting factors II, V, VII, and X, prothrombin times, and platelets should be assessed periodically to detect the presence of an impending blood dyscrasia. LDH and SGOT should be checked to monitor for liver toxicity. Serum creatinine, BUN, potassium, phosphate, and magnesium should be checked to monitor for renal function. Calcium should also be monitored for therapeutic effect. The individual who will be responsible for drawing these blood tests, the home IV chemotherapy nurse or a home service lab, should also be determined. Some mechanism must be arranged so that both the physician and the home IV chemotherapy nurse receive a copy of the test results. In most situations, the nurse must know the recent lab values before the next dose of IV chemotherapy can be safely administered. Many physicians write

Table 12.3   DRUGS WITH A LOW RISK OF REACTIONS

Cytosar	Mitomycin
Fluorouracil	Mustargen

Adapted from Brager 1984, 140–41

Table 12.4   DRUGS WITH FEW KNOWN REACTIONS

Carmustine	Leucovorin	Velban
Dacarbazine	Plicamycin	Vincristine
Dactinomycin	Streptozocin	
Ifosfamide	Thiotepa	

specific standing orders about how high the blood counts must be in order for the chemotherapy to be administered. Therefore, it is recommended that the home IV chemotherapy nurse receive a copy or at least a phone report of most test results.

The objective measures may also include some type of physical assessment, such as the size of a tumor or lymph node, palpation of the liver or spleen, abdominal or leg girths, and lung sounds. The nurse's skills in physical assessment may determine the feasibility of the program's assuming this type of responsibility.

The fifth area to be included in the admission criteria is that of family support. At least one physically and mentally competent family member or significant other must be available at the time of IV chemotherapy home administration. This person should also be present in the home for at least 6 to 8 hours after the chemotherapy has infused. This person may need to assist the client with supportive care during nausea and vomiting or to monitor a hydration IV with or without IV drip antiemetics. Additionally, if the client experiences an unusual delayed reaction, someone will be needed to assist the client and call for help. Therefore, someone with a reasonable capacity to learn and remember must be available.

The last item to be addressed in the admission criteria is reimbursement. The home IV chemotherapy program must obtain financial information from the client in order to determine reimbursement mechanisms. The insurance company or Medicare/Medicaid must be contacted regarding willingness to reimburse for the client's type of home IV chemotherapy. If the third party provider will not assume 100 percent of the cost, will the client be able to pay the remainder? All costs involved in home IV chemotherapy must be specified when inquiring about reimbursement: the drugs and IV supplies, the nurse's visit, the lab tests, and the safe handling of supplies for both the nurse and family.

In summary, client referral to a home IV chemotherapy program is based on several considerations. While the philosophy and mission statements describe the agency's direction, the admission criteria indicate a client's eligibility to enter the program. A sample admission criteria form is included as Figure 12.1.

Figure 12.1 Home IV chemotherapy program referral: admission criteria.

CLIENT
Name: _____

Address: _____

_____

Phone: _____

Age: _____

Illness: _____

Significant Other (must be present during and 8 hours after chemo.)
Name: _____

Address: _____

_____

Phone: _____

Name/Route/Schedule/Frequency

Antineoplastic Drugs*: _____

_____

_____

_____

Antiemetic Drugs: _____

_____

_____

IV Solutions and _____

Supportive Drugs: _____

Lab Tests Prior to Chemo: _____

_____

_____

Response Parameters: _____

_____

_____

MD F/U: _____

Plan _____

Emergency Drug†:
   Benadryl 50 mg IV push for extrapyramidal reactions and rashes.
   Cogentin 1–2 mg IV push for extrapyramidal reactions 2° to Haldol.
   Epinephrine 1:1000 IV push for anaphylactoid reactions, repeated in 10 minutes
   if insufficient response. Dose: 1–5 years = .1–.4 ml; 6–12 years = .5 ml; 12 years–
   adult = .5–.75 ml

Extravasation Drugs†:
   Decadron 4 mg/ml IV push for all vesicants except those below.
   Hyaluronidase 150 units/ml IV push for vincristine and velban.
   Sodium thiosulfate 100 mg/ml IV push for nitrogen mustard and mitomycin.
   Other: _____

PHYSICIAN

Name: _____

Address: _____

_____

Phone: W: _____

H: _____

ALTERNATE PHYSICIAN

Name: _____

Address: _____

_____

Phone: W: _____

H: _____

The goal of this chemotherapy is: cure, control, palliation. (Circle one)

The client's code status is: Full or DNR. (Circle one)

I, or my alternate, agree to be available by phone when the client is receiving IV chemotherapy at home. I understand that the home IV chemotherapy nurse will inform me of the time of administration so that I can make appropriate arrangements. Also, if my client has a central line or other catheter, I guarantee its proper placement in _____ as of _____. It is a _____ catheter and it
      anatomical location   date   type
was placed on _____.
              date

_____

Physician's Signature/Date

Client's Employer: Name: _____

Address: _____

Phone: _____

PRIMARY INSURANCE

Name: _____

Address: _____

_____

Phone: _____

Policy #: _____

% Coverage of: Drugs: _____

IV supplies: _____

Nurse's Visits: _____

Lab Tests: _____

Safe Handling Supplies: RN: _____

Client: _____

PRIMARY INSURANCE

Name: _____

Address: _____

_____

Phone: _____

Policy #: _____

% Coverage of: Drugs: _____

IV Supplies: _____

Nurse's Visits: _____

Lab Tests: _____

Safe Handling Supplies: RN: _____

Client: _____

GOVERNMENT ASSISTANCE

Medicare ID #: _____

Medicaid ID #: _____

Other: _____

State: _____

ID #: _____

*A copy of the client's signed consent form to receive these drugs must accompany this form. May not include asparaginase, cisplatin, or etopside.
†These drugs will be given as standing orders if physician signs this form.

Nursing Assessment

Figure 12.2 shows a sample nursing assessment form for obtaining the background data needed about the client and family for admission into the home IV chemotherapy program.

Client background

The first step for the home IV chemotherapy nurse is to review the admission criteria form. The nurse must determine whether the form is complete, the drug doses are within normal limits, the physician has signed the form, and the client's signed consent form is attached. The client's medical history should also be reviewed by the nurse. Special attention should be paid to the most recent lab values as they relate to the contraindications and side effects of the drugs ordered.

Next the nurse meets with the client and family to determine their eligibility for the home IV chemotherapy program. The nurse should review with them the contraindications of the drugs ordered and any existing symptoms that might compound the side effects of these drugs. The nurse should also obtain information on the client's and family's previous experience with IV therapy and/or chemotherapy. The nurse should inquire about family members and other support systems that might be able to offer assistance if needed. Also, after reviewing the goals of the program and its advantages and disadvantages, the nurse should ask the client and family how they feel about entering a home IV chemotherapy program. This initial meeting with the client and family should give the nurse an indication of the client's and family's motivation and ability to learn and participate in the program.

Venous Access

After interviewing the client and family, the nurse should ask the client's permission to inspect the client's veins for accessibility. If severe vesicants are ordered for several courses of chemotherapy and the client's veins are extremely poor, the nurse should discuss the option of a port or permanent venous catheter with the client and family. After obtaining the client's consent, the nurse should recommend to the physician that the client receive such a central line before treatment is begun in the home. If the physician disagrees, the nurse manager should also assess the client's venous access. Based on the manager's assessment, a decision should be made as to whether the client can be admitted into the program without the central line. An effort should be made to convince the physician of the necessity of a central line before the client is denied entry into the program for this reason. If the client already has an existing central line, port, or other catheter, the nurse should assess how well it is functioning and how well the client and/or family can care for it.

Figure 12.2   Home IV chemotherapy program nursing assessment.

1. Existing symptoms that are contraindications to the drugs ordered: _____
   _____

2. Existing symptoms that might compound the side effects of the drugs ordered: _____
   _____

3. Previous experience with IV therapy or chemotherapy: _____
   _____

4. Family members and support systems available (name/relationship/skill):
   _____
   _____
   _____
   _____

5. Client's ability to learn: Understands English? _____   Speaks English? _____
   Reads English? _____   Eyesight? _____   Hearing? _____
   Level of education? _____   Manual dexterity? _____
   _____   Motivation? _____
   Other comments: _____

6. Significant other's ability to learn: Understands English? _____   Speaks English? _____
   Reads English? _____   Eyesight? _____   Hearing? _____
   Level of education? _____   Manual dexterity? _____
   _____   Motivation? _____
   Other comments: _____

7. Venous access: Peripheral veins: Right arm: _____
   Left arm: _____   Recommend CVC? _____
   Central lines: If the client already has an existing permanent CVC catheter or other catheter
   or port, what is it and is it functioning properly? _____
   Can the client and/or SO care for it? _____
   _____

8. Pertinent medical history: _____
   _____
   _____

9. Pertinent lab data: _____
   _____

10. Client's performance status: _____
    _____

11. Client's/family's coping methods: _____
    _____

12. Conclusions: _____
    _____

                                                        _____
                                                        RN signature/Date

CLIENT/FAMILY TEACHING PLAN

Introduction

The information to be included in the client and family teaching plan depends on several factors. These factors include their previous experience with IVs and IV chemotherapy, the types of drugs ordered, the method of administration (IV push, IV drip, or continuous infusion), the rate of administration, the need for hydration and/or supportive therapy, the possibility of vesicant extravasation, the possibility of hypersensitivity reactions, the type of venous access, and the side effects expected. Below are behavioral objectives and content for topics basic to a home IV chemotherapy program. The nurse must individualize the teaching plan by choosing objectives and content relevant to each client and family.

What is Home IV Chemotherapy?

Objective: A nurse will describe the home IV chemotherapy program to the client and family, state its purpose, and review the mechanics of the program and the role of the nurse.

Content: Description of the program: Instead of receiving IV chemotherapy in the hospital, clinic, or doctor's office, the client is given the choice of receiving the same therapy in the home by an RN specially skilled in IV chemotherapy administration. Although the RN will assess the client with each chemotherapy administration, occasional visits to the doctor are still necessary for examinations, X rays, and scans.

Purpose: The purpose of the program is to administer IV chemotherapy in the home in a safe, skilled, and caring manner so that clients and families can achieve optimal well-being in familiar surroundings at a cost-effective price.

Mechanics of the program and role of the nurse:

- The client, family, and physician complete the Admission criteria form.
- An RN interviews the client and family and assesses the client's veins to determine eligibility for the program.
- An RN obtains a prescription for the IV and drug supplies and obtains them from a pharmacy where the drugs can be mixed under a vertical flow hood if at all possible. Alternatively, the RN and the client may decide to utilize a delivery service that will bring the drugs and IV supplies to the home before the nurse is scheduled to arrive.

- The RN arranges an appointment with the client and family to examine and interview the client, administer the IV chemotherapy, and observe the client for at least 30 minutes.
- The RN instructs the client and family on how to manage the IV site and/or the IV setup after the RN has gone.
- The RN informs the client and family of the 24-hour, 7-day-a-week availability of a home IV chemotherapy nurse.
- The RN makes a return appointment or phone call to assess the client's status and/or draw samples for interim lab work before the next IV chemotherapy is due.

Choosing Home IV Chemotherapy

Objective: The client and/or family will state the advantages and disadvantages of home IV chemotherapy.

Content: Advantages of home IV chemotherapy:

- Reduced cost if covered by insurance company
- Perhaps less nausea and vomiting with the ability to lie quietly in bed or on the couch
- Increased comfort and relaxation in familiar surroundings with family, friends, pets, and favorite distractions (TV, radio, stereo, etc.)
- Less inconvenience from making arrangements to go to the doctor
- No waiting; more flexibility in getting the treatment when it is convenient for the client
- No disturbance from other patients who are sick

Disadvantages of home IV chemotherapy:

- Increased personal cost if not covered by insurance company
- Less availability of immediate medical assistance if an unusual reaction to the chemotherapy occurs
- Less social contact with other clients and families
- Increased personal and family time in learning how to care for the home IV chemotherapy

Regulating an IV Drip Rate

Objective: The client and/or family will demonstrate (at least once) the regulation of an IV drip rate.

Content: Explain and identify all the IV set parts, including a piggyback setup.

Demonstrate how to tape all junctions to prevent tubing from coming apart. (Demonstrate how to reconnect the tubing in a sterile manner if this should happen.)

Demonstrate the adjustment of the IV flow rate with the regulator clamp.

Provide information on the number of drops to count in 15 seconds.

Demonstrate how to count drops and adjust the flow clamp until the proper rate is maintained.

Explain when to turn on the piggyback setup, remembering to readjust the flow rate (when applicable), and turn off the piggyback when completed.

Explain how the rate will change with a change in client's position.

Inspecting the Peripheral IV Site for Signs of Infiltration

Objective: The client and/or family will state a number of ways to determine when a peripheral IV has infiltrated.

Content: Observe for a slowing or stopping of the IV drip rate.

Observe the IV site for redness, change in temperature, swelling, discomfort, or leakage of fluid.

If these symptoms are observed, turn the chemotherapy off, slow down the main solution to two or three drops a minute, and call the home IV chemotherapy nurse.

Discontinuing a Peripheral IV or an IV from an Internal Port

Objective: The client and/or family will demonstrate (at least once) how to discontinue a peripheral IV.

Content: Explain the importance of clamping off the IV set before air gets close to the IV site.

Demonstrate how to heparinize an internal port.

With rubber gloves on, demonstrate how to apply gentle pressure to the IV site with a dry gauze pad while pulling out the needle.

With rubber gloves on, demonstrate the application of firm pressure at the IV site (with the arm in a nondependent position with a peripheral IV) for 3 to 5 minutes.

With rubber gloves on, demonstrate the application of an adhesive bandage after checking the IV site for bleeding and infiltration.

With rubber gloves on, demonstrate wrapping up the IV tubing in a protective pad and taping it securely for disposal in a 2-ply plastic trash bag.

With rubber gloves on, demonstrate disposal of the IV needle in a jar with a screw-on lid.

(*Note:* The jar with the needle should be placed in the two-ply plastic trash bag and disposed of in a garbage can with a lid on it.)

Chemotherapy Safe Handling at Home

Objective: The client and family will demonstrate (at least once) safe handling of the client's waste.

Content: Explain the rationale for safe handling procedures and determine the length of time the procedures will be necessary. (Refer to the last line of each drug in the "Nursing Implications" section of the drug charts in this book.)

Instruct the mobile client to have bowel movements and to urinate by sitting down on the commode and flushing the toilet, with the lid down, two or three times.

With rubber gloves on, demonstrate how to empty a urinal, bedpan, and/or emesis pan close to the commode water to avoid splashing. Also with rubber gloves on, demonstrate how to rinse out the urinal, bedpan, or emesis pan with a clean cup of water or household disinfectant, emptying them close to the water to avoid splashing. Remember to flush the toilet, with the lid down, two or three times.

Wearing rubber gloves and a full-length apron or old housecoat, demonstrate how to gather up soiled linens for washing twice in a washing machine on the hottest setting. (*Note:* the apron or housecoat should be washed twice along with the linen.)

With rubber gloves on, demonstrate how to cleanse the perineum of an incontinent or dependent client and how to arrange a protective pad and pillowcase under the client's buttocks.

Instruct client and family to call the nurse if a bag of chemotherapy should accidentally spill on the floor. Until the nurse arrives with a spill kit, the family should place protective pads with the absorbent side down over the spill.

Learning to Monitor the Side Effects of Chemotherapy

Objective: The client and/or family will state the common side effects of their chemotherapy and any necessary actions to prevent, reduce, or adapt to them.

Content: Review the National Cancer Institute (NCI) booklet "Chemotherapy and You: A Guide to Self-Help during Treatment" (NIH Publication #85-1126, 8/85), pointing out the specific drugs that the client is on in the back section of the book. Also, refer to the drug chart section of this book for more information, especially on drugs not included in the NCI booklet.

"Taking Time: Support for People with Cancer and the People Who Care About Them" (NIH Publication #85-2059, 7/85) in an effort to enhance client and family communication.

Review the NCI booklet "Eating Hints: Recipes and Tips for Better Nutrition during Cancer Treatment" (NIH Publication #86-2079, 8/86) in an effort to improve the client's and family's nutritional status.

Review two other NCI booklets if they are appropriate: "When Cancer Recurs: Meeting the Challenge Again" (NIH Publication #85-2709, 10/84) and "Advanced Cancer: Living Each Day (NIH Publication #85-856, 4/85).

Review The American Cancer Society (ACS) pamphlet "Understanding Blood Counts" (Franklin County Unit, Ohio Division) to assist the client and family in understanding infection and bleeding precautions and knowing when to call the physician or nurse.

Assist the client and family in making a list of phone numbers to keep by the phone: the home IV chemotherapy nurse or office, the chemotherapy physician and/or family physician, the nearest ambulance in case of an emergency, and a close friend, neighbor, or relative who could come over to help at a moment's notice.

Maintaining a Portable Infusion Pump at Home

Objective: The client and family will demonstrate (at least once) how to operate a portable pump for continuous infusion of chemotherapy at home.

Content: Explain all the parts of the pump and keep the directions handy as a reference in the home.

Demonstrate how the pump operates. Include:

- How to check periodically to see if the chemotherapy is infusing properly
- How to change the battery
- How to check and/or change the infusion rate
- If necessary, how to change the IV tubing and bag

Reinforce safe pump care (e.g., use of the carrying case, not getting it wet, etc.).

Provide the client and family with any additional names and phone numbers in case the pump malfunctions.

Maintaining a Permanent Catheter at Home

Objective: The client and family will demonstrate the skills needed to care for the client's permanent catheter at home.

Content: Demonstrate proper technique in dressing the catheter insertion site, according to the physician's orders.

Demonstrate proper aseptic technique in maintaining a patent catheter with normal saline or heparin injections into the catheter, according to the physician's orders.

State the appropriate actions to take in case of complications with the catheter, such as local infection, systemic fever, a tear in the catheter, the cap accidentally falling off, the shoulder swelling, etc.

Caring for a Vesicant Extravasation Site

Objective: The client and family will state how to care for an IV site where vesicant chemotherapy has extravasated.

Content: Define what an extravasation is.

Review the factors and events that resulted in the extravasation.

Review the actions that the RN takes when an extravasation occurs.

Instruct the client and family on signs of healing (a decrease in swelling and redness with tissue appearing nearly normal) and signs of worsening damage (an increase in redness and swelling with possible seeping of the skin and even tissue breakdown).

Emphasize the importance of notifying the physician as soon as the *first* signs of worsening damage appear. Inform the client to insist on seeing a plastic surgeon immediately.

Instruct client and family to keep an ice pack 30 minutes on the site and 30 minutes off until bedtime (or for a minimum of 8 hours), followed by 30 minutes of ice on the site every 4 to 6 hours until the site appears normal. *Exception:* Warm room temperatures or mild heat should be applied to extravasations that occur with vincristine or velban.

Documentation

Once the RN has completed the individualized teaching plan with the client and family, the instructions should be documented. Because much of the teaching will be similar from client to client, it would be time-saving and cost-effective for the nurses in the program to develop generic teaching/learning sheets. These can be made flexible enough to accommodate individualization. Figure 12.3 provides an example of a generic teaching/learning sheet for one objective and content area.

Figure 12.3   Home IV chemotherapy teaching/learning documentation record.

Regulating An IV Drip Rate

C = Client = _____
S = SO = _____

Content Areas	Teaching Method	States Understanding	Asks Questions	Demonstrates	Needs Practice	Proficient	Comments
1. Explain and identify all the IV set parts including a piggyback setup.	Demonstration of actual setup with written handout as reference.						_____ RN/Date
2. Demonstrate how to tape each juncture to avoid tubing coming apart.	Demonstration of actual setup with written handout as reference.						_____ RN/Date
3. Demonstrate adjustment of the IV flow rate with the regulator clamp.	Demonstration of actual setup with written handout as reference.						_____ RN/Date
4. Provide information on the number of drops to count in 15 seconds.	____ at ____ qtts ____ at ____ qtts ____ at ____ qtts						_____ RN/Date
5. Demonstrate how to count drops and adjust the flow clamp rate until the proper rate is maintained.	Demonstration of actual setup with written handout as reference.						_____ RN/Date
6. Explain when to turn on the piggy-	Demonstration of actual setup with						

back set, remembering to readjust the flow rate and to turn off the piggyback when done.	written handout as reference.							RN/Date
7. Explain how the rate will change with a change in the client's position.	Ask the client to stand up to demonstrate this.							RN/Date

Conclusions:

_____   _____
      Client/SO Signature/Date   RN Signature/Date

LEGALITIES OF HOME IV CHEMOTHERAPY ADMINISTRATION

Consent Forms

It is the physician's responsibility to obtain the client's signature on the consent form. In doing so, the physician is obligated to inform the client of the benefits and risks of the chemotherapy that is being recommended, explain the side effects that can be expected from the therapy and describe any alternative therapy options that are available to the client.

It is the nurse's responsibility to reinforce and clarify the physician's explanation, assist the client in seeking more information if requested, and inform the physician if the client is hesitant about any aspect of the consent or if the client wishes to withdraw consent.

Physician Coverage

As soon as the RN has arranged a date and time to administer IV chemotherapy in a client's home, the RN needs to contact the physician's office. The RN should make sure that the agency, primary, or alternate physician will be available at the scheduled date and time. Also, the nurse may need to contact the physician's office to obtain the latest interim lab values. Finally, the nurse may need to contact the physician after interviewing and examining the client regarding the client's eligibility to continue the present chemotherapy regimen.

Regardless of the issue or need, one of the most crucial elements in the IV home chemotherapy program is prompt and clear written and verbal communication between the physician and nurse.

Nurse Qualifications

Before nurses begin to administer IV chemotherapy, the home IV chemotherapy program needs to develop policies and procedures regarding:

- Which nurses are permitted to administer home IV chemotherapy
- How these nurses will receive their initial knowledge and skill competency in IV chemotherapy administration and in using a variety of venous access devices
- How these nurses will maintain continuing education on a regular basis
- How clinical peer review will be arranged for these nurses on a regular basis
- Which antineoplastic, antiemetic, and supportive drugs can be administered in the home
- Which emergency drugs can be administered as standing orders for anaphylactic or hypersensitive reactions
- Which antidote drugs can be administered as standing orders for accidental vesicant drug extravasations

The procedures must include:

- Specific techniques for administering vesicant and nonvesicant drugs through peripheral IVs, central catheters, other catheters, and ports
- Specific actions to take in case of anaphylactic or hypersensitive reactions
- Specific actions to take in case of accidental extravasation
- Specific actions to take if the client needs to be hospitalized
- Specific measures to take for safe handling precautions
- The various forms of documentation and how and when to use them

Since policies and procedures provide legal protection for the employing agency, it is important that the nurse practice according to these policies. However, because IV chemotherapy is a high-risk skill, the nurse is encouraged to purchase personal malpractice insurance for additional security.

PROCUREMENT OF SUPPLIES

Prescription Supplies

The supplies listed in Table 12.5 require a physician's prescription. The nurse will need to obtain these supplies from the pharmacy and take them to the clients' home unless a home IV delivery service is used.

Table 12.5   HOME IV CHEMOTHERAPY SUPPLIES REQUIRING A PRESCRIPTION OR PHYSICIAN'S ORDER

Antineoplastic IV drugs prepared in syringes or IV bags and ready for administration

Antiemetic IV drugs in syringes or IV bags ready for administration or in vials or ampules that can be drawn up in the home

Supportive IV drugs prepared in syringes or IV bags ready for administration or in vials or ampules that can be drawn up in the home

IV hydration solutions (with or without electrolytes added), IV tubings, syringes and needles, alcohol and povidone-iodine swabs

A continuous IV administration pump (if one of these pumps is not available in the pharmacy, the client may have to rent or purchase one from a local or national supplier)

Two 1-ml vials of epinephrine 1:1000, two 1-ml vials of Benadryl 50 mg, and a 2-ml vial of Cogentin 1 mg/1ml

Two 1-ml vials of Decadron 4 mg, two 1-ml vials of hyaluronidase 150 u, and two 1-ml vials of sodium thiosulfate 100 mg

21-gauge and 23-gauge butterfly needles

Several 5- or 10-ml syringes to check needle placement

21-gauge straight needles for placing on syringes and pushing through the side port of the IV line

TB syringes for aspirating extravasated drug

Note: All syringes and tubings should have Luer-Lok fittings (Barry and Booker 1985, 44).

Nonprescription Supplies

Both the nurse and the client/family will need to obtain nonprescription supplies from the local pharmacy, hospital supply department, or home IV delivery service. The supplies the nurse will need are listed in Table 12.6 and those the client and family may need are shown in Table 12.7.

NURSING CARE IN THE HOME

Before IV Chemotherapy Administration

Before leaving for the client's home, double-check the physician's availability, review drug orders with pertinent lab data, inquire about dose adjustments if the lab values are not within normal limits, and obtain drugs and necessary supplies from the pharmacy or verify previous delivery from a home delivery service.

Upon arriving at the client's home, interview the client and family about how they are feeling and what side effects the client experienced after the last dose of chemotherapy. Then do a brief physical assessment based upon the toxicities of the drugs the client is receiving.

For example, if the client was on Adriamycin, check for signs of early

Table 12.6   NURSE'S HOME IV CHEMOTHERAPY SUPPLIES (NONPRESCRIPTION)

Povidone-iodine
Alcohol swabs
Several types and widths of tape
Tourniquets
Sphygmomanometer
Stethoscope
Bottle of Hemastixs
Guaiac kit
Bottle of Chemstrips
Adhesive bandages
Scissors
Clean gauze pads
Sterile gauze pads
Chemical ice pack
Box of extra thickness latex gloves
A few pairs of extra thickness PVC gloves (if Mustargen is ordered)
A few disposable gowns (to assist in cleaning up an incontinent client still on safe
    handling precautions)
A chemotherapy spill kit in case of an accident
Several protective pads
A waterproof, hazardous-waste disposal container
Two-ply plastic trash bags
Hot-water bottle for dilating veins

Note: If therapy is to continue, some of these supplies may be purchased by the client and kept
    at home (e.g., alcohol swabs and gauze pads).

congestive heart failure. This physical assessment should include listening to lung sounds, taking the heart rate and blood pressure, feeling extremities for edema, and observing the client for shortness of breath. Also, if the client's platelet count was bordering on the limits of low normal, inspect the client closely for bruises or petechiae and ask the client to void so the urine can be tested with a Hemastix.

On the other hand, if the client was on vincristine, inquire about the client's bowel pattern and check the abdomen for bowel sounds if the client has not had a bowel movement in several days. With vincristine, also check the client's ability to button and unbutton a shirt or blouse, and ask the client about feelings of numbness or tingling in the fingers or toes.

Thus the nurse's interview questions and physical assessment are based upon the toxicities of the drugs that the client is receiving. If toxicity is present, the nurse must discuss this with the physician before administering the chemo-therapy.

Table 12.7   CLIENT'S AND FAMILY'S HOME IV CHEMOTHERAPY SUPPLIES (NONPRESCRIPTION)

If client is mobile:
IV pole or something to hang an IV bag on, like a coatrack or nearby curtain rod
2-ply plastic trash bags
Rubber household gloves (if the client and family are discontinuing the IV)

If client is not mobile:
Bedpan, urinal, and/or emesis basin
Rubber household gloves (for handling waste of incontinent client)
Full-length apron or housecoat (used to protect regular clothing when handling
   linens of incontinent client)
Protective pads
Access to a washing machine with a hot setting

Administration of IV Home Chemotherapy

1. Find a comfortable location for the client that is also convenient for the nurse.
2. Either select a vein and cleanse with povidone-iodine, or cleanse the catheter/injection cap juncture with povidone-iodine.
3. While the IV site or juncture is drying (a minimum of 2 minutes), prime the IV set with the maintenance IV solution.
4. Perform the venipuncture with a 21- or 23-gauge scalp vein or special port needle, or remove the injection cap from the catheter and hook up the maintenance IV solution.
5. Check the patency of the vein or catheter by aspirating gently for blood with a 5- or 10-ml syringe and 21-gauge straight needle inserted into the IV tubing's side port. Also, after the maintenance solution has infused for several minutes, the IV site, port site, or catheter site should be inspected closely for signs of infiltration—redness, swelling, discomfort, change in IV drip rate, or change in skin temperature. Peripheral IV sites should also be checked by occluding the vein a few inches above the needle site and observing for stoppage of the IV rate. These patency checks should be done every 2 or 3 minutes during and after IV push administration. Observation of the IV drip site should usually be done every 15 to 20 minutes. (For more detailed information on techniques of IV chemotherapy administration, refer to Brager and Yasko 1984, 63–81; Mourad and Glass 1985, 6–9; or Miller 1980, 8–16.)
6. Administer supportive drugs and/or antiemetics via IV push, IV drip, or orally.

7. With extra thickness gloves on and a protective pad and gauze under the IV tubing's side port, the IV push chemotherapy should be slowly and carefully injected. After each IV push drug is administered, each syringe should be flushed with about a fourth of a syringe of maintenance solution and reinfused into the client. This is done to rinse out the chemotherapy syringe before it is pulled out of the side port. Also, while the needle and syringe are being pulled from the side port, a couple of thicknesses of gauze should be used to absorb any droplets so they will not aerosolize or be spilled. Intact needles and syringes should be placed in a waterproof hazardous-waste container and taken back to the agency for proper hazardous-waste disposal (Barry and Booker 1985, 44). IV drip chemotherapy should be administered via piggyback into the IV maintenance tubing setup.

After IV Chemotherapy Administration

After the chemotherapy has been given, the maintenance solution should be allowed to flush for a minimum of 3 to 5 minutes. If the client needs hydration, the rest of the maintenance bag or hydration solution should be infused. The nurse may want to teach the client and/or family the technique of discontinuing the IV with a dry, clean gauze and the arm in a nondependent position. They should also be instructed to apply an adhesive bandage and dispose of the IV tubing and non-needle supplies in a protective pad that is securely wrapped with tape. The needle should be placed in a jar with a screw-on lid. Both the protective pad wrap and the jar are then disposed of in a two-ply trash bag. An additional reason for having the client and family learn how to discontinue an IV is to administer an IV drip antiemetic, which the nurse could piggyback into the maintenance/hydration setup. The family could then administer this antiemetic by turning on the piggyback at the time instructed by the nurse, probably 4 to 6 hours after chemotherapy administration.

If the client has a catheter, the nurse must have previous documentation of the client's or family's ability to discontinue the IV setup, screw on an injection cap, and inject heparin into the catheter before they can be allowed to perform this independently. Also, if the client has an internal port, the client and/or family will need to be instructed on injecting heparin into the extension tubing of the special needle before the needle is pulled from the port and an adhesive bandage applied.

Another home IV chemotherapy alternative is a portable continuous infusion pump. Usually all the nurse needs to do with this setup is to check for a blood return with the catheter and replace the bag of drug in the pump. The pump should be double-checked for accurate and complete infusion according to the rate at which it was set.

Documentation

Documentation of IV chemotherapy should include the medications administered; the IV solution used; the location of the IV site; the size and type of needle; how the patency was checked before, during, and after IV chemotherapy administration; and the appearance of the peripheral or internal port site when the nurse left the home. If the client or family discontinues the IV, the nurse should examine the site and record its appearance during the next home visit. Also, if the nurse did any initial or reinforcement teaching regarding chemotherapy or symptom management, this should be recorded as well. Finally, if any unusual problems arose, like an allergic reaction or extravasation of a vesicant, the nurse needs to chart in detail early detection of the problem, prompt actions taken (record in detail the times involved), when the physician was notified and what directions were given, how the client and family responded to the situation, and what aftercare instructions the client and family were given. Figure 12.4 is an example of a nursing flow sheet that can minimize the time needed to record important details. Progress notes should also be available to chart additional information or unusual problems and their resolution.

As a follow-up to home IV chemotherapy administration, the nurse may be the resource responsible for obtaining interim blood samples from the client, checking urine or stool for occult blood, checking for proteinuria, or transporting a 24-hour urine collection to the lab for creatinine clearance analysis. Regardless of whether the nurse collects the specimens, the results of the tests should be recorded by the nurse on the flow sheet. The nurse may also be responsible for follow-up care of problems related to chemotherapy.

REFERRALS

Since the nurse is the primary health care professional who interacts with the client and family, it is important that the nurse's ongoing assessment include whether the client and family may benefit from referral to additional resources. The nurse should explain pertinent programs available through most units of the American Cancer Society, such as I Can Cope, provision of free medical supplies and equipment (including hospital beds, bedside commodes, and wheelchairs), and some one-to-one counseling services. Many communities have local chapters of Make Today Count, a support group for persons with life-threatening illnesses. If finances are a concern, referral to a social worker in the local health department or a hospital social worker who has worked with the client previously may assist the client and family in utilizing all the benefits that are available to them. Often the stress of dealing with a chronic illness on a daily basis strains individual personalities as well as the entire family system. Depending on the interpersonal problems that arise, the

Figure 12.4 Home IV chemotherapy nursing flow sheet.

Side Effects	Date	Date	Date	Date	Date
WBC					
Platelets					
H/H					
Creatinine/BUN					
LDH					
SGOT/PT					
Hemastix/Guaiac					
Other: _____					
IV Needle/Site					
Patency Checks:					
1. Aspiration OK					
2. Site WNL					
3. Occlusion					
IV Solution Before					
IV Solution After					
Premed/Antiemetics					
Chemotherapy Drugs					

RN Signature					

nurse may suggest a referral to a local mental health center for appropriate counseling. Also, a client may need a referral to an agency for home care services such as a home health aide, a regular visiting nurse, or a physical therapist. Lastly, if the client's condition worsens and the prognosis is poor, the nurse may want to explain the services of hospice if one is available in the community to provide terminal and bereavement care.

DISCHARGE FROM THE HOME IV CHEMOTHERAPY PROGRAM

If the client is being referred to another agency, the nurse should review the client's home care records and write a summary of the care given in the home IV chemotherapy program. Important points to include are: family and social supports, client's illness, description of home chemotherapy given and side effects experienced, most effective antiemetics and supportive drugs, client's response to chemotherapy and current condition, and client's and family's knowledge of self-care. Depending on the detail needed by the receiving agency, parts of the client's home care record may be copied with the client's permission and sent with the letter of transfer. (The agency should develop a release form for the transfer of client's records.)

PATIENT EDUCATION CARE GUIDE

WHAT IS HOME IV CHEMOTHERAPY?

The IV chemotherapy that you are now receiving in the clinic, in your doctor's office, or in the hospital may also be given in your home. A registered nurse specially trained in IV chemotherapy administration can come to your home to give it to you. Although this nurse will check you over carefully before administering the chemotherapy each time, you still may have to visit your physician periodically for a complete medical checkup or to have X rays or scans done. Thus, the purpose of the home IV chemotherapy program is to give you chemotherapy in your home as often as possible, in a safe, skilled, and caring manner, so that you and your family can achieve optimal well-being in familiar surroundings at a cost-effective price.

Here's how the home IV chemotherapy program works:

- Your physician completes the top portion of an admission criteria form.
- You and your family complete the bottom portion of this form so our secretary can check on your insurance coverage for you.
- A home IV chemotherapy nurse will talk with you and your family about the program and about how you have felt taking previous chemotherapy. The nurse will also look at your arms to see the condition of your veins. If you already have a central venous catheter because of poor veins, the nurse will ask you some questions about how you care for your catheter.
- When your IV chemotherapy is due to be given, the home IV chemotherapy nurse will call you to see what time is most convenient for you to receive it.
- The nurse will either obtain your drugs and other IV supplies or have them delivered before coming to your home at the time arranged with you and your family.
- You must obtain at least two items before the nurse comes to your home:

  1. An IV pole (may be delivered by an IV supply company if desired) or something similar to hang an IV bag onto, like a coatrack or curtain rod near your couch, bed, or chair
  2. A two-ply plastic trash bag

- Also before the nurse arrives, you must arrange for one of your family members or a friend to be with you while you receive your IV chemotherapy and for at least 6 to 8 hours afterward.
- Upon arriving at your house, the nurse will ask you how you have been feeling and will examine you for any signs of lingering side effects from previous chemotherapy or problems from your disease. If you or the nurse have any concerns about how you are doing, the nurse will call your doctor to determine whether to go ahead and give you your chemotherapy or to do something else.
- Following are some ways that IV chemotherapy can be given in the home.

  1. *IV push:* The nurse starts an IV (in your arm or with your catheter) by hanging a solution of IV fluid, which is usually sugar or saltwater. The nurse may then give one or more syringes of medicine through the side port of the tubing hooked to the IV bag. This method of administration is called IV push. These medicines may include not

only your chemotherapy drugs but also medicines to keep you from throwing up and/or to make your kidneys work faster. After all the IV push medicines are given, the nurse will allow the IV bag of solution to drip in to flush out your veins before discontinuing the IV. The nurse will stay with you for at least half an hour after IV push chemotherapy is given to make sure you are all right.

2. *IV push followed by IV drip:* Everything is done the same as in 1 above except that the nurse may teach you and your family how to discontinue your IV. This may be necessary because you may need an extra bag of IV fluid to help flush the chemotherapy from your body. Or, if you usually get fairly sick to your stomach with the chemotherapy, the nurse may hang a minibag of antinausea medication next to the main bag of solution. Thus, 3 or 4 hours after the nurse has left, you can allow the minibag of medicine to drip into your IV to help keep you from getting so sick. After this minibag and the main bag of IV solution have dripped in, you may then discontinue the IV.

3. *IV drip:* Everything is the same as in 1 above except that some of the chemotherapy may be given in minibags. This is called IV drip. IV drip is sometimes given in large bags, too. The nurse may start the minibag of chemotherapy and then teach you and your family how to turn it off when it is done. The main IV bag will then drip in to flush out your veins before you and your family discontinue the IV.

4. *Continuous infusion:* If your IV chemotherapy needs to run in over 24 hours for several days, your IV may be hooked up to a very tiny bag or a syringe of IV chemotherapy that is pumped in slowly by a small portable pump that fits on your belt, in your pocket, or in a pouch over your shoulder. The nurse will teach you how to check the pump to make sure that it is working. The nurse will then return to your home when the IV chemotherapy bag or syringe needs to be replaced. Or, if appropriate, the nurse may teach you how to change your IV bag or syringe.

- The home IV chemotherapy nurse will return to your home when your chemotherapy is due or if you are having problems and would like a nurse to check you. The nurse may also make a home visit if you need blood drawn or other tests done. The nurse will make sure that your physician gets a report of the results.

- If you have any questions or concerns related to your chemotherapy, feel free to call a home IV chemotherapy nurse, who is available by beeper 24 hours a day, 7 days a week. The nurse is also available to talk to you and your family about other resources and agencies that may assist you in dealing with your illness and treatments.

CHOOSING HOME IV CHEMOTHERAPY

Home IV chemotherapy is a convenient way to receive cancer treatment, but it is not for everyone. Several factors need to be considered. For example, some IV chemotherapy drugs have severe side effects and cannot be given in the home. Or, you may be sensitive to a particular drug and need to be closely monitored while it is given. Or, if your heart, kidneys, liver, or lungs are at all weak, your doctor may want to watch you closely while you receive your chemotherapy. Therefore, the first step in deciding whether you want to enter the home IV chemotherapy program is to talk it over with your doctor to see if it is a safe option for you. If your doctor tells you that home IV chemotherapy is medically OK for you, you and your family should discuss the following advantages and disadvantages of home IV chemotherapy before making your decision. You may also want to ask your nurse for more information if you have any questions about the program. You and your family should discuss these issues with your doctor and nurse so that you can make the best decision for you.

Advantages of Home IV Chemotherapy

1. Home IV chemotherapy may be cheaper than chemotherapy given in the hospital, clinic, or physician's office. In one study in Boston, "the average cost of an outpatient course of chemotherapy showed more than a 90% savings compared with costs of a five-day hospital stay" (Holmes 1985, 168). However, you need to make sure the home IV chemotherapy program calls your insurance companies to verify that they will pay for the particular type of home IV chemotherapy that you will be getting.

2. You should feel more comfortable and relaxed if you receive your IV chemotherapy in your own home. You can have your family, friends, and even your pets close by to support you and offer you encouragement. You can also have your favorite distractions, like TV, radio, and stereo, to help keep your mind off the IV chemotherapy.

3. The nurse will come to your house so you do not have to worry about driving to and parking at a medical facility. If you have small children, you will not have to worry about or pay for baby-sitters.

4. Because the nurse will arrange a time that is convenient for you and will come to your home, you will not have to spend time waiting. Also, if your family members work, they will not have to miss work, since the nurse can arrange to visit you after they come home.

5. Sometimes other patients receiving IV chemotherapy get sick in the waiting room or treatment room. If this bothers you, you can avoid it by having treatments in the privacy of your own home.

Julie Holman, a patient in the home chemotherapy program in Houston, Texas, says: "Learning and doing things for myself have made me feel very competent. There's no joy in being completely dependent on other people. The independence is the biggest advantage to home care. . . . For me, cancer treatment has been a chronic problem. The less it can interfere with my normal life-style, the more acceptable I consider my treatment to be . . ." (Dana 1985, 17).

Disadvantages of Home IV Chemotherapy

1. If your insurance companies will not cover all the expenses of your particular type of IV chemotherapy, you may have to assume part or all of the cost if you really want your IV chemotherapy at home. Although having chemotherapy at home may be cheaper than other places, it is still a fairly expensive procedure.

2. Because a doctor will not be close by while you are receiving the chemotherapy, there is a slightly increased risk involved if you should experience an unusual reaction. Although the nurse is specially trained in IV chemotherapy and does carry emergency drugs that can be given to you, a nurse is not as qualified as a doctor to handle emergency situations. Nonetheless, as a safety precaution, the nurse will make sure you keep important numbers by your phone, such as the telephone number of your doctor, the nearest ambulance, the nearest hospital, and a close friend or neighbor who could come over at a moment's notice.

3. Sometimes people with cancer feel lonely and isolated from other people. Getting out of the house to go to the hospital, a clinic, or a doctor's office may be a needed opportunity for you and your family to socialize with other people.

4. With some types of IV chemotherapy that are given in the home, you and your family may have to spend some time learning how to take care of an IV.

REGULATING AN IV DRIP RATE

Because it is important that the IV fluids go into your body at a particular rate, it is important that you and your family learn how to perform this procedure correctly. If you should get too much fluid too fast, it could cause your heart to beat too fast or cause your lungs to collect extra fluid. If you should not get enough fluid in the time that you are supposed to, it could cause your kidneys to function less well. This handout has been developed with step-by-step directions so that you can refer to it as you learn how to regulate an IV drip rate.

Step 1: Become familiar with the important parts of the two types of IV tubings. One type is the long IV tubing set that is hooked to the main IV bag of salt or sugar water. The other type of IV tubing is much shorter and is sometimes called "piggyback" tubing. It is connected into the longer IV site at the top port. Both these tubings have regulator clamps that can squeeze the tubing so the IV fluid cannot get through as fast.

Step 2: Double-check to make sure that all connections on the IV tubing are taped securely so that the IV tubing does not accidentally come apart. This could be harmful to you because blood could leak out of your IV site. Also, if the sterile IV system is opened, germs may have a chance to get in and cause infection. (*Note:* Persons with central venous catheters may also get air into their blood if the tubing comes apart. This can be very harmful and may require a trip to the emergency room.)

(**Step 2a:** If your IV does come apart, it is important to clean the ends of the needle or catheter and the IV tubing with alcohol before hooking them back together. While you are cleaning the ends, your IV should be clamped off so that IV fluid will not drip onto the floor. The catheter or IV needle tubing should also be clamped or pinched off so that you will not bleed or get air into your system. Thus, it is better to be safe than sorry by making sure all your IV tubing connections are taped securely.)

Step 3: The nurse will figure out how fast the IV drops must drip in order for the IV fluid to run into your body at the correct rate. The nurse will tell you the rate in terms of how many drops need to drip in 15 seconds. To help you remember this number, the nurse will write it on the main IV bag. Using a watch with a second hand, count the drops that drip into the IV chamber for 15 seconds. If there are too many, push the clamp a little tighter to squeeze the IV tubing and slow the drop rate. Then count the drops for another 15 seconds. If you tightened the regulator clamp too much, loosen it to allow more IV fluid to go through the tubing. Then count the drops for another 15 seconds. Keep tightening or loosening the clamp and counting the drops for 15 seconds until the rate is within 2 or 3 drops of what the nurse told you it should be. Under certain circumstances the nurse may recommend that a pump be used to regulate the IV rate.

Step 4: The nurse may leave a minibag of medicine on the piggyback tubing for you to turn on at a certain time. In this case, you need to do two things: (1) Turn the piggyback tubing clamp wide open. (2) Count the drops dripping from the minibag into the IV chamber to make sure the rate is what the nurse told you it should be. The nurse will write this number on the minibag to help you remember it. Note that if the numbers on the main IV bag and the minibag are the same, you should not have to readjust the regulator clamp. If the rates are different for each bag you will have to recount the drops from the minibag until it is flowing at the correct rate.

When the minibag is empty, the main bag will start running in again on its own. However, as soon as you can after the minibag has run dry, you need to clamp off the minibag tubing. At this time, you should recount the drops from the main IV bag to make sure the rate is correct.

Step 5: Because IVs run on the principle of gravity, the drop rate will decrease if the person with the IV stands up. Therefore, if you are going to be standing up for over 3 or 4 minutes, you need to recount and readjust the drop rate. You will need to repeat this process if you sit or lie back down.

In summary, regulating the IV drip rate is a very important process. It is important that you and your family learn how to do it correctly for your safety.

INSPECTING THE PERIPHERAL IV SITE FOR SIGNS OF INFILTRATION

Infiltration is a word used to describe the collection of fluid outside your vein. When an IV is in your arm, the concern is that the end of the needle stay within your vein. If the end of the needle should get outside your vein, the IV fluid will flow into your fatty tissue instead of into your bloodstream. The needle may move outside your vein because of movement in your arm or hand or because the tape over the needle becomes loosened. Therefore, it is important that you not move the arm or hand with the IV in it too much and that you reinforce the tape if it becomes loosened.

While the IV is running into your arm or hand, it is important that you check the IV drop rate every 15 to 20 minutes to make sure that it has not slowed down or stopped. This may happen if the IV fluid is running into your fatty tissue instead of into your vein and bloodstream. If the IV rate has slowed down or stopped, first check to see if the IV tubing is pinched or if the regulator clamp has been accidentally closed. If these things appear to be all right, check the IV site closely for the following signs:

- Redness
- Swelling
- Skin warmer or cooler than the surrounding skin
- Leaking of fluid from the needle
- Discomfort

If you find any of these signs, turn off any IV drip chemotherapy, slow down the IV drip rate to 2 or 3 drops per 15 seconds and call the home IV chemotherapy nurse. The nurse will probably come to your home to take the IV out and start a new one. Depending upon the medicines that you received through your IV, the nurse may show you how to apply warm or cold compresses to the old IV site to make it feel more comfortable.

DISCONTINUING A PERIPHERAL IV OR AN IV FROM AN INTERNAL PORT

When the fluid in your IV bag begins to get low, it is important to watch it closely so that air does not get into your system. This will not happen if you clamp off the IV tubing when the fluid is no longer dripping into the IV chamber. If air begins to move into the IV tubing, clamp off the IV tubing right away to prevent the air from getting closer to your IV site. (*Note:* If you have an internal port, you need to heparinize it according to your doctor's orders before removing the IV needle.)

After the IV has been clamped off, your assistant should place a protective pad next to you and gently remove the tape from the IV needle. Your assistant may need to hold the needle still with one hand while removing the tape with the other. After all the tape is off, your assistant should put on a pair of rubber household gloves and place a clean piece of gauze over the end of the needle where it goes into the skin. While gently pulling out the needle, your assistant should apply pressure to the needle hole to keep blood from leaking out. The IV needle should be placed on the protective pad. Then firm pressure should be applied to the IV site for 3 to 5 minutes (no peeking before the time is up—it may cause a bruise). If the IV was in your hand or arm, hold your hand or arm up in the air to decrease the pressure of the blood trying to leak out of the IV site hole.

After the IV site hole has been pressed with the gauze for 3 to 5 minutes, the gauze can be removed. All you should see is a tiny red hole in the skin. If blood is still leaking from the hole, apply pressure with the gauze for another 3 to 5 minutes. After the bleeding has stopped, an adhesive bandage should be placed over the IV site hole so it will not get infected. The adhesive bandage may be removed after 24 hours.

Now that the IV site is taken care of, the IV needle and tubing need to be disposed of properly. Your assistant should pick up the IV needle and tubing from the protective pad and untape and disconnect the IV needle from the tubing. The needle should be placed in a glass jar with a lid on it. The lid should be screwed on tightly. Next, the IV tubing and bag should be placed in the protective pad and wrapped up securely with tape. The protective pad with the IV bag and tubing in it and the jar with the IV needle in it should be placed in a 2-ply plastic trash bag. This bag should be placed in a metal garbage can where it will not be smashed or broken into by animals. Your assistant should then wash gloved hands with soap and water for 1 to 2 minutes before removing the gloves. The gloves should be allowed to dry and be kept for use the next time.

CARING FOR A VESICANT EXTRAVASATION SITE

Vesicant is a word used to describe IV drugs that irritate fatty tissue, sometimes to the point of causing skin sores. *Extravasation* is a term used to describe the leaking of these irritating drugs into the fatty tissue. A vesicant extravasation occurs when an IV needle slips out of a vein and into the fatty tissue while irritating drugs are being administered. A vesicant extravasation may also occur if there is a nearby hole in the vein from which the drugs can leak into the fatty tissue.

Your nurse will make every effort to start your IV carefully and tape it securely so that if you are given a vesicant drug, it will not extravasate into the fatty tissue. While giving you a vesicant drug, the nurse will be checking for a blood return every 2 to 3 minutes to make sure the IV needle is still in the vein. The nurse may also shut off your vein 1 to 2 inches above the needle to see if the IV stops dripping. This is a second check to make sure the IV needle is inside the vein and not in the fatty tissue. The third check involves what you are feeling at the IV site. If you feel any burning, pain, or discomfort, it is important that you let the nurse know right away.

Sometimes, despite all the safety measures that are taken, a vesicant extravasates from a vein, simply because the veins are weak or fragile. If this should happen, the nurse will stop giving you the drug, stop the IV and disconnect it, and place a small syringe on the end of your IV needle to suck out as much of the drug as possible. The nurse will then put some other medicine through the IV needle in an attempt to decrease the irritating effects of the vesicant drug. Next, the nurse will take the IV needle out, hold the IV site hole for 3 to 5 minutes, and apply an adhesive bandage over the hole.

Depending on the type of vesicant drug that extravasated, the nurse will tell you to do one of two things:

1. Keep a cold pack on the IV site for 30 minutes, off for 30 minutes, then on again for another 30 minutes. Keep this cycle up until you go to bed (at least 8 hours). Set an alarm clock for 4 hours and get up once in the night to put the cold pack on for 30 minutes. Put the cold pack on again the next morning as soon as you get up. Reapply the cold pack every 4 to 6 hours during the day until the area looks normal—that is, until the redness, swelling, and discomfort are gone.
2. Keep the IV site area warm by keeping it covered with a light dressing (like a washcloth) gently taped over the area. Do not apply a heating pad or hot-water bottle or anything that would be heavy on the IV site. Keep the area warm until the IV site looks normal—that is, until the redness, swelling, and discomfort are gone.

Besides doing *one* of the above, you need to watch the area closely. If the redness or swelling gets worse or if the skin begins to peel or seep fluid, call the home IV chemotherapy nurse right away. The nurse will advise you to see your physician and perhaps a plastic surgeon as soon as possible to avoid further damage to your tissues. Your physician may order a special cream for you to apply to the area to help it heal.

BIBLIOGRAPHY

Barry, L. K., and R. Booker. 1985. Promoting the responsible handling of antineoplastic agents in the community. *Oncology Nursing Forum* 12 (Sept./Oct.): 41–46.

Barstow, J. 1985. Safe handling of cytotoxic agents in the home. *Home Healthcare Nurse* 3 (Sept./Oct.): 46–47.

Brager, B. L., and J. Yasko. 1984. *Care of the Client Receiving Chemotherapy.* Reston Publishing Company, Inc.

Bubela, N. 1981. Technical and psychological problems and concerns arising from the outpatient treatment of cancer with direct intraarterial infusion. *Cancer Nursing* 4 (Aug.): 305–9.

Dana, W. 1985. Outpatient and home chemotherapy: offering the cancer patient a more normal life. Summary and excerpts from multidisciplinary roundtable workshop, January 16, University of Texas, M.D. Anderson Hospital, and Tumor Institute, Houston, Texas.

DeMoss, C. J. 1980. Giving intravenous chemotherapy at home. *American Journal of Nursing* 80 (Dec.): 2188–89.

Holmes, W. 1985. SQ chemotherapy at home. *American Journal of Nursing* 85 (Feb.): 168–69.

Mourad, L. A., and E. Glass. 1985. *Guide to the Administration of IV Chemotherapy Agents,* 2d ed. Columbus, Ohio: The Ohio State University Comprehensive Cancer Center Cancer Control Program.

Perri, J., and K. A. Erikson. 1983. Nursing issues for hepatic arterial infusion therapy. *Seminars in Oncology* 10 (June): 191–98.

Pughe, H. 1985. A way to go home. *Nursing Mirror* 160 (June 12): 38–41.

Rees, G. J. G. 1985. Cost-effectiveness in oncology. *The Lancet* (Dec. 21/28): 1405–8.

Rowland, C. G. 1985. Home continuous infusion therapy. *The Practitioner* 229 (Oct.): 889–92.

Schaffner, A. 1984. Safety precautions in home chemotherapy. *American Journal of Nursing* 84 (March): 346–47.

Slevin, M. L., et al. 1983. Subcutaneous infusion of cytosine arabinoside: a practical alternative to intravenous infusion. *Cancer Chemotherapy Pharmacology* 10:112–14.

UNIT VI

INTRAVENOUS MEDICATION CARE GUIDES

Generic Name: ACETAZOLAMIDE SODIUM

Trade Name: DIAMOX

Classification: Anticonvulsant, carbonic inhibitor, diuretic, alkalizer (systemic, urinary), sulfonamide derivative

Actions: A potent carbonic anhydrase inhibitor and nonbacteriostatic sulfonamide, acetazolamide rapidly decreases the secretion of aqueous humor, thus decreasing intraocular pressure; suppresses abnormal paroxysmal discharge from the central nervous system and depresses the tubular reabsorption of sodium, potassium, and bicarbonate. This action produces diuresis, alkalinazation of the urine, and a mild degree of metabolic acidosis.

Indications: For treatment of glaucoma (preoperatively and in acute crisis) and convulsive disorders and as a diuretic in the treatment of congestive heart failure or drug-induced edema (steroids).

Dosage:
Acute Narrow-Angle Glaucoma: 250 mg every 4 hours. May bolus dose: 500 mg.
Convulsive Disorders: Pediatric and adult: 8–30 mg/kg/day. Optimal dose range: 375–1000 mg/24 hours. When used in conjunction with other anticonvulsants, start with 250 mg/24 hours and titrate as indicated.
Congestive Heart Failure: 5 mg/kg, usually 250–375 mg daily on alternate days. *Not recommended for pediatric use.*

Preparation: Supplied in powder form. Reconstitute with 5 ml of sterile water for injection.

Home Stability: [*Stable for 1 week under refrigeration; 24 hours at room temperature.*]

Compatibilities: Compatible with solutions containing dextrose, saline, KCl, Ringer's, or lactated Ringer's. Do not mix with *any* other medications.

Administration:
Neonatal: Not indicated.
Pediatric: 250–500 mg over 5–6 minutes at the injection site.
Adult: 250–500 mg over 5–6 minutes at the injection site; for higher doses, dilute 250 mg in 50 ml.

Contraindications: Hypersensitivity to sulfonamides; renal and hepatic dysfunction; Addison's disease or other types of adrenocortical insufficiency; hyponatremia; hypokalemia; hyperchloremic acidosis; prolonged administration to clients with hyphema or chronic noncongestive narrow-angle glaucoma. Use with caution in clients with diabetes mellitus, hypercalciuria, gout, and obstructive pulmonary disease, and in digitalized clients.

Side Effects:
Primary: Rash, renal calculus, casts in the urine, fever, bone marrow depression, thrombocytopenic purpura, pancytopenia, agranulocytosis.
Secondary: Mild paresthesia, tingling feelings in extremities, anorexia, drowsiness and confusion, transient myopia.

Nursing Implications: Assess for hypersensitivity reactions.

Monitor intake and output when used to reduce edema.

Weigh clients under standard conditions daily.

Maintain adequate fluid intake during therapy to reduce risk of kidney stone formation.

Transient nearsightedness may occur following initiation of therapy. Notify physician for dosage reduction.

Advise clients to report any unusual side effects.

Monitor diabetics closely for increase in blood glucose. Change in management of the diabetic may be indicated.

Generic Name: ACYCLOVIR

Trade Name: ZOVIRAX

Classification: Antiviral

Actions: Synthetic acyclic purine nucleoside analogue with activity against HSV-1, HSV-2, varicella-zoster, Epstein-Barr virus, and cytomegalovirus.

Indications: For treatment of initial and recurrent mucosal and cutaneous herpes simplex type 1 and 2 infections in immunosuppressed clients and of severe initial clinical episodes of herpes genitalis in clients who are not immunocompromised.

Dosage:

Neonatal: 750 mg/m²/day divided into 3 doses every 8 hours for 7 days.

Pediatric: See neonatal dosage.

Adult: 15 mg/kg/day divided into 3 doses every 8 hours for 7 days.

General: For severe initial clinical episodes of herpes genitalis administer the same dosage for 5 days. *Reduce dosage or increase interval between doses for acute or chronic renal-impaired clients.*

Preparation: Supplied as a powder. Reconstitute a 500-mg vial with 10 ml of sterile water for injection (50 mg/ml). Shake well to dissolve completely. Withdraw the desired dosage and reconstitute further in a compatible solution to provide a concentration less than 7 mg/ml. *Do not use any bacteriostatic water containing parabens as this may cause precipitation.*

Home Stability: Initial reconstituted solution of 50 mg/ml is stable for 12 hours. Final concentration is stable for 24 hours. Refrigeration of reconstituted solutions may result in formation of a precipitate that will redissolve at room temperature.

Compatibilities: Compatible with most IV solutions.

Administration:

Neonatal: Dilute to a concentration of less than 7 mg/ml and infuse using an infusion pump over at least 60 minutes.

Pediatric: See neonatal administration.

Adult: See neonatal administration. *The incidence of renal tubular damage is increased if the solution is infused in less than 1 hour or given by IV bolus.*

Contraindications: Known hypersensitivity to the drug.

Side Effects:

Primary: Acute renal failure, inflammation or phlebitis at the injection site following extravasation of IV fluid, transient increases of serum creatinine, rash, hives.

Secondary: Encephalopathic changes such as lethargy, obtundation, tremors, confusion, hallucinations, agitation, seizures, or coma. Elevated serum creatinine, usually following rapid IV infusion; thrombocytosis, jitters.

Nursing Implications: Prior to and during therapy, culture and sensitivity tests should be completed.

Monitor for allergic reactions.

Monitor baseline and periodic renal, hepatic, and hematologic functions.

Administration must be accompanied by adequate hydration, because maximum urine concentration occurs within the first 2 hours following infusion.

Monitor intake and output every 8 hours. Reassess fluid balance prior to administration of drug. Notify physician if urinary output decreases.

Monitor infusion for signs of thrombophlebitis or extravasation.

Generic Name: ALBUMIN (HUMAN)

Trade Name: ALBUMINAR-5, ALBUTEIN, BUMINATE, PLASBUMIN

Classification: Blood volume expander

Actions: Expands blood volume, preventing marked hemoconcentration, reducing edema, and raising serum protein levels.

Indications: Shock, burns, hypoproteinemia, nephrosis, hepatic cirrhosis, cerebral edema.

Dosage:
Neonatal: 3–4 ml/pound.
Pediatric: 5–25 g/day.
Adult: 5–75 g/day, with a maximum dose of 250 g in 48 hours.

Preparation: Available as 5% solution (5 g/100 ml) in 50-, 250-, 500-, and 1000-ml vials and as a 25% solution (25 g/100 ml) in 20-, 50-, and 100-ml vials.

Home Stability: Not applicable.

Compatibilities: Compatible with dextrose, sodium chloride and lactated Ringer's and often admixed into TPN solutions. Infuse saline before and after to clear tubing of maintenance IV fluid.

Administration:
Neonatal: Variable, depending on patient response, usually one-fourth the adult rate.

Pediatric: Variable depending on patient response, usually one-fourth to one-half the adult rate.

Adult: Depending on patient response, may range from 50 g as rapidly as tolerated to 1 ml/minute.

Contraindications: Anemia, cardiac failure, history of allergic reaction to infused albumin, normal or increased intravascular volume.

Side Effects:
Primary: Circulatory failure, dyspnea, circulatory overload, precipitous hypotension, pulmonary edema.
Secondary: Fever, nausea, salivation, vomiting.

Nursing Implications: Monitor pulse rate and rhythm, blood pressure, and hemodynamic parameters (if available) during therapy. Assess for signs of circulatory overload.

Assess for regular venous distension, peripheral edema, dyspnea, wheezing, rales, and rhonchi during therapy.

Monitor daily weights, intake/output, and skin turgor.

Monitor hemoglobin, hematocrit, electrolyte, and serum protein levels during therapy.

Assess for signs of bleeding during and after therapy.

Assess for signs of allergic reactions 5 and 15 minutes after initiation of therapy.

Generic Name: ALPHAPRODINE HYDROCHLORIDE

Trade Name: NISENTIL

Classification: Narcotic analgesic, Schedule II controlled substance

Actions: Drugs in this class act to relieve moderate to severe pain and provide preoperative sedation. A patient's perception of pain is altered by preventing or changing the transmission of painful stimuli along the sensory pathways in the central nervous system. These pathways are specific to the perception and emotional response of the patient to pain. In addition, these drugs suppress the respiratory and cough centers of the brain and have an antiperistaltic effect on the smooth muscle of the intestine. Because of their actions, narcotics can produce physical and psychological dependence. When used to treat severe pain, as that associated with terminal illness, they should be given around the clock to maximize pain relief and reduce anxiety.

Indications: For management of moderate to severe pain due to a diversity of causes. Should not be used in cases of mild pain or pain that can be relieved by non-narcotic analgesics. Use in pediatrics limited to analgesia during dental procedures.

Dosage:
Neonatal: Not recommended.
Pediatric: 0.3–0.6 mg/kg for dental procedures.
Adult: 0.4–0.6 mg/kg IV or 0.4–1.2 mg/kg subcutaneously. The lower range is recommended initially to assess patient response. Maximum initial IV dose: 30 mg. Initial SC dose: 60 mg. Total maximum dose: 240 mg in 24 hours.

Preparation: Supplied in injectable form. Strengths available are 40 mg/ml and 60 mg/ml.

Compatibilities: Should not be administered directly with diazepam, aminophylline, barbiturates, phenytoin, heparin, sodium bicarbonate, or methicillin.

Administration:
Neonatal: Not recommended.
Pediatric: Should be used only for analgesia during dental procedures, and a narcotic antagonist should be available for use as necessary.
Adult: IV or SC. Do not give IM. Drug should be diluted before IV administration. IV route is used when rapid onset of analgesia and shorter duration of action is needed. Give slow IV push to decrease the chance of adverse reactions. After SC administration effects will be noted in about 10 minutes and last 1–2 hours.

Contraindications: Known sensitivity to narcotic analgesics; during delivery of a premature infant; in clients taking MAO inhibitors or those who have taken them within 14 days. Use with caution in clients with head injuries, increased intracranial pressure, shock, CNS and respiratory depression, COPD, or in clients receiving other narcotic analgesics.

Side Effects:
Primary: Respiratory depression and apnea during IV administration. In patients with known sensitivity to narcotic analgesics, hypotension, bradycardia, nausea, vomiting, dizziness, sedation, sweating.
Secondary: Constipation owing to effect on the smooth muscle of the bowel. Urinary retention, pain at injection site, and phlebitis after IV administration. Physical dependence.

Nursing Implications: Because of the chance for respiratory depression, a narcotic antagonist should be available for rapid administration, especially if the route of choice is IV. Naloxone is the antagonist most often used.

Monitor vital signs frequently: for IV dose, every 5–10 minutes, for SC dose, every 15–30 minutes.

Supportive equipment should be readily available in case of cardiac or respiratory arrest. A patent airway should be maintained.

Monitor infants when the drug is used during labor and delivery.

Monitor intake and output when this drug is given repeatedly, because it may cause urinary retention.

To augment the use of narcotic analgesics, give before severe pain occurs. Nursing actions also include the use of emotional support and patient comfort measures. Because of depression of respiratory centers, postoperative use in management of pain should include turning, coughing, and deep breathing to prevent pulmonary complications.

Patients should be warned to avoid activities requiring alertness.

Assist patient with ambulation. This medication may cause orthostatic hypotension.

Generic Name: AMIKACIN SULFATE

Trade Name: AMIKIN

Classification: Antibiotic (aminoglycoside)

Actions: Semisynthetic aminoglycoside derivative from kanamycin with neuromuscular blocking action. Inhibits protein synthesis in bacterial cell and is bactericidal. Effective against a wide variety of gram-negative bacilli: *Escherichia coli,* Enterobacter, *Klebsiella pneumoniae,* and most strains of *Pseudomonas aeruginosa,* Proteus, Serratia, *Providencia stuartii, Citrobacter freundii,* and Acubetibacter. Also effective against *Mycobacterium tuberculosis* and atypical Mycobacterium, penicillinase and non-penicillinase-producing Staphylococci.

Indications: Bacteremia and septicemia, including neonatal sepsis; serious infections such as infections of the urinary or respiratory tract, bones, joints, and central nervous system, including meningitis; burns and postoperative infections.

Dosage:
Neonatal: Loading dose: 10 mg/kg of body weight. Maintenance dose: 5 mg/kg every 8 hours or 7.5 mg/kg every 12 hours.
Pediatric: 5 mg/kg every 8 hours or 7.5 mg/kg every 12 hours.
Adult: Usual dose is up to 15 mg/kg of body weight per 24 hours in 2 or 3 equal doses at equally divided intervals. May administer up to 1.5 g/day in heavier clients.
General: Duration of therapy: 7–10 days.
Dosage is highly individualized and should be based on therapeutic drug monitoring.
Desirable peak serum level: 15–30 µg/ml.
Trough serum level: 5–10 µg/ml.
Toxic serum level (peak): >35 µg/ml.

Preparation: Supplied as a colorless solution, which does not require refrigeration, in the following concentrations:
    50 mg/1-ml vial
    100 mg/2-ml vial
    250 mg/1-ml vial
    500 mg/2-ml vial or disposable syringe
    1000 mg/4-ml vial

Home Stability: Stable at room temperature as prepared by manufacturer for at least 2 years.

Compatibilities: Compatible with solutions containing dextrose, saline, KCl, Ringer's, or lactated Ringer's. Compatible with aminophylline, calcium, epinephrine, levarterenol, and pentobarbital. Not compatible with total parenteral nutrition or heparin.

Administration:
Neonatal: Infuse over 1–2 hours. Administer at appropriate IV site based on infusion rate. Dilution should be based on fluid volume needs.
Pediatric: Infuse over 30–60 minutes. Administer at appropriate IV site based on infusion rate. Dilution should be based on fluid volume needs.
Adult: Dilute in 100–200 ml of IV solution and administer over 30–60 minutes.

Contraindications: Known amikacin sulfate sensitivity. Use with caution in clients with impaired renal function, eighth cranial nerve impairment, dehydration, fever, myasthenia gravis, parkinsonism, or hypocalcemia. The neuromuscular blocking effect of amikacin is enhanced with concurrent administration of potent diuretics, pancuronium, succinylcholine, aminoglycosides, or anesthetics. This drug may inactivate the aminoglycoside; administer at least 2 hours apart if ordered concurrently.

Side Effects:
Primary:
Nephrotoxicity: Proteinuria and presence of red and white blood cells in the urine, granular casts, azotemia, oliguria, urinary frequency, frank hematuria, increase in BUN and serum creatinine, decrease in creatinine clearance and specific gravity, renal damage and failure.
Ototoxicity: *Auditory*—high-frequency hearing loss; complete hearing loss (occasionally permanent); tinnitus; fullness, ringing, or buzzing in ears. *Vestibular*—dizziness and vertigo, ataxia, nausea and vomiting, nystagmus.
Neurotoxicity: Drowsiness, headache, unsteady gait, clumsiness, paresthesias, tremors, muscle twitching and weakness, convulsions, neuromuscular blockade with respiratory depression.
Secondary: Nausea, vomiting, stomatitis, skin

rash, urticaria, pruritus, generalized burning sensation, drug fever, arthralgia, eosinophilia, anemia, leukopenia, granulocytopenia, thrombocytopenia, unusual thirst, difficulty breathing, superinfections, peripheral neuritis.

Nursing Implications: Monitor serum blood levels initially and throughout therapy.

Document the *exact* time of medication administration for determination of blood levels.

Assess renal function prior to initial administration via baseline BUN, creatinine and creatinine clearance, specific gravity, and urine analysis.

Monitor renal function throughout therapy via assessment of BUN, creatinine and creatinine clearance, specific gravity, urine analysis, and strict intake and output.

Encourage hydration of client to reduce chemical irritation to renal tubules.

Assess eighth cranial (vestibulocochlear) nerve function prior to initial administration and throughout therapy and upon discharge via audiometric tests and assessment of vestibular disturbance.

Monitor for overgrowth infection as evidenced by diarrhea, anogenital itching, vaginal discharge, stomatitis, or glossitis.

Antidote: Peritoneal dialysis or hemodialysis will assist in removal of the drug from the bloodstream.

Generic Name: AMINOCAPROIC ACID

Trade Name: AMICAR

Classification: Coagulant

Actions: Inhibits plasminogen activator substances and to a lesser degree plasmin activity. Increases fibrinogen activity in clot formation by inhibiting the enzyme required for destruction of the formed fibrin.

Indications: Hemorrhage resulting from overactivity of the fibrinolytic system, systemic hyperfibrinolysis, and urinary fibrinolysis.

Dosage:
Neonatal and Pediatric: Not applicable.
Pediatric: Not applicable.
Adult: Initial dose: 5 g followed by 1–1.25 g/hour for 6–8 hours. Maximum dose: 30 g/24 hours.

Preparation: 1 g/4 ml of solution.

Home Stability: Not applicable.

Compatibilities: May infuse with normal saline, dextrose in saline, or in water, or Ringer's.

Administration:
Neonatal: Not applicable.
Pediatric: Not applicable.
Adult: Dilute initial dose in 250 ml of solution and infuse over 1 hour. For subsequent doses, dilute 1 g in 50–100 ml of solution and infuse 1 g/hour.

Contraindications: Disseminated intravascular coagulation; evidence of thrombosis during first and second trimester of pregnancy. Use with caution in clients with cardiac, hepatic, or renal disease.

Side Effects:
Primary: Cramps, diarrhea, dizziness, headache, grand mal seizure, malaise, nausea, skin rash, stuffy nose, tearing, thrombophlebitis, tinnitus.
Secondary: None.

Nursing Implications: Monitor lab studies to determine the amount of fibrinolysis present.

Monitor blood pressure and pulse rate and rhythm frequently. Rapid infusion may cause hypotension, bradycardia, or arrhythmias.

Infuse blood products as ordered by the physician in conjunction with aminocaproic acid therapy.

Assess IV site frequently for redness, heat, tenderness, or pain. Assess for Homans' sign every 4 hours during therapy. Notify physician of any signs of thrombophlebitis.

Generic Name: AMIODARONE HYDROCHLORIDE

Trade Name: CORDARONE

Classification: Group III antiarrhythmic

Actions: Prolongs the refractory period and repolarization.

Indications: Ventricular and supraventricular arrhythmias, including WPW syndrome, atrial fibrillation and flutter, ventricular tachycardia.

Dosage:
Neonatal: Not applicable.
Pediatric: Not applicable.
Adult: Loading dose of 5–10 mg/kg followed by continuous IV infusion to equal 10 mg/kg/day for 3–5 days.

Home Stability: Not applicable.

Compatibilities: Infuse with dextrose or saline solutions.

Administration:
Neonatal: Not applicable.
Pediatric: Not applicable.
Adult: Via intravenous infusion.

Contraindications: Hypersensitivity to amiodarone. Use with caution in patients with preexisting bradycardia or sinus node disease, conduction disturbances, severely depressed ventricular function, or marked cardiomegaly.

Side Effects:
Primary: Corneal microdeposits, altered liver enzymes, pneumonitis, photosensitivity.
Secondary: Peripheral neuropathy, extrapyramidal symptoms, bradycardia, hypotension, altered thyroid function, hepatic dysfunction, muscle weakness.

Nursing Implications: Continuous cardiac monitoring during IV therapy.

Monitor blood pressure and heart rate and rhythm frequently. Notify doctor of any significant change.

Recommend instillation of methylcellulose ophthalmic solution to minimize development of corneal microdeposits, usually seen 1–4 months after initiation of therapy.

Monitor hepatic and thyroid function tests.

Assess for symptoms of pneumonitis: exertional dyspnea, nonproductive cough, and pleuritic chest pain. Monitor pulmonary function tests and chest X rays.

Side effects are very common and even more prevalent at higher doses: resolution may take up to 4 months following discontinuation of drug.

Infuse via intravenous infusion pump.

Generic Name: AMMONIUM CHLORIDE

Trade Name: AMMONIUM CHLORIDE INJECTION

Classification: Diuretic

Actions: Urinary and systemic acidifying agent or diuretic. Used in the treatment of metabolic alkalosis to increase the number of free hydrogen ions, which in turn decreases pH.

Indications: Metabolic alkalosis and hypochloremia.

Dosage: Highly individualized depending on condition under treatment.

Preparation: Injectable 2.14% (0.4 mEq/ml) or 26.75% (5 mEq/ml).

Administration: *Slow* IV infusion, checking pH frequently because there is a chance for metabolic acidosis to occur.

Contraindications: Impaired renal or hepatic function and respiratory acidosis.

Side Effects:
Primary: Metabolic acidosis, headache, confusion, bradycardia, irregular respirations with some periods of apnea.
Secondary: Rash, pallor, pain at injection site.

Nursing Implications: Take vital signs and assess presenting symptoms.
Monitor resolution of symptoms and document. Monitor IV infusion carefully to prevent too rapid administration and extravasation.
Monitor laboratory results closely.
Assess patient for signs of ammonia toxicity. These include pallor, irregular respirations, vomiting, cardiac arrhythmias, convulsions, and coma.

Generic Name: AMOBARBITAL SODIUM

Trade Name: AMYTAL SODIUM

Classification: Barbiturate/sedative

Actions: Short-acting central nervous system depressant, hypnotic, and anticonvulsant.

Barbiturates act at the level of the thalamus to depress cortex functioning, which decreases motor activity and produces sedation.

Indications: For sedation and relief of anxiety; hypnotic effects; as preanesthetic medication; to control seizures secondary to eclampsia, chorea, meningitis, tetanus, drug poisoning, and epilepsy; for narcoanalysis and narcotherapy; as a diagnostic aid in schizophrenia.

Dosage:
Neonatal: Not indicated.
Pediatric:
Children Under 6 Years: 3–5 mg/kg per dose. Safety in children under 6 years has not been established.
Children Over 6 Years: 65 mg–250 mg. Maximum dosage: 500 mg. For convulsions: 5–8 mg/kg. Dosage should be determined by client indication and response.
Adult: 65–500 mg. Maximum single dosage: 1 g. Dosage should be determined by client indication and response.

Preparation: Supplied in ampules of 125, 250, and 500 mg. Reconstitute each 125 mg with 1.25 ml of sterile water for injection to make a 10% solution. Further dilution may be indicated. Rotate vial gently after diluent is added; do not shake. Dissolution may take several minutes. Do not use a solution that has not cleared within 5 minutes or one that contains a precipitate. Use reconstituted solution within 30 minutes.

Home Stability: Not indicated.

Compatibilities: It is compatible with aminophylline and hydrocortisone.

Administration:
Neonatal: Not indicated.
Pediatric: Inject at a rate not to exceed 60 mg/m^2/minute at the IV site. More rapid injection may result in apnea or hypotension.
Adult: Inject at a rate not to exceed 100 mg/minute at the IV site. More rapid injection may result in apnea or hypotension.

Contraindications: Known hypersensitivity, impaired liver function, family or client history of porphyria, impaired respiratory function, history of sedative/hypnotic addiction. Safety in pregnancy has not been established; may cause respiratory depression in the infant if used during labor.

Side Effects:
Primary: Somnolence, agitation, ataxia, CNS depression, anxiety, dizziness, respiratory depression, hypotension, bradycardia.
Secondary: Skin rashes, constipation, nausea, vomiting, tissue necrosis from extravasation, headache, fever.

Nursing Implications: Monitor vital signs every 5 minutes for 1 hour after injection. Do not leave the patient unattended.

Have supportive equipment available in case of respiratory depression.

Maintain a safe environment for client in light of depressant effects—raise side rails of bed and assist with ambulation.

Do not administer closely with a narcotic analgesic.

Generic Name: AMPHOTERICIN B

Trade Name: FUNGIZONE

Classification: Antibiotic, antifungal

Actions: Antibiotic effective against many species of fungi. Not effective against bacteria, rickettsai, or viruses.

Indications: Progressive, potentially fatal fungal infections such as cryptococcosis; blastomycosis; disseminated moniliasis, coccidioidomycosis, and histoplasmosis; mucormycosis (phycomycosis); sporotrichosis; aspergillosis. May be effective in the treatment of American (mucocutaneous) leishmaniasis but is not the drug of choice.

Dosage:
Neonatal: Test dose of 0.1 mg/kg over 6 hours. Increase the dose over the next 4 days if there are no adverse reactions. Do not exceed 1 mg/kg/ 24 hours.
Pediatric: See neonatal dosage.
Adult: Test dose of 1 mg may be given over 30 minutes in an infusion. Increase the dose up to 1 mg/kg/day or 1.5 mg/kg on alternate days if there are no adverse reactions. Usual dose is 0.25 mg/kg/day.

Preparation: Supplied as a powder in vials of 50 mg. Reconstitute by adding 10 ml of sterile water for injection to the vial for a concentration of 5 mg/ml. Shake immediately after reconstitution. *Do not use diluents containing bacteriostatic agents or saline.*

Stability: Store powder and reconstituted solution in the refrigerator. Discard reconstituted solution after 7 days. Protect against exposure to light. Do not use if solution is not clear.

Compatibilities: Compatible only with dextrose for infusion vehicle. Do not mix with any solution having a pH less than 6. Do not mix with any other medication except heparin or hydrocortisone to decrease the risk of infusion phlebitis.

Administration:
Neonatal: Further reconstitute the solution to a final concentration of 1:50 with 5% dextrose. Administer by slow IV infusion using an infusion pump over 6 hours at a concentration of 0.1 mg/ml. Physician should specify IV infusion rate. An in-line filter with a mean pore diameter of 1 micron should be used to assure passage of the drug.
Pediatric: See neonatal administration.
Adult: See neonatal administration.

Contraindications: Known hypersensitivity, unless the possible lifesaving benefits of the drug outweigh the reaction. Safety for use in pregnancy has not been established.

Side Effects:
Primary: Renal damage (hypokalemia, azotemia, renal tubular acidosis, nephrocalcinosis), fever with shaking chills, headache, anorexia, weight loss, nausea, vomiting, dyspepsia, malaise, muscle and joint pains, pain at injection site with phlebitis and thrombophlebitis, normochromic and normocytic anemia.
Secondary: Anuria, cardiac toxicity (arrhythmias, cardiac arrest, hypertension, hypotension), blood dyscrasias (thrombocytopenia, leukopenia or leukocytosis, agranulocytosis, eosinophilia), hemorrhagic gastroenteritis, rash, pruritus, loss of hearing, tinnitus, vertigo, blurred vision or diplopia, peripheral neuropathy, convulsions, anaphylaxis, acute liver failure.

Nursing Implications: Prior to and during therapy, culture and sensitivity tests should be completed.
Assess the client every 15–30 minutes for signs of side effects. Assess vital signs and slow the infusion to a keep-the-vein-open rate or discontinue the infusion if any severe adverse reaction occurs.
Assess the IV site every 15 minutes for signs of extravasation.
Assess intake-output ratio hourly. Report any decrease in urinary output or change in the appearance of the urine. Monitor for signs of electrolyte imbalance.
Monitor baseline and periodic renal, hepatic, and hematologic functions.

Prolonged therapy is usually necessary, and unpleasant reactions are common. Therefore this drug can be administered in the home health setting with stabilized patients and careful clinical monitoring.

Do not administer concurrently with other nephrotoxic antibiotics and antineoplastic agents.

Administer corticosteroids as ordered to decrease febrile reactions, and antipyretics as ordered if fever occurs.

Generic Name: AMPICILLIN SODIUM

Trade Name: OMNIPEN-N, POLYCILLIN-N, SK AMPICILLIN-N, TOTACILLIN-N

Classification: Antibiotic (penicillin)

Actions: Broad-spectrum synthetic penicillin, bactericidal against enterococci and several gram-negative strains, which include *Escherichia coli*, *Neisseria gonorrhoeae* and *meningitidis*, *Hemophilus influenzae*, *Proteus mirabilis*, Salmonella, and Shigella.

Indications: Moderate to severe infections such as those of urinary, respiratory, and gastrointestinal tracts and skin and soft tissues; gonococcal infections; bacterial meningitis; otitis media; prophylactic treatment of bacterial endocarditis.

Dosage:
Neonatal: 50–300 mg/kg/day every 8–12 hours.
Pediatric: 50–300 mg/kg/day every 4–6 hours.
Adult: 50–300 mg/kg/day every 4–6 hours.

Preparation: Supplied as a powder in the following vial sizes: 125 mg, 250 mg, 500 mg, 1 g, 2 g. Reconstitute with sterile water.

Home Stability: Use within 1 hour of reconstitution. Once added to IV fluid, stability is extended to 2–8 hours. In sodium chloride stability equals 72 hr under refrigeration.

Compatibilities: Compatible with solutions containing dextrose, saline, KCl, and Ringer's or lactated Ringer's. Compatible with heparin, cimetidine, hydrocortisone, and total parenteral nutrition. Do not mix with any other antibiotic.

Administration:
Neonatal: Infuse over 10–30 minutes by IV push or IV Y-site. More rapid infusion can result in seizures.
Pediatric: See neonatal administration.

Adult: Infuse over 10–30 minutes by IV push, IV Y-site, or IV piggyback. More rapid infusion can result in seizures.

Contraindications: Hypersensitivty to penicillin derivatives or cephalosporins; pregnancy. Individuals with a history of allergic problems are more susceptible to untoward reactions.

Side Effects:
Primary: Hypersensitivity reactions such as anaphylaxis, exfoliative dermatitis, rashes, urticaria.
Secondary: Pseudomembranous colitis, diarrhea, abdominal pain, nausea, vomiting, headache, seizures, phlebitis, superinfections, morbilliform rash (ampicillin rash), anemia, thrombocytopenia, leukopenia, agranulocytosis.

Nursing Implications: Prior to and during therapy, culture and sensitivity tests should be completed.

Monitor for allergic reactions.

Sodium concentration must be taken into consideration in clients on a sodium-restricted diet.

Assess for ampicillin rash daily. It usually develops after 5–14 days of therapy. The rash is dull red, macular or maculopapular, and mildly pruritic. It begins on light-exposed or pressure areas such as the knees, elbows, palms, and soles, then spreads over the body symmetrically. Therapy does not have to be discontinued, but close assessment for other signs of anaphylaxis is indicated.

Assess for pseudomembranous colitis. Monitor onset, duration, and character of stools, weight, temperature, and associated symptoms.

Monitor baseline and periodic renal, hepatic, and hematologic functions.

Monitor for superinfection. Assess for the onset of black, hairy tongue; oral lesions (stomatitis, glossitis); rectal or vaginal itching; vaginal discharge; loose, foul-smelling stools; unusual odor to urine.

Generic Name: AMRINONE LACTATE

Trade Name: INOCOR

Classification: Cardiac inotropic agent

Actions: Appears to produce a positive inotropic effect by increasing myocardial cell stores of C-AMP. Vasodilatory effects, reducing both preload and afterload, appear to be the result of a direct relaxation of vascular smooth muscle.

Indications: For short-term treatment of congestive heart failure.

Dosage:
Neonatal: Not applicable.
Pediatric: Not applicable.
Adult: Initial bolus of 0.75 mg/kg. Maintenance infusion begun at 5 μg/kg/minute and titrated to patient's response. An additional bolus of 0.75 mg/kg may be given 30 minutes after initiation of therapy if indicated.

Preparation: Supplied as clear yellow sterile solution in 20-ml ampules.

Home Stability: Not applicable.

Compatibilities: Must be mixed in solutions containing only saline: not compatible with solutions containing dextrose. Inocor infusion may be Y-connected to infusions of dextrose solutions.

Administration:
Neonatal: Not applicable.
Pediatric: Not applicable.
Adult: Bolus may be given undiluted over 2–3 minutes. Infusion should be diluted to a concentration of 1:3 mg/ml and used within 24 hours.

Contraindications: Hypersensitivity to amrinone lactate or bisulfites. Concurrent use with Norpace should be undertaken with caution. Use in patients after myocardial infarction is not recommended.

Side Effects:
Primary: Thrombocytopenia, hepatic toxicity.
Secondary: Nausea, vomiting, abdominal pain, anorexia, arrhythmia, hypotension, hypersensitivity reactions.

Nursing Implications: Continuous cardiac monitoring is essential during treatment: report arrhythmias and changes in heart rate.

Monitoring of hemodynamic parameters is beneficial in assessing patient's response. Therapeutic effects should result in an increase in cardiac output and a decrease in pulmonary arteriole wedge pressure.

Continuous monitoring of blood pressure is preferred; otherwise, blood pressure should be checked at least every 5 minutes after the bolus and after any change in infusion levels until stabilized.

Assess heart tones, jugular venous distension, peripheral edema, lung sounds, dyspnea, and capillary refill every 4 hours and as needed to ascertain the effect of treatment.

Electrolyte changes and renal function should be monitored frequently.

Fluid status should be monitored via intake and output, daily weights and pulmonary arterial wedge and central venous pressures.

Infuse via infusion pump.

Generic Name: ANTIHEMOPHILIC FACTOR (HUMAN)

Trade Name: FACTORATE, FACTORATE GENERATION II, HEMOFIL, HEMOFIL T, HUMAFAAC, KOATE, PROFILATE

Classification: Coagulant

Actions: Coagulation Factor VIII, necessary for the completion of coagulation.

Indications: For treatment of classical hemophilia A, for control of unexpected hemorrhagic episodes during emergency or elective surgery, and prophylactically to prevent hemorrhage in known hemophiliac patients.

Dosage: Completely individualized. Suggested doses are as follows:

Prophylaxis of Spontaneous Hemorrhage: 10 IU/kg to increase Factor VIII by 20 percent. Minimum of 30 percent of normal is indicated.

Minor Hemorrhage and Minor Surgery: 15–25 IU/kg to increase Factor VIII by 30–50 percent of normal. Maintain with 10–15 IU/kg every 8–12 hours.

Severe Hemorrhage: 40–50 IU/kg to increase Factor VIII to 80–100 percent of normal. Maintain with 20–25 IU/kg every 8–12 hours.

Major Surgery: Sufficient dose to increase Factor VIII to 80–100 percent of normal given 1 hour before surgery. Confirm with antihemophitin factor level assays just before surgery. Give a second dose, one-half of the first, in 5 hours. Maintain Factor VIII at 30 percent of normal for 10–14 days.

Preparation: Varies in number of units. All provide diluent and administration equipment.

Home Stability: Not applicable.

Compatibilities: Infuse in a separate line; do not mix with other drugs.

Administration: Prepare using the provided diluent and administration set. Infuse preparation with less than 34 IU/ml at a rate of 10–20 ml over 3 minutes. Infuse preparations with more than 34 IU/ml at a maximum rate of 2 ml/minute.

Contraindications: None when used as indicated.

Side Effects: Backache, erythema, fever, headache, hepatitis, hives. May transmit the AIDS virus.

Nursing Implications: Monitor Factor VIII assays before and during therapy. Notify physician for dosage adjustments.

Monitor partial thromboplastin time. Notify physician for possible dosage adjustments.

Must be refrigerated and administered within 3 hours of reconstitution. Use plastic syringes to prevent binding to glass surfaces.

Monitor for side effects. Most subside within 15–20 minutes. Notify physician of the development of side effects.

May transmit hepatitis and AIDS. Use special care to avoid accidental punctures with equipment.

Generic Name: ANTI-INHIBITOR COAGULANT COMPLEX

Trade Name: AUTOPLEX, FEIBA IMMUNO

Classification: Coagulant

Indications: For control of hemorrhagic episodes in hemophiliacs with Factor VIII inhibitors at levels above 2–10 Bethesda units.

Dosage: Dosage range is 25–100 Factor VIII correctional units/kg, repeated in 6–12 hours, not to exceed 200 units/kg/24 hours. Dosage is individualized according to patient response.

Preparation: Dried or freeze-dried concentrate prepared from human plasma with diluent provided.

Home Stability: Not applicable.

Compatibilities: Infuse in a separate line; do not mix with other drugs.

Administration: Prepare using the provided diluent and administration set. Infuse at a rate of 10 ml/minute or less. If side effects occur, discontinue until symptoms subside and restart at 2 ml/minute.

Contraindications: Disseminated intravascular coagulation, signs of fibrinolysis, known hypersensitivity. Use with extreme caution in patients with liver disease.

Side Effects: Anaphylaxis, bradycardia, chest pain, chills, cough, decreased fibrinogen concentration, decreased platelet count, fever, flushing, headache, hypertension, hypotension, prolonged partial thromboplastin time, prolonged prothrombin time, prolonged thrombin time, respiratory distress, tachycardia, urticaria.

Nursing Implications: Monitor prothrombin time before and after treatment. Posttreatment time must be two-thirds of preinfusion value if therapy is to continue. Other clotting factor tests do not correlate with actual patient response. Inaccurate dosing may lead to overdose and disseminated intravascular coagulation.

Identification of Factor VIII inhibitor level is mandatory previous to administration.

Refrigerate before reconstitution.

Monitor blood pressure, pulse rate and respiratory rate and effort frequently during therapy.

Monitor infusion rate and patient response carefully. Symptoms of a too rapid infusion include headache, flushing, and changes in blood pressure or pulse rate.

May transmit hepatitis or AIDS. Use special care to avoid accidental punctures with equipment.

Generic Name: ANTIVENIN (CROTALIDAE) POLYVALENT

Trade Name: SAME AS GENERIC

Classification: Antivenin

Actions: Provides passive immunity to the venom of pit vipers native to North, Central, and South America, Asia, and the tropics. Pit vipers include rattlesnakes, copperheads, and water moccasins. Will not neutralize the venom of true vipers such as cobras, puff adders, and coral snakes. Should be given as soon as possible after the snakebite—most effective when administered within 4 hours. Effectiveness decreases with time after snakebite. Value of administration after 12 hours is questionable.

Indications: For treatment of envenomization from the pit viper family.

Dosage: Dosage is not based on size or weight. Therefore it may be necessary to administer a larger dose to a child or small adult because of the smaller amount of body fluid.

Initial Parenteral Dosage:
Minimal envenomization: 2–4 vials.
Moderate envenomization: 5–9 vials.
Severe envenomization: 10–15 vials.

Further doses are based on patient's response to the initial dose and assessment of the severity of the poisoning (e.g., continuing progress of swelling, a fall in hematocrit, or hypotension). The additional dose would be contents of 1–5 vials.

Preparation: Injectable form yields 10 ml of serum. This should be used immediately after reconstitution. A 1-ml vial of 1:10 normal horse serum is available for use in sensitivity testing. The combination package includes a vacuum vial of serum, a 10-ml vial of bacteriostatic water, and a 1-ml vial of normal horse serum.

Compatibilities: Reconstitute with 10 ml of bacteriostatic water. May be diluted with normal saline or D_5W for IV administration.

Administration: Prior to administration, patient should be tested for a reaction to horse serum.

During administration, emergency equipment and medications should be immediately available in case of anaphylactic reaction.

IV administration is the preferred route, especially for moderate and severe envenomization. If it must be administered IM, a large muscle mass should be the site of administration.

Infuse initial 5–10 ml of diluted 1:1 or 1:10 serum over 3–5 minutes. Observe patient closely for reaction. If no reactions occur, continue infusion at the maximum safe rate based on age and weight of the patient, severity of envenomization, and type and amount of parenteral fluids needed. The time interval between bite and start of therapy must also be considered.

Side Effects:

Primary: Within 30 minutes after serum administration: shock, anaphylaxis, anxiety, flushing, urticaria, itching, weakness, faintness, and numbness or tingling around the mouth, tongue, fingers, toes, or bite area.

Secondary: Delayed serum-sicknesslike reaction may occur 5–24 days after administration: malaise, fever, urticaria, nausea, vomiting, and joint pain.

Nursing Implications: Observe bite area closely for edema. This may progress and involve the entire extremity very quickly. Measure extremity proximally to the bite and at several other sites close to the trunk. Repeat every 5–15 minutes. Also possible are ecchymosis, skin discoloration, vesicules, and petechiae. In some cases necrosis may develop.

Monitor laboratory results closely—the poison may cause destruction of erythrocytes, and pulmonary edema can develop because of changes in capillary permeability.

Attempt to estimate the severity of envenomization before administration. Assessment should include size and species of snake, location and number of bites, time the snake's fangs were in the body, type of first-aid treatment given, and protective effect of clothing or shoes. The amount of antivenin administered depends on this information; therefore, observations of the patient's condition should be carefully documented.

Monitor vital signs and blood pressure frequently. Document intake and output.

Emergency equipment and medications should be available for use. This is especially important during administration of antivenin.

Systemic signs and symptoms of envenomization include (but are not limited to) weakness, faintness, nausea, sweating, hypotension, prolongation of bleeding and clotting times, hematuria, and vomiting. In a fatal poisoning, death is usually due to pulmonary edema due to capillary permeability changes and erythrocyte destruction.

Generic Name: ARGININE HYDROCHLORIDE

Trade Name: R-GENE

Classification: Pituitary function (diagnostic agent)

Actions: Dibasic amino acid that stimulates the release of prolactin and growth hormone from the pituitary gland and the release of insulin and glucagon from the pancreas. The exact mechanism of action is not known. When administered to patients with known or suspected impaired pituitary function, there is lower than normal or no increase in plasma concentrations of growth hormone. Arginine also increases blood glucose levels and elevates serum gastrin.

Indications: To test growth hormone reserve and detect growth hormone deficiency in conditions such as panhypopituitarism, pituitary dwarfism, craniopharyngioma, pituitary trauma, hypophysectomy, and in problems with stature and growth. It may also be used to evaluate growth hormone production in acromegaly and gigantism.

Dosage:
Neonatal: Not applicable.
Pediatric: 500 mg/kg (up to 30 g) as a one-time dose.
Adult: 30 g as a one-time dose.

Preparation: Supplied as a clear, colorless solution, which does not require refrigeration, in the concentration of 10 g/100 ml.

Home Stability: Must be stored in containers with a vacuum.

Compatibilities: Compatible with solutions containing saline.

Administration:
Neonatal: Not applicable.
Pediatric: Infuse at a constant rate over 30 minutes.

Adult: Infuse at a constant rate over 30 minutes.

Contraindications: Known allergic tendencies. Use with caution in patients with renal disease or anuria. May be hazardous in patients with electrolyte imbalance because of its high chloride concentration. The following drugs may also affect growth hormone production and thus could interfere with interpretation of growth hormone levels following administration of arginine hydrochloride: estrogen and estrogen-progestin oral contraceptives, medroxyprogesterone acetate, and norethindrone.

Side Effects:
Primary: Nausea, vomiting.
Secondary: Flushing, headache, numbness, local venous irritation.

Nursing Implications: Stress and exercise can affect growth hormone production. Therefore, the patient should have a normal night of sleep, and distress and apprehension should be minimized before and during the test as much as possible.

The patient should fast overnight.

A plasma growth hormone level should be done prior to initiation of the arginine hydrochloride infusion and 30, 60, 90, and 120 minutes after the infusion is begun.

Document the *exact* time of medication administration for interpretation of plasma growth hormone levels.

An infusion pump is recommended, because if the infusion period is prolonged beyond 30 minutes, stimulation to the pituitary may be diminished and thus the test may be nullified.

Assess pancreatic function prior to administration via baseline blood sugar and at 120 minutes after administration.

If nausea and vomiting occur, it is usually within 30–120 minutes of administration and resolves within 3 hours of administration.

Generic Name: ASPARAGINASE

Trade Name: ELSPAR, ERWINIA

Classification: Antineoplastic (miscellaneous agent)

Actions: Some tumor cells do not possess the ability to synthesize the nonessential amino acid asparagine. Since asparagine is required for protein synthesis and cell division, the tumor cells must obtain asparagine from the patient's blood supply. Asparaginase is an enzyme produced from *Escherichia coli* and from the plant parasite *Escherichia carotovora* that renders blood asparagine ineffective. Thus, tumor cells dependent on a blood supply of asparagine are deprived of this amino acid. The absence of asparagine interrupts tumor cell function, primarily at the G_1 phase of the cell cycle, and keeps the tumor cell from dividing, resulting in cell death. It is cell-cycle specific at the G_1 phase.

Indications: Acute lymphocytic leukemia, melanoma, acute and chronic myelocytic leukemia, and some lymphomas.

Dosage:
Neonatal: Not applicable.
Pediatric: Sample regimens: 200 IU/kg/day IV every day for 28 days; 6000 IU/m²/day, IM every 3 days × 9; 6000 IU/m² every other day for 3/4 weeks. A number of doses and schedules have shown some therapeutic effectiveness.
Adult: 1–20,000 IU/m² every 10–14 days. A number of doses and schedules have shown some therapeutic effectiveness.

Preparation: Elspar is derived from *Escherichia coli* and is supplied in vials of 10,000 IU that should be diluted with 2–5 ml of nonpreserved normal saline or sterile water. The reconstituted drug should be clear and should not be used if cloudy. Vials in solution should not be shaken to avoid loss of potency.
Erwinia is obtained from *Escherichia carotovora* and is supplied in 10,000-IU/2-ml vials that can be diluted up to 35 IU/ml in either nonpreserved saline or sterile water.

Home Stability: Unopened Elspar vials should be refrigerated. Erwinia vials are stable for 4 years in the refrigerator and 2 years at room temperature. Reconstituted Elspar can be stored at room temperature for 1 week but should be used within 8 hours. Erwinia is stable for 20 days at room temperature or in the refrigerator. However, asparaginase should *never* be administered at home because of the possibility of anaphylactic reactions, even when problems have not occurred with previous administrations.

Compatibilities: Compatible with either normal saline or dextrose. May reduce cytotoxicity of methotrexate. As with most antineoplastic agents, it is advisable not to administer asparaginase with other admixture solutions.

Administration:
Neonatal: Not applicable.
Pediatric: Infuse by slow IV push over 30 minutes or more. A physician and emergency supplies and equipment should be immediately available in case of a life-threatening anaphylactic reaction. (Because Elspar is derived from a bacterium, some of the proteins may be antigenic, thus resulting in such an immune response.)
A maximum of 2 ml should be given at IM sites. Significantly less anaphylactoid reactions have occurred with IM administration, but a physician and emergency supplies and equipment should be immediately available. Intrathecal doses of 100–5000 IU/day and intraventricular administration have also been tried.
Adult: Same as pediatric administration, except hypersensitivity reactions are more common in adults.

Contraindications: Pregnancy. An intradermal skin test of 2 IU/0.1 ml asparaginase is recommended at least 1 week after the last dose. The site should be observed for a wheal or flare reaction for at least 1 hour. Although this test may be negative, it does not guarantee that a reaction will not occur during the next administration of asparaginase.
Sensitivity reactions can also be lessened by administering dilute IV solutions, by administering the IV very slowly, or by beginning at a very low dose and gradually increasing the dose (e.g., every 10–15 minutes) until the total dose is infused. Administering vincristine or prednisone

along with or immediately after asparaginase may increase the risk of hypersensitivity reactions.

Severe or recurring reactions usually indicate a necessity to change from the one form of asparaginase to the other (Elspar to Erwinia or vice versa). An antihistamine and/or epinephrine oil given subcutaneously should also be given to lessen the chance of further reactions.

Patients with a past history of, or current, pancreatitis should not be given asparaginase because of the risk of acute, and possibly fatal, hemorrhage.

Side Effects:
Primary:

Immunologic: Hypersensitivity reactions with an itching rash, fever, aches, and chills occur in 20–35 percent of patients. A small portion of these reactions are life-threatening, including laryngeal constriction, decreased blood pressure, sweating, swelling, difficulty breathing, and loss of consciousness. The potential for reactions increases with each dose.

Hematopoietic: Mild anemia is possible.

Gastrointestinal: Malaise, anorexia, moderate nausea and vomiting, abdominal cramps.

Hepatic: Elevated liver function tests, including SGPT, SGOT, bilirubin, and alkaline phosphatase are common within 2 weeks after administration. Acute pancreatitis may result in increased serum amylase and hyperglycemia. Diabetic ketoacidosis has been seen in children.

Neurotoxicity: Lethargy and somnolence occur mostly in adults, and coma has occurred.

Nephrotoxicity: Increased BUN or other nitrogenous compounds in the blood and increased uric acid levels.

Reproductive: Possible teratogenesis.

Secondary: Weight loss; decreased albumin levels may be severe, resulting in anasarca; cholesterol levels and clotting factors may be reduced, but severe bleeding is usually not a problem; disorientation, confabulation, easy suggestibility, and loss of recent memory. Risk of infertility and secondary malignancy is unknown.

Nursing Implications: Do not administer asparaginase without a physician present or nearby and emergency equipment and supplies immediately available.

Observe closely for hypersensitivity and anaphylactic reactions; monitor vital signs frequently.

Assess level of consciousness frequently. Reassure patient and family that changes in mental status are temporary and can be treated.

Administer antiemetics as needed.

Monitor liver function tests, glucose, albumin, amylase, BUN, uric acid and cholesterol levels, prothrombin time, and partial thromboplastin time.

Inform patient of the possibility of birth defects if pregnancy occurs during asparaginase therapy.

Safe-handling precautions should continue for 9 days after the last dose of asparaginase.

Generic Name: ATROPINE SULFATE

Trade Name: ATROPINE SULFATE INJECTION

Classification: Cholinergic blocking agent

Actions: Blocks the vagal effects on the sino-atrial node.

Indications: Symptomatic bradycardia and bradyarrhythmias (junctional or escape rhythms).

Dosage:
Neonatal: Not applicable.
Pediatric: 0.1 mg/kg up to maximum of 0.4 mg; may be repeated every 4–6 hours.
Adult: 0.5–1.0 mg by IV push, repeated every 5 minutes to a maximum of 2 mg. Doses less than 0.5 mg can cause bradycardia.

Preparation: Supplied in dosette vials of 400 μg/ml, 1 mg/ml, and 1.2 mg/ml and in jet syringes of 0.5 mg/5 ml and 1.0 mg/10 ml, both with a 22-gauge, 1½-inch needle.

Home Stability: Not applicable.

Compatibilities: May push into lines infusing dextrose, saline, or lactated Ringer's solution. Incompatible with sodium bicarbonate.

Administration:
Neonatal: Not applicable.
Pediatric: No need for dilution. Give by IV push over 1 minute.
Adult: See pediatric administration.

Contraindications: Hypersensitivity. May produce extrapyramidal symptoms if given concurrently with methotrimeprazine. Other anticholinergic drugs may increase vagal blockage.

Side Effects:
Primary: Headache, restlessness, insomnia, dizziness, tachycardia, palpitations, angina, mydriasis, blurred vision, dry mouth, constipation, urinary retention, thirst.
Secondary: Leukocytosis, ataxia, disorientation, hallucinations, delirium, nausea, vomiting, hot and flushed skin.

Nursing Implications: Continuous cardiac monitoring is essential. Document heart rate and rhythm pre- and postadministration; immediately notify physician of patient's response.

Monitor blood pressure pre- and postadministration.

Assess level of consciousness, capillary refill, and skin color and temperature along with vital signs.

Be prepared to initiate emergency measures (external or transvenous pacing, cardiopulmonary resuscitation) if bradycardia becomes symptomatic or if heart rhythm deteriorates further.

Most common side effect is a dry mouth and thirst. This may be alleviated by sucking on hard candy or with pilocarpine syrup.

Monitor closely for urinary retention, especially in males with benign prostatic hypertrophy.

Physostigmine salicylate is the antidote for atropine sulfate.

Generic Name: AZATHIOPRINE

Trade Name: IMURAN

Classification: Antiarthritic

Actions: Used to produce immunosuppression in renal transplant patients and to treat active rheumatoid arthritis. It is a slow-acting drug, so its effects may be seen for a period of time after the drug is discontinued. The exact mechanism of action is unknown.

Indications: To prevent rejection in renal transplant patients. Used in treatment of severe, active rheumatoid arthritis when other measures have failed.

Dosage:
Pediatric and Adult:
Transplantation: Initial dose: 3–5 mg/kg/day. Maintenance: 1–3 mg/kg/day.
Rheumatoid Arthritis: 1 mg/kg single dose. May increase dose in 6–8 weeks and then at 4-week intervals until desired response is reached. Dose can be increased to a maximum of 2.5 mg/kg/day in increments of 0.5-mg/kg/day. Maintenance level should be lowest effective dose.

Preparation: Injectable 100 mg/vial.

Administration: May be by IV route initially but should be changed to oral as soon as possible. Length of infusion will vary.

Contraindications: Hypersensitivity, pregnancy.

Side Effects: Severity of effects is proportional to dose; decreasing the dose will reverse its effects.
Primary: Leukopenia, thrombocytopenia, anemia, nausea and vomiting.
Secondary: Skin rashes, alopecia, fever.

Nursing Implications: General health status should be assessed regularly. Lab work should also be drawn as appropriate.

Monitor intake and output, urine specific gravity, and electrolyte balances in the renal transplant patient.

Observe for signs of infection because of immunosuppressive action of this drug. Prevent exposure to possible contaminants.

Patient and family should be taught to avoid contact with possible contaminants (i.e., upper respiratory conditions and any communicable diseases).

Document drug response in the arthritic patient—pain relief, joint movement, and drug tolerance.

Pregnancy during therapy is not recommended.

Generic Name: AZLOCILLIN

Trade Name: AZLIN

Classification: Antibiotic (penicillin)

Actions: Extended-spectrum synthetic penicillin, bactericidal against *Pseudomonas aeruginosa,* gram-positive cocci such as *Streptococcus faecalis,* gram-negative bacilli such as *Escherichia coli, Hemophilus influenzae, Proteus mirabilis, Bacteroides fragilis,* and other anaerobes. Not effective against penicillinase-producing strains of Staphylococci.

Indications: Serious infections of the lower respiratory tract, urinary tract, skin and skin structures, bone and joints; bacterial septicemia caused primarily by *Pseudomonas aeruginosa;* acute pulmonary exacerbation of cystic fibrosis. Usually administered concurrently with an aminoglycoside.

Dosage:
Neonatal: Safety in neonates not established. Older than 1 month, 75 mg/kg every 4 hours.
Pediatric: 75 mg/kg every 4 hours.
Adult: 200–300 mg/kg/day every 4–6 hours. Maximum adult dose, 24 g. Dosage should be decreased in renal-impaired clients: 2–3 g every 8–12 hours.
General: Usual duration of therapy is 10–14 days.

Preparation: Supplied as a powder. Reconstitute with sterile water, 0.9% sodium chloride, or 5% dextrose. Each gram of azlocillin should be reconstituted with at least 10 ml of diluent.

Home Stability: Solutions are stable at room temperature for 24 hours. Concentrations up to 100 mg/ml are stable for 24 hours when refrigerated below 8°C (46.4°F).

Compatibilities: Compatible with solutions containing dextrose, saline, KCl, Ringer's, or lactated Ringer's. Do not administer in the same IV tubing with any other drug.

Administration:
Neonatal: IV push or IV Y-site over 5 minutes or more. To minimize vein irritation, dilute to a 10% solution.
Pediatric: See neonatal administration.
Adult: IV piggyback. Dilute with compatible IV solution to 50–100 ml and infuse over 30 minutes. Rapid injection can cause transient chest pain.

Contraindications: Hypersensitivity to penicillin derivatives or cephalosporins. Individuals with a history of allergic problems are more susceptible to untoward reactions. Safety in pregnancy has not been established.

Side Effects:
Primary: Hypersensitivity reactions such as anaphylaxis, urticaria, arthralgia, myalgia, drug fever, chills, and chest discomfort. Superinfections, pain, and thrombosis of the IV site.
Secondary: Headache, dizziness, neuromuscular hyperirritability, seizures, diarrhea, abdominal pain, nausea, vomiting, anemia, thrombocytopenia, leukopenia, neutropenia, prolonged prothrombin and bleeding times, hypokalemia; increased alkaline phosphatases, LDH, bilirubin, creatinine, BUN, SGPT, and SGOT; hypernatremia.

Nursing Implications: Prior to and during therapy, culture and sensitivity tests should be completed.
Monitor for allergic reactions.
Sodium concentration must be taken into consideration in clients on a sodium-restricted diet.
Monitor baseline and periodic renal, hepatic, and hematologic functions.
Monitor intake-output ratio and pattern, particularly in clients with impaired renal function.
Monitor for superinfection. Assess for the onset of black, hairy tongue; oral lesions (stomatitis, glossitis); rectal or vaginal itching; vaginal discharge; loose, foul-smelling stools; unusual odor to urine.
Monitor clotting time, platelet aggregation, prothrombin and partial prothrombin time.

Generic Name: BENZTROPINE MESYLATE

Trade Name: COGENTIN

Classification: Cholinergic blocking agent

Actions: Inhibits the neurotransmission of impulses in the parasympathetic nervous system at the junction between postganglionic nerve endings and effector organs by inhibiting the effects of acetylcholine.

Indications: Adjunct in the therapy of all forms of parkinsonism; control of extrapyramidal disorders due to neuroleptic drugs.

Dosage:
Neonatal: Not applicable.
Pediatric: Not applicable.
Adult: Initial dosage: 0.5–1.0 mg, up to 6 mg/24 hours. For acute dystonic reactions: 1–2 mg.

Preparation: 2-ml ampules (1 mg/ml).

Home Stability: Not applicable.

Compatibilities: May infuse with solution containing dextrose, saline, any combination of dextrose and saline, Ringer's and lactated Ringer's solutions.

Administration:
Neonatal: Not applicable.
Pediatric: Not applicable.
Adult: May give undiluted over 1 minute.

Contraindications: Hypersensitivity, use in children under 3 years of age, narrow-angle glaucoma. Use with caution in clients with prostatic hypertrophy, tendency to tachycardia, and in the elderly or pregnant.

Side Effects:
Primary: Constipation, dry mouth.
Secondary: Tachycardia, paradoxical bradycardia, palpitations, disorientation, hallucinations, restlessness, irritability, incoherence, headache, sedation, depression, muscular weakness, dilated pupils, blurred vision, photophobia, vomiting, nausea, epigastric distress, urinary hesitancy or retention.

Nursing Implications: Monitor vital signs frequently.

Assess for development of side effects, particularly in elderly or debilitated patients. Warn patients to avoid activities that require alertness until effects on central nervous system are determined. Intermittent constipation, distension, and abdominal pain may indicate onset of paralytic ileus. Cool drinks, ice chips, hard candy, or sugarless gum can relieve dry mouth. Encourage fluids to help prevent constipation.

Monitor intake and output for development of urinary retention.

Discontinuation of drug should be done slowly.

Physostigmine salicylate will reverse symptoms of anticholinergic intoxication. Diazepam will reduce central nervous system excitation.

Generic Name: BIPERIDEN LACTATE
Trade Name: AKINETON

Classification: Cholinergic blocking agent

Actions: Inhibits the neurotransmission of impulses in the parasympathetic nervous system at the junction between postganglionic nerve endings and effector organs by inhibiting the effects of acetylcholine.

Indications: Acute episodes of drug-induced extrapyramidal disturbances.

Dosage:
Neonatal: Not applicable.
Pediatric: Not applicable.
Adult: 2 mg every 30 minutes, not to exceed 8 mg daily.

Preparation: 1-ml ampules containing 5 mg of biperiden.

Home Stability: Not applicable.

Compatibilities: May infuse with D_5W.

Administration:
Neonatal: Not applicable.
Pediatric: Not applicable.
Adult: May give undiluted at a rate of 2 mg over 1 minute.

Contraindications: Hypersensitivity. Use with caution in patients with narrow-angle glaucoma, prostatic hypertrophy, cardiac arrhythmias, and those who are taking narcotic analgesics, antipsychotics, tricyclic antidepressants, and antihistamines.

Side Effects:
Primary: Constipation, dry mouth.
Secondary: Transient orthostatic hypotension, disorientation, restlessness, irritability, incoherence, blurred vision, vomiting, nausea, epigastric distress, urinary hesitancy or retention.

Nursing Implications: Keep patient supine during administration of drug, then assist patient in changing position and getting out of bed.
Monitor vital signs frequently.
Assess for development of side effects, particularly in elderly or debilitated patients. Warn patients to avoid activities that require alertness until effects on central nervous system are determined. Cool drinks, ice chips, hard candy, or sugarless gum can relieve dry mouth. Encourage fluids to help prevent constipation.
Monitor intake and output for development of urinary retention.
Discontinuation of drug should be done slowly.
Physostigmine salicylate will reverse symptoms of anticholinergic intoxication. Diazepam will reduce central nervous system excitation.

Generic Name: BLEOMYCIN SULFATE

Trade Name: BLENOXANE

Classification: Antineoplastic antibiotic

Actions: Binds to DNA, keeps it from replicating, and causes breaks in its strands. Also decreases RNA and protein synthesis to some extent. Produces these effects mostly in the G_2 and M phases of the cell cycle and is therefore cell-cycle specific. It also seems to keep cells from moving out of the G_2 phase and thus can be synchronized with other drugs that affect the cell cycle.

Indications: Squamous cell carcinomas, Hodgkin's and non-Hodgkin's lymphoma, mycosis fungoides, testicular cancer, and lung cancer.

Dosage:
Neonatal: Not applicable.
Pediatric: 10–20 u/m² IV or IM or SC 1–2 times per week or 15 mg/m² daily for 4 days by continuous infusion or 60 u/day intra-arterially to local tumors, but not greater than 400 u cumulative dose with normal renal function.
Adult: Same as pediatric dosage, except that cumulative doses may need to be reduced in the elderly.

Preparation: Supplied as a white or yellowish powder of 15 u per ampule, which can be stored at 1–35°C for 18 months. The ampule can be dissolved in 1–5 ml of sterile water, D_5W, or normal saline.

Home Stability: If a bacteriostatic diluent is used, the solution is stable for 1 month in the refrigerator or 2 weeks at room temperature.

Compatibilities: Compatible with either normal saline or dextrose. Decreases the efficacy of digoxin and phenytoin. Avoid admixture with ascorbic acid solutions. As with most antineoplastic agents, it is advisable not to administer bleomycin with other admixture solutions.

Administration:
Neonatal: Not applicable.
Pediatric: By IV push over 10 minutes, IV drip by continuous infusion, IM, or SC.

Dilute 15–240 u in 100 ml and instill into the pleural cavity via a thoracotomy tube to control pleural effusions. The tube should be kept clamped for the first 24 hours and then allowed to drain for 2–3 days before removing.
Dilute 30–120 u in 30–60 ml of sterile water, instill into the bladder via catheter, and retain for 2 hours before draining.
Dilute 60 mg/m² in appropriate solution for intraperitoneal administration.
Dilute small doses in a small amount of normal saline and inject into superficial tumors.
Dilute up to 60 u daily in a large amount of solution and infuse intra-arterially for squamous cell cancers of the cervix and head/neck as well as melanoma.
Apply a 1–3.5% ointment to superficial tumors and cover with a dry sterile dressing.
Adult: See pediatric administration.

Contraindications: Pregnancy. Check for bleomycin sensitivity for the first two doses—especially in patients with lymphomas—by administering a test dose of 1–2 u IM. Observe the patient over 2–4 hours for an anaphylactic reaction or high fever before giving the full dose. Consider dose reductions for patients with a serum creatinine greater than 1.5 or a creatinine clearance less than 40 mg/minute. Use with caution in patients with compromised pulmonary function. Cumulative lifetime doses should not exceed 400 IU.

Side Effects:
Primary:
Pyrogenic: Fever to 103–105°F, with or without chills occurs in about one-fourth to one-half of all patients and can be reduced with acetaminophen given a few hours before and every 4 hours as needed after bleomycin administration. Sweating, dehydration, and decreased blood pressure resulting in renal failure and death have been reported.
Pulmonary: Irreversible pulmonary fibrosis can occur, especially with cumulative doses of more than 400–450 IU in patients with previous radiation therapy to the chest, a history of pulmonary disease or smoking, or over age 70. Pulmonary function tests and chest X rays should be done periodically during the course of therapy to detect early lung toxicity, which can occur at lower

doses and which can be life-threatening if the drug is not discontinued. Early clinical symptoms include dry cough, dyspnea, rales, infiltrates, and pneumonitis. Postoperative respiratory failure has occurred in patients who received more than 200 mg/m^2 of bleomycin preoperatively.

Cutaneous: Hyperpigmentation, swelling, and redness and peeling of the skin on palms, fingers, and arm and leg joints may occur, because bleomycin concentrates in the skin. Thickening or ridges in the nailbeds may be evident, and some patients can count their therapies by the number of ridges in their fingernails. Alopecia usually begins after several weeks and is reversible.

Immunologic: Hypersensitivity reactions with itching, rash, periorbital edema, and bronchospasm.

Reproductive: Teratogenesis is probable.

Secondary: Stomatitis, mild nausea, vomiting, anorexia, fatigue, weight loss, Raynaud's phenomenon, increased blood pressure, increased bilirubin, pain at the tumor site, and mild bone marrow depression with high doses. Risk of infertility and secondary malignancy is unknown.

Nursing Implications: Administer a test dose of 1–2 u before the first course of bleomycin and observe the patient closely over 2–4 hours for high fever and anaphylactoid reactions. When the test dose is given, a physician should be nearby and emergency equipment and supplies immediately available. Pretreatment with corticosteroids may decrease risk of allergic reactions.

Obtain an order to give prophylactic acetaminophen before administration and as needed afterward. Antihistamines may also be useful in decreasing febrile reactions. Encourage fluids to keep patients with fever well hydrated.

Remind physician to order periodic pulmonary function tests and chest X rays.

Observe for and tell patient to report cough, shortness of breath, or pleuritic pain. Check lung sounds for fine rales.

Record the cumulative dose with each drug administration.

Instruct patient on the possibility of skin and fingernail changes as well as alopecia.

Monitor renal function by assessment of serum creatinine and creatinine clearance.

Inform patient of the possibility of birth defects if pregnancy occurs while taking bleomycin.

Safe-handling precautions are necessary for only 1 day with bleomycin.

Generic Name: BRETYLIUM TOSYLATE

Trade Name: BRETYLOL

Classification: Antiarrhythmic

Actions: Exact mechanism of action is not known, but bretylium results in an increase in ventricular fibrillation threshold, an increase in action potential duration and effective refractory period, and a decrease in the disparity in action potential duration between normal and infarcted myocardium.

Indications: Ventricular fibrillation and life-threatening ventricular arrhythmias that have failed to respond to other antiarrhythmic therapy.

Dosage:
Neonatal: Safety of bretylium for neonates has not yet been determined.
Pediatric: Safety of bretylium for children has not yet been determined.
Adult:
Ventricular Fibrillation: 5 mg/kg by IV push. If necessary increase dose to 10 mg/kg and repeat every 15–30 minutes until 30 mg/kg have been given.
Other Ventricular Arrhythmias: 5–10 mg/kg given over at least 8 minutes, diluted in at least 50 ml: may repeat in 1–2 hours if needed.
Maintenance: Infuse diluted solution at 1–2 mg/minute.

Preparation: 10-ml ampules containing 500 mg bretylium tosylate.

Home Stability: Not applicable.

Compatibilities: Compatible with solutions containing dextrose, or saline, or lactated Ringer's.

Administration:
Neonatal: Not applicable.
Pediatric: Not applicable.
Adult:
Ventricular Fibrillation: Give by IV push only.
Maintenance: Dilute in at least 50 ml and give over at least 8 minutes.

Contraindications: Digitalis-induced arrhythmias. Use with caution in patients with fixed cardiac output, aortic stenosis, and pulmonary hypertension. Decrease dosage in patients with renal impairment. Bretylium potentiates pressor amines (sympathomimetics).

Side Effects:
Primary: Severe hypotension, bradycardia, orthostatic hypotension.
Secondary: Severe nausea, vomiting (with rapid infusion), anginal pain, recurrence of arrhythmias.

Nursing Implications: Continuous cardiac monitoring is essential. Document heart rate and rhythm before and after bretylium dose: immediately notify physician of patient's response.

Monitor blood pressure before and after bretylium dose and every 5 minutes until stable following successful conversion of heart rhythm.

Assess level of consciousness, capillary refill, and skin color and temperature along with vital signs.

Be prepared to initiate and/or continue resuscitative measures if ventricular arrhythmias persist or recur.

Keep patient supine until tolerance to hypotension develops.

Infuse maintenance dose via automatic infusion pump.

Generic Name: **BROMPHENIRAMINE MALEATE**

Trade Name: **DIMETANE-TEN HISTAJECT**

Classification: Antihistamine

Actions: Competes with histamine for H_1-receptor sites on effector cells.

Indications: Symptomatic treatment of allergic manifestations.

Dosage:
Neonatal: Not applicable.
Pediatric: 0.5 mg/kg/24 hours divided into 3–4 doses.
Adult: 5–20 mg every 6–12 hours (not to exceed 40 mg per day).

Duration of Therapy: Oral forms available for maintenance therapy.

Preparation: 10 mg/ml concentration.

Home Stability: Not applicable.

Compatibilities: Compatible with solutions of 5 percent dextrose or 0.9 percent sodium chloride.

Administration:
Neonatal: Not applicable.
Pediatric: May give diluted (in 5% dextrose or 0.9% sodium chloride) or undiluted. Administer slowly.
Adult: See pediatric administration.

Contraindications: Acute asthmatic attack, hypersensitivity to antihistamines, use in newborns or nursing mothers, concurrent MAO inhibitor therapy. Use with caution in elderly patients, and in patients with prostatic hypertrophy, narrow-angle glaucoma, hyperthyroidism, cardiovascular or renal diseases, hypertension, or asthma.

Side Effects:
Primary: Agranulocytosis, drowsiness, stimulation, dry mouth and throat. Transient hypotension, syncope, sweating, and a local reaction may accompany IV administration.
Secondary: Thrombocytopenia, dizziness, tremors, irritability, insomnia, palpitations, anorexia, nausea, vomiting, urinary retention, urticaria, rash.

Nursing Implications: Patient should be recumbent during infusion and be monitored for possible reactions.

Advise patient to avoid the use of alcohol and other central nervous system depressants during therapy and to avoid activities requiring alertness.

Monitor blood work for signs of blood dyscrasias.

Sugarless gum or hard candy may help alleviate dry mouth.

Allergy skin tests are not accurate if brompheniramine has been given within 4 days of the testing.

Generic Name: BUMETANIDE

Trade Name: BUMEX

Classification: Diuretic

Actions: Inhibits sodium and chloride reabsorption in the ascending limb of the loop of Henle, with a lesser effect on the proximal tubule.

Indications: For treatment of edema associated with congestive heart failure, hepatic and renal disease, including the nephrotic syndrome.

Dosage:
Neonatal: Not applicable.
Pediatric: Not applicable.
Adult: 0.5–1.0 mg; may repeat at 2–3-hour intervals, not to exceed 10 mg/day.

Preparation: 2-ml ampules, 0.25 mg/ml.

Home Stability: Not applicable.

Compatibilities: May infuse with dextrose, saline, or lactated Ringer's.

Administration:
Neonatal: Not applicable.
Pediatric: Not applicable.
Adult: Dilute in 5–10 ml and give over 1–2 minutes.

Contraindications: Hypersensitivity, anuria. Patients allergic to sulfonamides may show hypersensitivity to bumetanide. Do not use in patients in hepatic coma or with severe electrolyte disturbances until corrected. Discontinue with marked increase in BUN or creatinine or if oliguria develops in patients with progressive renal disease. Avoid giving concurrently with ototoxic or nephrotoxic drugs. The actions of bumetanide are inhibited by indomethacin and probenecid. Bumetanide may potentiate the effects of various antihypertensive drugs.

Side Effects:
Primary: Volume depletion, dehydration, muscle cramps, dizziness, hypotension, headache, nausea, encephalopathy, hyponatremia, hypochloremia, hypokalemia, hyperuricemia, increased serum creatinine, hyperglycemia.
Secondary: Impaired hearing; pruritus; EKG changes; weakness; hives; rash; vomiting; abdominal, arthritic, or musculoskeletal pain.

Nursing Implications: Because of potential for volume and electrolyte depletion, leading to profound water loss, dehydration, reduction in blood volume, and circulatory collapse, monitor intake and output, serum electrolytes, blood pressure, and pulse rate frequently.

Assess for signs of hypokalemia (muscle weakness and cramping). Teach patients about potassium-rich foods (citrus fruits, tomatoes, bananas, dates, apricots). Monitor patients receiving digitalis carefully because of increased risk of digitalis toxicity.

Caution patient to change position slowly because of orthostatic hypotension.

Monitor BUN and creatinine for signs of deteriorating renal function.

Administer bumetanide in the morning to prevent nocturia.

Monitor blood glucose levels, especially in diabetics.

Monitor serum uric acid levels, especially in patients with a history of gout.

Diuresis starts within minutes and reaches maximum levels within 15–30 minutes: half-life is 1–11/2 hours.

The diuretic action of 1 mg of bumetanide is roughly equivalent to that of 40 mg of furosemide.

Generic Name: BUTORPHANOL TARTRATE

Trade Name: STADOL

Classification: Potent analgesic with narcotic agonist and antagonist effects

Actions: Relieves moderate to severe pain and provides preoperative sedation. (A patient's perception of pain is altered by preventing or changing the transmission of painful stimuli along the sensory pathways in the central nervous system. These pathways are specific to the perception and emotional response of the patient to pain.) In addition, this drug suppresses the respiratory and cough centers of the brain. This drug is less likely to cause physical dependence than narcotic analgesics, but it is more potent in action than morphine, meperedine, or pentazocine.

Indications: For management of moderate to severe pain from a diversity of causes. It should not be used in cases of mild pain or pain that can be relieved by other less potent non-narcotic analgesics.

Dosage:
Neonatal: Not recommended for children under 18 years.
Pediatric: Not recommended for children under 18 years.
Adult:
IM: 1–4 mg every 3–4 hours. Do not exceed 4 mg for a single dose.
IV: 0.5–2.0 mg every 3–4 hours.

Preparation: Injectable form contains 1mg/ml and 2 mg/ml.

Administration:
Neonatal: Not recommended for children under 18 years.
Pediatric: Not recommended for children under 18 years.
Adult: By IM or slow IV push; SC route is not recommended. Naloxone should be readily available for administration in cases of severe respiratory depression.

Contraindications: Hypersensitivity, in delivery of premature infants. Limited use in patients sensitive to morphine. Use with caution in patients with head injuries, increased intracranial pressure, shock, central nervous system and respiratory depression, chronic obstructive pulmonary disease, ventricular dysfunction, acute myocardial infarction, coronary insufficiency, renal or hepatic dysfunction, and those receiving narcotic analgesics.

Side Effects:
Primary: Sedation, headache, nausea, clamminess, palpitations, blood pressure instability, respiratory depression.
Secondary: Dizziness, lethargy, lightheadedness, nervousness, unusual dreams, blurred vision, dry mouth.

Nursing Implications: Because of the chance for respiratory depression, a narcotic antagonist should be available for rapid administration, especially if the route of choice is IV. Naloxone is the antagonist most often used.

Monitor vital signs frequently. For IV or IM dose, every 5–10 minutes; for SC dose, every 15–30 minutes.

Supportive equipment should be readily available in case of cardiac or respiratory arrest. A patent airway should be maintained.

Monitor infants when the drug is used during labor and delivery.

To augment the use of potent analgesics, give before severe pain occurs. Nursing actions also include the use of emotional support and patient comfort measures. Because of depression of the respiratory centers, postoperative use in the management of pain should include turning, coughing, and deep breathing to prevent pulmonary complications.

Patients should be warned to avoid activities that require alertness. They should also be assisted with ambulation.

Generic Name: CALCIUM CHLORIDE

Trade Name: CALCIUM CHLORIDE

Classification: Electrolyte replacement

Actions: An essential electrolyte for many physiological processes, including muscle contraction, renal function, transmission of nerve impulses, blood coagulation, and mineralization of bones and teeth. Most calcium in the body is stored in the teeth and bones. This stored calcium serves as a reservoir if serum levels fall below normal.

Indications: Given by IV during cardiac resuscitation to improve myocardial contractions. Calcium chloride is preferred to calcium gluconate during resuscitation because it produces more predictable results. Also used to treat hypocalcemia as evidenced by low serum levels, tetany, muscle spasms, and electrocardiographic changes (such as prolonged QT intervals and lengthened S-T segments). It is common for neonates to develop hypocalcemia, especially those with respiratory distress syndrome, hypoxia, or sepsis, those receiving diuretics and bicarbonate, and those who are premature. Neonatal symptoms also include irritability, jitteriness, and hypotonia.

Dosage:
Neonatal: 0.2–0.5 ml/kg (average dose: 0.3 ml/kg). May repeat dose in 10–20 minutes.
Pediatric: See neonatal dosage.
Adult: 500 mg–1 g depending on requirements of patient.

Preparation: Injectable form available in 10% solution (100 mg/ml) for IV or intracardiac administration only.

Compatibilities: For infusion mix with D_5W or normal saline. Incompatible with bicarbonate, chelates, tetracycline hydrochloride, and phosphate salts.

Administration:
Neonatal, Pediatric, and Adult: This form of calcium should be given by IV method *only*. It will cause severe tissue necrosis. Administer with care in the digitalized patient. Administration rate should not exceed 0.5–1.0 ml/minute, and the patient's EKG should also be monitored during administration. In neonates, administration through an umbilical artery catheter is a possible precipitating factor in necrotizing enterocolitis.

Contraindications: Hypercalcemia, digitalis toxicity, ventricular fibrillation.

Side Effects:
Primary: Too rapid administration can cause hypercalcemia, which will result in vasodilation, bradycardia, hypotension, and cardiac arrhythmias and arrest.
Secondary: Vein irritation after administration; tingling sensations and a chalky calcium taste, burning, and necrosis and sloughing of tissue will follow extravasation.

Nursing Implications: Assess patient for signs and symptoms of hypocalcemia. Document observations.

Monitor for side effects during administration, especially bradycardia, hypotension, and cardiac arrhythmias. Patient should be on cardiac monitor.

Calcium chloride *must* be administered by IV method to prevent severe tissue damage.

Avoid too rapid administration, especially to an infant via umbilical artery catheter. Stop or slow infusion if side effects are noted.

Continuing assessment should include resolution of the symptoms of hypocalcemia. Document observations.

Generic Name: CALCIUM GLUCEPTATE

Trade Name: SAME AS GENERIC

Classification: Electrolyte replacement

Actions: An essential electrolyte for many physiological processes, including muscle contraction, renal function, transmission of nerve impulses, blood coagulation, and mineralization of bones and teeth. Most calcium in the body is stored in the teeth and bones. This stored calcium serves as a reservoir if serum levels fall below normal.

Indications: Given by IV during cardiac resuscitation to improve myocardial contractions. Calcium chloride is preferred to calcium gluceptate during resuscitation because it produces more predictable results. Also used to treat hypocalcemia as evidenced by low serum levels, tetany, muscle spasms, and EKG changes (such as prolonged QT intervals and lengthened S-T segments). It is common for neonates to develop this condition, especially those with respiratory distress syndrome, prematurity, hypoxia, or sepsis and those receiving diuretics and bicarbonate. Neonatal symptoms also include irritability, jitteriness, and hypotonia.

Dosage:
Neonatal: During exchange transfusions, 0.5 ml IV after each 100 ml of blood.
Pediatric: By mouth: 45–65 mg/kg daily in divided doses. By IV: Same as neonatal dosage.
Adult: 5–20 ml by IV. Dose is based on serum calcium level.

Preparation: Injectable form available in 1.1 g/5 ml.

Compatibilities: For infusion, mix with D_5W or normal saline. Incompatible with bicarbonate, chelates, tetracycline hydrochloride, and phosphate salts.

Administration:
Neonatal: By IV slowly during exchange transfusions.
Pediatric: See neonatal administration.
Adult: By slow IV injection. Rate not to exceed 1 to 2 ml/min. May be given IM if IV route impossible. IM injection should be given into the gluteal region.

Contraindications: Hypercalcemia, digitalis toxicity, ventricular fibrillation.

Side Effects:
Primary: Too rapid administration can cause hypercalcemia, which will result in vasodilation, bradycardia, hypotension, and cardiac arrhythmias and arrest.
Secondary: Vein irritation after administration; tingling sensations and a chalky calcium taste, burning, necrosis, and sloughing of tissue will follow extravasation.

Nursing Implications: Assess patient for signs and symptoms of hypocalcemia. Document observations.

Monitor for side effects during administration, especially bradycardia, hypotension, and cardiac arrhythmias. Patient should be on cardiac monitor.

Avoid too rapid administration, especially to an infant via umbilical artery catheter. Stop or slow infusion if side effects are noted.

Continuing assessment should include resolution of the symptoms of hypocalcemia. Document observations.

Generic Name: CALCIUM GLUCONATE

Trade Name: CALCET

Classification: Electrolyte replacement

Actions: An essential electrolyte for many physiological processes, including muscle contraction, renal function, transmission of nerve impulses, blood coagulation, and mineralization of bones and teeth. Most calcium in the body is stored in the teeth and bones. This stored calcium serves as a reservoir if serum levels fall below normal.

Indications: Given by IV during cardiac resuscitation to improve myocardial contractions. Calcium chloride is preferred to calcium gluconate during resuscitation because it produces more predictable results. Recent ACLS guidelines do not recommend the use of calcium during pediatric resuscitation. Also used to treat hypocalcemia as evidenced by low serum levels, tetany, muscle spasms, and EKG changes (such as prolonged QT intervals and lengthened S-T segments). It is common for neonates to develop this condition, especially those with respiratory distress syndrome, hypoxia, or sepsis, those receiving diuretics and bicarbonate, and those who are premature. Neonatal symptoms also include irritability, jitteriness, and hypotonia.

Dosage:
Neonatals:
Severe Hypocalcemia and Resuscitation: 1–2 ml/kg/dose. Maximum of 5 ml in the premature and 10 ml in the full-term infant.
Asymptomatic Hypocalcemia: 5–10 ml/kg/day.
Pediatric: See neonatal dosage.
Adult: 5–20 ml as patient's condition requires. Range of 1–15 g daily.

Preparation: Injectable form available in 10% solution (100 mg/ml) in 10-ml vials.

Compatibilities: For infusion, mix with D_5W or normal saline. Incompatible with bicarbonate, chelates, tetracycline, and phosphate salts.

Administration:
Neonatal: Slowly by IV. Monitor EKG during infusion for severe hypocalcemia—give over 5–10 minutes. May also be administered over several hours.
Pediatric: See neonatal administration.
Adult: Do not exceed 0.5–2 ml/minute by IV infusion.
General: The IM route is not recommended for any age.

Side Effects:
Primary: Too rapid administration can cause hypercalcemia, which will result in vasodilation, bradycardia, hypotension, and cardiac arrhythmias and arrest.
Secondary: Vein irritation after administration; tingling sensations and a chalky calcium taste, burning, and necrosis and sloughing of tissue will follow extravasation.

Nursing Implications: Assess patient for signs and symptoms of hypocalcemia. Document observations.

Monitor for side effects during administration, especially bradycardia, hypotension, and cardiac arrhythmias. Patient should be on a cardiac monitor.

Calcium gluconate *must* be administered by IV method to prevent severe tissue damage.

Avoid too rapid administration, especially to infants via umbilical artery catheter. Stop or slow infusion if side effects are noted.

Continuing assessment should include resolution of the symptoms of hypocalcemia. Document observations.

Generic Name: CARBENICILLIN DISODIUM

Trade Name: GEOPEN, PYOPEN

Classification: Antibiotic (penicillin)

Actions: Extended-spectrum semisynthetic penicillin with bactericidal effect against the following gram-positive and gram-negative organisms: *Pseudomonas aeruginosa,* Proteus, *Escherichia coli,* Enterobacter, Hemophilus, *Streptococcus pneumoniae, Neisseria gonorrhoeae,* and *Streptococcus faecalis.*

Indications: Severe infections such as septicemia, genitourinary infections, acute and chronic respiratory infections, and infections of the soft tissue, abdominal cavity, skin, and female pelvis. Also used in clients with impaired immunologic systems, usually in conjunction with an aminoglycoside.

Dosage:

Neonatal:

Under 2000 g: Loading Dose: 100 mg/kg/day. Maintenance Dose: 75 mg/kg/day every 8 hours for 7 days.

Over 2000 g: Loading Dose: 100 mg/kg/day. Maintenance Dose: 75 mg/kg/day every 6 hours for 3 days.

Pediatric: Loading Dose: 100 mg/kg/day. Maintenance Dose: 50–500 mg/kg/day every 4–6 hours. Maximum dosage recommended: 40 g/day.

Adult: 200–500 mg/kg/day in 4–6 divided doses or continuous infusion. Maximum dosage recommended: 40 g/day.

Preparation: Supplied as a powder in the following vial sizes: 1-g, 2-g, and 5-g vials and in 2-g, 5-g, and 10-g piggyback units. Reconstitute with sterile water for injection as follows:

VIAL SIZE	VOLUME DILUENT	CONCENTRATION
1 g	1.4 ml	500 mg/ml
2 g	3.0 ml	500 mg/ml
5 g	7.0 ml	500 mg/ml

Home Stability: Refrigerate reconstituted solution. Stable in IV solution for 72 hours under refrigeration or 24 hours at room temperature.

Compatibilities: Compatible with solutions containing dextrose, saline, KCl, Ringer's, or lactated Ringer's. Compatible with total parenteral nutrition. Do not mix with any other drugs.

Administration:

Neonatal: Dilute to 100 mg/ml and administer by IV push over 5–10 minutes. Do not administer at a rate greater than 200–500 mg/minute.

Pediatric: Dilute to 100 mg/ml and administer by IV push or IV Y-site over 5–10 minutes. Do not administer at a rate greater than 200–500 mg/minute.

Adult: Dilute to 1 g/20 ml and infuse over 30–60 minutes.

Contraindications: Hypersensitivity to penicillin derivatives or cephalosporins. Individuals with a history of allergic problems are more susceptible to untoward reactions. Safety in pregnancy has not been established.

Side Effects:

Primary: Hypersensitivity reactions such as skin rash, pruritus, anaphylaxis, urticaria, and febrile reactions; superinfections; pain; thrombosis of the IV site.

Secondary: Neutropenia, leukopenia, eosinophilia, thrombocytopenia, hypokalemia; increase in SGOT, SGPT, alkaline phosphatase, serum bilirubin, creatinine, and BUN; decrease in hematocrit and hemoglobin; seizures; neuromuscular hyperirritability; nausea, vomiting, diarrhea; abnormal taste sensations.

Nursing Implications: Prior to and during therapy, culture and sensitivity tests should be completed.

Monitor for allergic reactions.

Monitor baseline and periodic renal, hepatic, and hematologic functions, especially in long-term therapy.

Monitor for superinfection. Assess for the onset of black, hairy tongue; oral lesions (stomatitis, glossitis); rectal or vaginal itching; vaginal discharge; loose, foul-smelling stools; unusual odor to urine.

Monitor infusion site hourly for signs of thrombophlebitis.

Sodium concentration must be taken into consideration in clients on a sodium-restricted diet.

Monitor intake and output pattern and ratio. Assess for bleeding. Observe for frank bleeding, nosebleed, bleeding gums, hemoptysis, hematuria, purpura, petechiae, easy bruising, or ecchymosis. Guaiac all stools. Drug should be discontinued if bleeding occurs.

Generic Name: CARMUSTINE

Trade Name: BiCNU

Classification: Antineoplastic nitrosurea, alkylating agent

Actions: Inhibits a number of enzyme reactions that lead to the formation of DNA. Also inhibits DNA repair and the production of some cellular proteins and interferes with the synthesis of RNA proteins. Although cell-cycle nonspecific but has some increased activity in the G_2 phase. Crosses the blood-brain barrier.

Indications: Tumors of the central nervous system, multiple myeloma, refractory Hodgkin's disease, non-Hodgkin's lymphoma, and mycosis fungoides.

Dosage:
Neonatal: Not applicable.
Pediatric: 75–100 mg/m^2 IV for 2 days or 200 mg/m^2 IV × 1 q 6–8 weeks; 0.5–3.0 mg/ml in 30% alcohol or aqueous solution topically every day for 14 days; 200 mg/m^2 intra-arterially into the hepatic artery.
Adult: See pediatric dosage.

Preparation: Supplied as a powder in 30-ml amber vials along with a separate vial of absolute alcohol diluent. After the 30-ml ampule of powder is mixed with 3 ml of the alcohol and then another 27 ml of sterile water, the clear, colorless solution contains 3.3 mg/ml of carmustine.

Home Stability: Unopened vials last for 3 years in the refrigerator. The 3.3-mg/ml solution is stable in glass containers for 24 hours at 4°C or for 8 hours at 25°C when protected from light. However, if this solution is diluted in 500 ml of D$_5$W or normal saline and protected from light, it is stable for 48 hours. The aqueous topical solution of 0.5–0.6 mg/ml has a half-life of 19 days if kept refrigerated and protected from light.

Compatibilities: Stable in D$_5$W and normal saline. Some studies indicate that vitamin A, caffeine, and amphotericin B increase the effectiveness of carmustine. Cimetidine augments the effects of bone marrow suppression of carmustine. Carmustine decreases the effects of phenytoin. As with most antineoplastic agents, it is advisable not to administer carmustine with other admixture solutions.

Administration:
Neonatal: Not applicable.
Pediatric: Infuse in 100–250 D$_5$W over 1–2 hours. Apply the topical solution as a total body paint using extra thickness Latex gloves, gown, and goggles to avoid splashing the solution in the eyes.
Adult: See pediatric administration.

Contraindications: Pregnancy, previous allergy to carmustine.

Side Effects:
Primary:
Hematopoietic: The WBC and platelet nadir is delayed, occurring 3–5 weeks after administration of carmustine and lasting for 1–3 weeks.
Gastrointestinal: Severe nausea and vomiting usually begin about 2 hours after administration and last for 4–6 hours.
Cutaneous: A burning sensation or pain at the IV site can occur as a result of venospasm with the alcohol diluent if carmustine is infused too rapidly. Thrombophlebitis may occur after several days. Tissue damage may occur with extravasation. Facial flushing may also occur with rapid administration. Brown stains appear if this drug is spilled on the skin.
Reproductive: Teratogenesis.
Secondary: Abnormal elevations of SGOT, alkaline phosphatase, serum bilirubin, and BUN; pulmonary fibrosis, especially when given with cyclophosphamide; neuroretinitis when given with procarbazine; gynecomastia; renal toxicity with prolonged use. Risk of secondary malignancy, especially leukemia, is relatively high. Risk of infertility is unknown.

Nursing Implications: Dilute the drug in 500 ml D$_5$W or normal saline to preserve its stability.
Administer it slowly to minimize vein pain.
Monitor site every 10–15 minutes for signs of infiltration.
Monitor for a delayed decrease in WBCs and platelets.

Premedicate and continue antiemetics for at least 8 hours after administration.

Avoid skin and eye contact with the drug.

Inform patient of the possibility of birth defects if pregnancy occurs while taking carmustine.

Safe-handling precautions are necessary for only 1 day with carmustine.

Generic Name: CEFAMANDOLE NAFATE

Trade Name: MANDOL

Classification: Antibiotic (cephalosporin)

Actions: Semisynthetic second-generation cephalosporin antibiotic with antibacterial action against a wide range of gram-positive and gram-negative organisms and anaerobes. Effective against *Streptococcus pneumoniae* and *pyogenes, Hemophilus influenzae,* Klebsiella, *Staphylococcus aureus,* beta-hemolytic streptococci, *Escherichia coli,* Proteus, and Enterobacter.

Indications: Serious infections of the urinary, respiratory, and biliary tracts, bones, joints, skin, and soft tissues; septicemia; peritonitis.

Dosage:
Neonatal: Limited experience with neonates.
Pediatric: 50–100 mg/kg/day in divided doses every 4–8 hours.
Adult: 500–2000 mg every 4–8 hours. Based on severity of infection.
General: Lower doses are needed by renal-impaired clients.

Preparation: Supplied as a powder. Reconstitute with sterile water for injection, bacteriostatic water for injection, 0.9% sodium chloride, or bacteriostatic sodium chloride in the following concentrations:

VIAL SIZE	VOLUME DILUENT	CONCENTRATION
500 mg	1.8 ml	250 mg/ml
1 g	3.5 ml	250 mg/ml
2 g	7.0 ml	250 mg/ml

CO_2 is produced in the vials after reconstitution. Positive pressure may be noticed when drawing doses out of the vial after standing.

Home Stability: After reconstitution, solution is stable for 24 hours at room temperature and 96 hours refrigerated.

Compatibilities: Compatible with solutions containing dextrose, saline, and KCl. Do not mix with any other antibiotic. Not compatible with total parenteral nutrition.

Administration:
Neonatal: Dilute to 100 mg/ml and administer by IV push over 3–5 minutes.
Pediatric: Dilute to 100 mg/ml and administer by IV push or IV Y-site over 3–5 minutes.
Adult: Dilute to 100 mg/ml and administer by IV piggyback over 15–30 minutes.

Contraindications: Hypersensitivity to cephalosporins or penicillin derivatives. Individuals with a history of allergic problems are more susceptible to untoward reactions. Safe use in pregnancy, prematures, and infants has not been established. Use with caution in clients with renal impairment or history of GI disease.

Side Effects:
Primary: Hypersensitivity reactions such as skin rash, pruritus, anaphylaxis, urticaria, and febrile reactions. Superinfections, pain, and thrombosis of the IV site.
Secondary: Nausea; vomiting; abdominal cramps; diarrhea; pseudomembranous colitis; neutropenia; thrombocytopenia; hypoprothrombinemia; positive Coombs' test; increase in SGOT, SGPT, alkaline phosphatase, BUN; decreased creatinine and creatinine clearance.

Nursing Implications: Prior to and during therapy, culture and sensitivity tests should be completed.

Monitor for allergic reactions.

Monitor baseline and periodic renal function and prothrombin time. Assess for bleeding.

Monitor for superinfection. Assess for the onset of black, hairy tongue; oral lesions (stomatitis, glossitis); rectal or vaginal itching; vaginal discharge; loose, foul-smelling stools; unusual odor to urine.

Monitor infusion site hourly for signs of thrombophlebitis.

Observe clients closely for the first half-hour after initial dose for a wheal or redness at IV site indicating allergic reaction.

Report onset of diarrhea to the physician.

Monitor intake-output ratio. Report oliguria, hematuria, and changes in intake-output ratio.

Use glucose oxidase reagents to check urine glucose. False positive reactions can occur with Clinitest.

Generic Name: CEFAZOLIN SODIUM

Trade Name: ANCEF, KEFZOL

Classification: Antibiotic (cephalosporin)

Actions: Semisynthetic first-generation cephalosporin antibiotic with antibacterial action against a wide range of gram-positive and gram-negative organisms and anaerobes. Effective against *Streptococcus pneumoniae* and *pyogenes*, *Hemophilus influenzae*, Klebsiella, *Staphylococcus aureus*, beta-hemolytic streptococci, *Escherichia coli*, Proteus, and Enterobacter.

Indications: Serious infections of the urinary, respiratory, and biliary tracts, bones, joints, skin, and soft tissues; septicemia; peritonitis. Prophylactic use in preoperative procedures, especially open heart surgery.

Dosage:
Neonatal: Not recommended for infants less than 1 month old.
Pediatric: 25–100 mg/kg/24 hours in divided doses every 6–8 hours.
Adult: 750–4000 mg/24 hours every 6–8 hours. Maximum dosage: 6–12 g/24 hours.
General: Lower dosage may be indicated for renal-impaired clients.

Preparation: Supplied as a powder. Reconstitute with sterile water for injection, bacteriostatic water for injection, 0.9% sodium chloride, or bacteriostatic sodium chloride in the following concentrations:

VIAL SIZE	VOLUME DILUENT	CONCENTRATION
250 mg	2.0 ml	125 mg/ml
500 mg	2.0 ml	240 mg/ml
1 g	2.5 ml	330 mg/ml

Home Stability: After reconstitution solution is stable for 24 hours at room temperature and 96 hours refrigerated.

Compatibilities: Compatible with solutions containing dextrose, saline, and KCl. Do not mix with any other antibiotic. Not compatible with total parenteral nutrition.

Administration:
Neonatal: Dilute to 100 mg/ml and administer by IV push over 3–5 minutes.
Pediatric: Dilute to 100 mg/ml and administer by IV push or IV Y-site over 3–5 minutes.
Adult: Dilute to 100 mg/ml and administer by IV piggyback over 15–30 minutes.

Contraindications: Hypersensitivity to cephalosporins or penicillin derivatives. Individuals with a history of allergic problems are more susceptible to untoward reactions. Safe use in pregnancy and premature and full-term infants has not been established. Use with caution in clients with renal impairment or history of GI disease.

Side Effects:
Primary: Hypersensitivity reactions such as skin rash, pruritus, anaphylaxis, urticaria, and febrile reactions. Superinfections, pain, and thrombosis of the IV site.
Secondary: Nausea; vomiting; abdominal cramps; diarrhea; pseudomembranous colitis; neutropenia; thrombocytopenia; hypoprothrombinemia; positive Coombs' test; increase in SGOT, SGPT, alkaline phosphatase, BUN; decreased creatinine and creatinine clearance.

Nursing Implications: Prior to and during therapy, culture and sensitivity tests should be completed.

Monitor for allergic reactions.

Monitor baseline and periodic renal function and prothrombin time. Assess for bleeding.

Monitor for superinfection. Assess for the onset of black, hairy tongue; oral lesions (stomatitis, glossitis); rectal or vaginal itching; vaginal discharge; loose, foul-smelling stools; unusual odor to urine.

Monitor infusion site hourly for signs of thrombophlebitis.

Observe clients closely for the first half-hour after initial dose for a wheal or redness at IV site indicating allergic reaction.

Report onset of diarrhea to the physician.

Monitor intake-output ratio. Report oliguria, hematuria, and changes in intake-output ratio.

Use glucose oxidase reagents to check urine glucose. False positive reactions can occur with Clinitest.

Generic Name: CEFOPERAZONE SODIUM

Trade Name: CEFOBID

Classification: Antibiotic (cephalosporin)

Actions: Long-acting semisynthetic extra-broad-spectrum third-generation cephalosporin with antibacterial action against a wide range of gram-positive and gram-negative organisms and anaerobes. Effective against *Pseudomonas aeruginosa, Hemophilus influenzae, Proteus mirabilis, Escherichia coli,* Enterobacter, and Klebsiella.

Indications: For treatment of serious infections of the urinary, respiratory, and biliary tracts, bones, joints, skin, and soft tissues; infections of the pelvis; septicemia; peritonitis.

Dosage:
Neonatal: Safe use in children has not been established.
Pediatric: Safe use in children has not been established.
Adult: 1–2 g every 12 hours. For severe infections, 6–12 g divided into equal doses every 6, 8, or 12 hours. Dosage may need to be adjusted in renal-impaired clients.

Preparation: Supplied as a powder. Reconstitute with sterile water for injection, bacteriostatic water for injection, 0.9% sodium chloride, or bacteriostatic sodium chloride. Each gram should be initially diluted with 5 ml, then diluted to a concentration of 50 mg/ml.

Home Stability: After reconstitution, solution is stable for 24 hours at room temperature and 5 days refrigerated.

Compatibilities: Compatible with solutions containing dextrose, saline, and KCl. Do not mix with any other antibiotic. Not compatible with total parenteral nutrition.

Administration:
Neonatal: Not indicated.
Pediatric: Not indicated.
Adult: Dilute to 50 mg/ml and administer by IV Y-site over 3–5 minutes.

Contraindications: Hypersensitivity to cephalosporins or penicillin derivatives. Individuals with a history of allergic problems are more susceptible to untoward reactions. Safe use in pregnancy and premature and full-term infants has not been established. Use with caution in clients with renal impairment or history of gastrointestinal disease.

Side Effects:
Primary: Hypersensitivity reactions such as skin rash, pruritus, anaphylaxis, urticaria, and febrile reactions. Superinfections, pain, and thrombosis of the IV site.
Secondary: Nausea, vomiting, abdominal cramps, diarrhea, pseudomembranous colitis, leukopenia, granulocytopenia, neutropenia, thrombocytopenia, eosinophilia, positive Coombs' test, increase in BUN, serum creatinine.

Nursing Implications: Prior to and during therapy, culture and sensitivity tests should be completed.
Monitor for allergic reactions.
Monitor baseline and periodic renal function and prothrombin time. Assess for bleeding.
Monitor for superinfection. Assess for the onset of black, hairy tongue; oral lesions (stomatitis, glossitis); rectal or vaginal itching; vaginal discharge; loose, foul-smelling stools; unusual odor to urine.
Monitor infusion site hourly for signs of thrombophlebitis.
Observe clients closely for the first half-hour after initial dose for a wheal or redness at IV site indicating allergic reaction.
Report onset of diarrhea to the physician.
Monitor intake-output ratio. Report oliguria, hematuria, and changes in intake-output ratio.
Monitor electrolyte balance, especially sodium level.
Use glucose oxidase reagents to check urine glucose. False positive reactions can occur with Clinitest.
Ingestion of alcohol during and 72 hours after therapy may cause a disulfiram reaction.

Generic Name: CEFOTAXIME SODIUM

Trade Name: CLAFORAN

Classification: Antibiotic (cephalosporin)

Actions: Semisynthetic third-generation cephalosporin with antibacterial action against a variety of gram-negative and gram-positive organisms: Streptococcus, Peptostreptococcus, *Streptococcus pneumoniae* and *pyogenes,* Staphylococcus, *Staphylococcus aureus* and *epidermidis, Escherichia coli,* Klebsiella, *Hemophilus influenzae,* Proteus, and Enterobacter.

Indications: For treatment of serious infections of the lower respiratory and urinary tract, gynecological infections, bacteremia, septicemia, intra-abdominal infections, infections of the skin and soft tissue of susceptible organisms, infections of the central nervous system, meningitis, ventriculitis.

Dosage:
Neonatal:
0–1 Week: 25–50 mg/kg every 12 hours.
1–4 Weeks: 25–50 mg/kg every 8 hours.
Pediatric: (under 50 kg): 25–180 mg/kg divided every 4–6 hours.
Adult: 1–2 g every 4–8 hours, not to exceed 12 g daily.
General: Lower doses may be needed for renal-impaired clients.

Preparation: Supplied as a powder in 500-mg, 1-g, and 2-g vials. Reconstitute with sterile water for injection, bacteriostatic water for injection, 0.9% sodium chloride, or bacteriostatic sodium chloride. Each strength should be diluted with 10 ml.

Home Stability: After reconstitution, solution is stable for 24 hours at room temperature and 10 days refrigerated.

Compatibilities: Compatible with solutions containing dextrose, saline, KCl, Ringer's, or lactated Ringer's. Do not mix with any other antibiotic. Not compatible with total parenteral nutrition.

Administration:
Neonatal: Administer reconstituted vial by IV push over 3–5 minutes.
Pediatric: Administer reconstituted vial by IV push or IV Y-site over 3–5 minutes.
Adult: Dilute to 50–100 mg/ml and administer by IV piggyback over 15–30 minutes.

Contraindications: Hypersensitivity to cephalosporins or penicillin derivatives. Individuals with a history of allergic problems are more susceptible to untoward reactions. Safe use in pregnancy has not been established. Use with caution in nursing mothers and clients with renal impairment or history of GI disease.

Side Effects:
Primary: Hypersensitivity reactions such as skin rash, pruritus, anaphylaxis, urticaria, and febrile reactions. Superinfections, pain, and thrombosis of the IV site.
Secondary: Nausea, vomiting, abdominal cramps, diarrhea, pseudomembranous colitis, leukopenia, granulocytopenia, neutropenia, thrombocytopenia, eosinophilia, positive Coombs' test, increase in BUN, serum creatinine.

Nursing Implications: Prior to and during therapy, culture and sensitivity tests should be completed.

Monitor for allergic reactions.

Monitor baseline and periodic renal function and prothrombin time. Assess for bleeding.

Monitor for superinfection. Assess for the onset of black, hairy tongue; oral lesions (stomatitis, glossitis); rectal or vaginal itching; vaginal discharge; loose, foul-smelling stools; unusual odor to urine.

Monitor infusion site hourly for signs of thrombophlebitis.

Observe clients closely for the first half-hour after initial dose for a wheal or redness at IV site indicating allergic reactions.

Report onset of diarrhea to the physician.

Monitor intake-output ratio. Report oliguria, hematuria, and changes in intake-output ratio.

Use glucose oxidase reagents to check urine glucose. False positive reactions can occur with Clinitest.

Generic Name: CEFOXITIN SODIUM

Trade Name: MEFOXIN

Classification: Antibiotic (cephalosporin)

Actions: Semi synthetic second-generation cephalosporin antibiotic with antibacterial action against a wide range of gram-positive and gram-negative organisms and anaerobes. Effective against *Streptococcus pneumoniae* and *pyogenes*, *Hemophilus influenzae*, Klebsiella, *Staphylococcus aureus*, beta-hemolytic streptococci, *Escherichia coli*, Proteus, Enterobacter, Providentia, *Neisseria gonorrhoeae*, Bacteroides, and Clostridium.

Indications: For treatment of serious infections of the genitourinary, gynecological, respiratory, and biliary tracts, bones, joints, skin, and soft tissues; intra-abdominal infections; septicemia, peritonitis.

Dosage:
Neonatal: Not indicated for children under 3 months of age.
Pediatric: 80–160 mg/kg/day divided into 4–6 equal doses. Maximum dosage: 12 g/day.
Adult: 1–3 g every 6–8 hours depending on the severity of the disease. Maximum dosage: 12 g/day.
General: Lower doses are needed by renal-impaired clients.

Preparation: Supplied as a powder. Reconstitute with sterile water for injection, bacteriostatic water for injection, 0.9% sodium chloride, or bacteriostatic sodium chloride in the following concentrations:

VIAL SIZE	VOLUME DILUENT	CONCENTRATION
1 g	2.0 ml	400 mg/ml
2 g	4.0 ml	400 mg/ml

Home Stability: After reconstitution, solution is stable for 24 hours at room temperature and 7 days refrigerated.

Compatibilities: Compatible with solutions containing dextrose, saline, KCl, lactated Ringer's, and sodium bicarbonate. Do not mix with any other antibiotic. Not compatible with total parenteral nutrition.

Administration:
Neonatal: Not applicable.
Pediatric: Dilute to 100 mg/ml and administer by IV push or IV Y-site over 3–5 minutes.
Adult: Dilute to 100 mg/ml and administer by IV piggyback over 15–30 minutes.

Contraindications: Hypersensitivity to cephalosporins or penicillin derivatives. Individuals with a history of allergic problems are more susceptible to untoward reactions. Safe use in pregnancy and premature and full-term infants has not been established. Use with caution in clients with renal impairment or history of gastrointestinal disease.

Side Effects:
Primary: Hypersensitivity reactions such as skin rash, pruritus, anaphylaxis, urticaria, and febrile reactions. Superinfections, pain, and thrombosis of the IV site.
Secondary: Nausea; vomiting; abdominal cramps; diarrhea; neutropenia; leukocytopenia; hemolytic anemia; positive Coombs' test; increase in SGOT, SGPT, alkaline phosphatase, BUN, LDH, serum creatinine; nephrotoxicity; oliguria.

Nursing Implications: Prior to and during therapy, culture and sensitivity tests should be completed.
Monitor for allergic reactions.
Monitor baseline and periodic renal function.
Monitor for superinfection. Assess for the onset of black, hairy tongue; oral lesions (stomatitis, glossitis); rectal or vaginal itching; vaginal discharge; loose, foul-smelling stools; unusual odor to urine.
Monitor infusion site hourly for signs of thrombophlebitis.
Observe clients closely for the first half-hour after initial dose for a wheal or redness at IV site indicating allergic reaction.
Report onset of diarrhea to the physician.
Monitor intake-output ratio. Report oliguria, hematuria, and changes in intake-output ratio.
Use glucose oxidase reagents to check urine glucose. False positive reactions can occur with Clinitest.

Generic Name: CEFTIZOXIME

Trade Name: CEFIZOX

Classification: Antibiotic (cephalosporin)

Actions: Broad spectrum third-generation cephalosporin with antibacterial action against a variety of gram-negative and gram-positive organisms: staphylococci, *Streptococcus pneumoniae*, beta-hemolytic streptococci, *Escherichia coli*, *Hemophilus influenzae*, Klebsiella, *Neisseria meningitidis*, *Proteus mirabilis* and *vulgaris*, *Morganella morganii*, *Proteus vulgaris*, *Providencia rettgeri*, Enterobacter, Citrobacter, *Pseudomonas aeruginosa*, Serratia, Acinetobacter, Clostridium, Peptococcus, Peptostreptococcus, *Bacteroides fragilis*.

Indications: For the treatment of serious infections of the lower respiratory tract and urinary tract; gynecological infections; bacteremia; septicemia; intra-abdominal infections; infections of the bone, joints, skin, and soft tissue of susceptible organisms.

Dosage:
Neonatal: Not recommended for use in children.
Pediatric: Not recommended for use in children.
Adult: 500 mg–4 g every 8–12 hours. In life-threatening infections: 2–12 g/day in divided doses initially; then dosage decreased based on clinical response. Lower doses may be needed for renal-impaired clients.

Preparation: Supplied as a powder in 1- and 2-gram vials. Reconstitute with sterile water for injection, bacteriostatic water for injection, 0.9% sodium chloride, or bacteriostatic sodium chloride. Each gram should be diluted with 10 ml.

Home Stability: After reconstitution, solution is stable for 8 hours at room temperature and 48 hours if refrigerated.

Compatibilities: Compatible with solutions containing dextrose, saline, KCl, Ringer's, or lactated Ringer's. Do not mix with any other antibiotic. Not compatible with total parenteral nutrition.

Administration:
Neonatal: Not recommended.
Pediatric: Not recommended.
Adult: Dilute to 50–100 mg/ml and administer by IV push over 3–5 minutes or by IV piggyback over 30 minutes.

Contraindications: Hypersensitivity to cephalosporins or penicillin derivatives. Individuals with a history of allergic problems are more susceptible to untoward reactions. Safe use in pregnancy has not been established. Use with caution in nursing mothers and clients with renal impairment or history of GI disease.

Side Effects:
Primary: Hypersensitivity reactions such as skin rash, pruritus, anaphylaxis, urticaria, and febrile reactions. Superinfections, pain, and thrombosis of the IV site.
Secondary: Nausea, vomiting, abdominal cramps, diarrhea, pseudomembranous colitis, leukopenia, granulocytopenia, neutropenia, thrombocytopenia, eosinophilia, positive Coombs' test, increase in BUN or serum creatinine.

Nursing Implications: Prior to and during therapy, culture and sensitivity tests should be completed.
Monitor for allergic reactions.
Monitor baseline and periodic renal function and prothrombin time. Assess for bleeding.
Monitor for superinfection. Assess for the onset of black, hairy tongue; oral lesions (stomatitis, glossitis); rectal or vaginal itching; vaginal discharge; loose, foul-smelling stools; unusual odor to urine.
Monitor infusion site hourly for signs of thrombophlebitis.
Observe clients closely for the first half-hour after initial dose for a wheal or redness at IV site indicating allergic reactions.
Report onset of diarrhea to the physician.
Monitor intake-output ratio. Report oliguria, hematuria, and changes in intake-output ratio.
Use glucose oxidase reagents to check urine glucose. False positive reactions can occur with Clinitest.

Generic Name: CEFUROXIME

Trade Name: ZINACEF

Classification: Antibiotic (cephalosporin)

Actions: Semisynthetic second-generation cephalosporin antibiotic with antibacterial action against a wide range of gram-positive and gram-negative organisms and anaerobes. Effective against *Streptococcus pneumoniae* and *pyogenes, Hemophilus influenzae,* Klebsiella, *Staphylococcus aureus, Neisseria meningitides* and, *gonorrhoeae, Proteus mirabilis, Escherichia coli.*

Indications: For treatment of serious infections of the urinary and respiratory tracts, skin, and soft tissues; septicemia; peritonitis; meningitis; gonorrhea.

Dosage:
Neonatal: Not indicated for children under 3 months of age.
Pediatric: 50–100 mg/kg/day in divided doses every 6–8 hours. Bacterial meningitis: 200–240 mg/kg/day.
Adult: 750 mg–1.5 g every 8 hours.
Life-threatening Infections: 1.5 g every 6 hours.
Bacterial Meningitis: Up to 3 g every 8 hours.
General: Lower doses are needed by renal-impaired clients.

Preparation: Supplied as a powder. Reconstitute with sterile water for injection, bacteriostatic water for injection, 0.9% sodium chloride, or bacteriostatic sodium chloride in the following concentrations:

VIAL SIZE	VOLUME DILUENT
975 mg	9.0 ml

Home Stability: After reconstitution, solution is stable for 24 hours at room temperature and 48 hours refrigerated.

Compatibilities: Compatible with solutions containing dextrose, saline, and KCl. Do not mix with any other antibiotic. Not compatible with total parenteral nutrition.

Administration:
Neonatal: Not indicated for children under 3 months of age.

Pediatric: Dilute to 100 mg/ml and administer by IV push or IV Y-site over 3–5 minutes.
Adult: Dilute to 100 mg/ml and administer by IV piggyback over 15–30 minutes.

Contraindications: Hypersensitivity to cephalosporins or penicillin derivatives. Individuals with a history of allergic problems are more susceptible to untoward reactions. Safe use in pregnancy and premature and full-term infants has not been established. Use with caution in clients with renal impairment or history of GI disease.

Side Effects:
Primary: Hypersensitivity reactions such as skin rash, pruritus, anaphylaxis, urticaria, and febrile reactions. Superinfections, pain, and thrombosis of the IV site.
Secondary: Nausea; vomiting; abdominal cramps; diarrhea; pseudomembranous colitis; neutropenia; leukopenia; eosinophilia; positive Coombs' test; increase in SGOT, SGPT, alkaline phosphatase, BUN, serum creatinine, bilirubin; decreased creatinine clearance.

Nursing Implications: Prior to and during therapy, culture and sensitivity tests should be completed.
Monitor for allergic reactions.
Monitor baseline and periodic renal function and prothrombin time. Assess for bleeding.
Monitor for superinfection. Assess for the onset of black, hairy tongue; oral lesions (stomatitis, glossitis); rectal or vaginal itching; vaginal discharge; loose, foul-smelling stools; unusual odor to urine.
Monitor infusion site hourly for signs of thrombophlebitis.
Observe clients closely for the first half-hour after initial dose for a wheal or redness at IV site indicating allergic reactions.
Report onset of diarrhea to the physician.
Monitor intake-output ratio. Report oliguria, hematuria, and changes in intake-output ratio.
Use glucose oxidase reagents to check urine glucose. False positive reactions can occur with Clinitest.

Generic Name: CEPHALOTHIN SODIUM

Trade Name: KEFLIN

Classification: Antibiotic (cephalosporin)

Actions: Semisynthetic first-generation broad-spectrum cephalosporin antibiotic with antibacterial action against a wide range of gram-positive and gram-negative organisms. Effective against nonpenicillinase- and penicillinase-producing staphylococci, beta-hemolytic streptococci, *Streptococcus pneumoniae* and *viridans*, *Hemophilus influenzae*, Klebsiella, *Proteus mirabilis*, *Escherichia coli*, Salmonella, Shigella.

Indications: For treatment of serious infections of the urinary, gastrointestinal, and respiratory tracts, bones, joints, skin, and soft tissues; septicemia; meningitis; endocarditis. Also used for perioperative prophylaxis.

Dosage:
Neonatal:
Premature and Full-term Infants Less Than 7 Days Old: 40 mg/kg/day every 12 hours.
Full-term Infants More Than 7 Days Old: 60 mg/kg/day every 8 hours.
Pediatric: 80–150 mg/kg/day every 4–6 hours in divided doses.
Adult: 500–1000 mg every 4–6 hours. Maximum dosage: 12 g/24 hours.
General: Lower doses are needed by renal-impaired clients.

Preparation: Supplied as a powder. Reconstitute with sterile water for injection, bacteriostatic water for injection, 0.9% sodium chloride, or bacteriostatic sodium chloride in the following concentrations:

VIAL SIZE	VOLUME DILUENT	CONCENTRATION
1000 mg	4.6 ml	200 mg/ml
2000 mg	9.1 ml	200 mg/ml

Home Stability: After reconstitution, solution is stable for 24 hours refrigerated. Crystals should dissolve as vial warms to room temperature.

Compatibilities: Compatible with solutions containing dextrose, saline, and KCl and with total parenteral nutrition. Do not mix with any other antibiotic.

Administration:
Neonatal: Dilute to 100 mg/ml and administer by IV push over 3–5 minutes.
Pediatric: Dilute to 100 mg/ml and administer by IV push or IV Y-site over 3–5 minutes.
Adult: Dilute to 100 mg/ml and administer by IV piggyback over 15–30 minutes.

Contraindications: Hypersensitivity to cephalosporins or penicillin derivatives. Individuals with a history of allergic problems are more susceptible to untoward reactions. Safe use in pregnancy has not been established. Use with caution in clients with renal impairment or history of GI disease.

Side Effects:
Primary: Hypersensitivity reactions such as skin rash, pruritus, anaphylaxis, urticaria, and febrile reactions. Superinfections, pain, and thrombosis of the IV site.
Secondary: Dizziness; vertigo; headache; fatigue; malaise; nausea; vomiting; anorexia; abdominal cramps; diarrhea; pseudomembranous colitis; neutropenia; leukopenia; pancytopenia; agranulocytopenia; thrombocytopenia; hypoprothrombinemia; hemolytic anemia; positive Coombs' test; increased SGOT, SGPT, alkaline phosphatase, BUN, serum creatinine, bilirubin; nephrotoxicity; oliguria; renal failure; decreased creatinine clearance.

Nursing Implications: Prior to and during therapy, culture and sensitivity tests should be completed.
Monitor for allergic reactions.
Monitor baseline and periodic renal function and prothrombin time. Assess for bleeding.
Monitor for superinfection. Assess for the onset of black, hairy tongue; oral lesions (stomatitis, glossitis); rectal or vaginal itching; vaginal discharge; loose, foul-smelling stools; unusual odor to urine.
Monitor infusion site hourly for signs of thrombophlebitis.
Observe clients closely for the first half-hour

after initial dose for a wheal or redness at IV site indicating allergic reaction.

Report onset of diarrhea to the physician.

Monitor intake-output ratio. Report oliguria, hematuria, and changes in intake-output ratio.

Use with caution in clients on sodium-restricted diets.

Use glucose oxidase reagents to check urine glucose. False positive reactions can occur with Clinitest.

Generic Name: CEPHAPIRIN

Trade Name: CEFADYL

Classification: Antibiotic (cephalosporin)

Actions: Semisynthetic first-generation broad-spectrum cephalosporin antibiotic with antibacterial action against a wide range of gram-positive and gram-negative organisms. Effective against nonpenicillinase- and penicillinase-producing staphylococci, beta-hemolytic streptococci, *Streptococcus pneumoniae* and *viridans, Hemophilus influenzae,* Klebsiella, *Proteus mirabilis, Escherichia coli,* Salmonella, Shigella.

Indications: For treatment of serious infections of the urinary, gastrointestinal, and respiratory tracts, joints, skin, and soft tissues; septicemia; meningitis; endocarditis; osteomyelitis.

Dosage:
Neonatal: Not indicated for children less than 3 months of age.
Pediatric: 40–80 mg/kg/day divided equally every 6 hours. Up to 100 mg/kg/day in severe infections.
Adult: 500 mg–1 g every 4–6 hours. Up to 12 g/day for life-threatening infections.
General: Lower doses are needed by renal-impaired clients.

Preparation: Supplied as a powder. Reconstitute with 10 ml of sterile water for injection, bacteriostatic water for injection, 0.9% sodium chloride, or bacteriostatic sodium chloride for every gram of drug.

Home Stability: After reconstitution, solution is stable for 12 hours at room temperature and for 10 days refrigerated.

Compatibilities: Compatible with solutions containing dextrose, saline, and KCl. Do not mix with any other antibiotic. Not compatible with total parenteral nutrition.

Administration:
Neonatal: Dilute to 100 mg/ml and administer by IV push over 3–5 minutes.
Pediatric: Dilute to 100 mg/ml and administer by IV push or IV Y-site over 3–5 minutes.
Adult: Dilute to 100 mg/ml and administer by IV piggyback over 15–30 minutes.

Contraindications: Hypersensitivity to cephalosporins or penicillin derivatives. Individuals with a history of allergic problems are more susceptible to untoward reactions. Safe use in pregnancy has not been established. Use with caution in clients with renal impairment or history of GI disease.

Side Effects:
Primary: Hypersensitivity reactions such as skin rash, pruritus, anaphylaxis, urticaria, and febrile reactions. Superinfections, pain, and thrombosis of the IV site.
Secondary: Dizziness; vertigo; headache; fatigue; malaise; nausea; vomiting; anorexia; abdominal cramps; diarrhea; pseudomembranous colitis; neutropenia; leukopenia; pancytopenia; agranulocytopenia; thrombocytopenia; hypoprothrombinemia; hemolytic anemia; positive Coombs' test; increased SGOT, SGPT, alkaline phosphatase, BUN, serum creatinine, bilirubin; nephrotoxicity; oliguria; renal failure; decreased creatinine clearance.

Nursing Implications: Prior to and during therapy, culture and sensitivity tests should be completed.

Monitor for allergic reactions.

Monitor baseline and periodic renal function and prothrombin time. Assess for bleeding.

Monitor for superinfection. Assess for the onset of black, hairy tongue; oral lesions (stomatitis, glossitis); rectal or vaginal itching; vaginal discharge; loose, foul-smelling stools; unusual odor to urine.

Monitor infusion site hourly for signs of thrombophlebitis.

Observe clients closely for the first half-hour after initial dose for a wheal or redness at IV site indicating allergic reactions.

Report onset of diarrhea to the physician.

Monitor intake-output ratio. Report oliguria, hematuria, and changes in intake-output ratio. Use with caution in clients on sodium-restricted diets.

Use glucose oxidase reagents to check urine glucose. False positive reactions can occur with Clinitest.

Generic Name: CEPHRADINE

Trade Name: VELOSEF

Classification: Antibiotic (cephalosporin)

Actions: Semisynthetic first-generation broad-spectrum cephalosporin antibiotic with anti-bacterial action against a wide range of gram-positive and gram-negative organisms. Effective against Staphylococcus, *Streptococcus pneumoniae* and *faecalis,* beta-hemolytic streptococci, *Escherichia coli, Hemophilus influenzae,* Klebsiella, *Neisseria gonorrhoeae* and *meningitidis,* Shigella, Clostridium, Peptococcus, Peptostreptococcus.

Indications: For treatment of serious infections of the urinary, gastrointestinal, and respiratory tracts, bones, skin, and soft tissues. Also used for perioperative prophylaxis and septicemia.

Dosage:
Neonatal: 50–100 mg/kg/day in equally divided doses every 6 hours.
Pediatric: 50–100 mg/kg/day in equally divided doses every 6 hours.
Adult: 2–4 g in equally divided doses every 6 hours.
Bone Infections: 1 g every 6 hours.
Uncomplicated Pneumonia, Skin, Skin-structure, and Urinary Tract Infections: 500 mg every 6 hours.
Severe Infections: Maximum dosage: 8 g/day in equal doses every 4 hours.
Perioperative Prophylaxis: 1 g 30–60 minutes before surgery, followed by 1 g every 4–6 hours for 1–2 doses or up to 24 hours postoperatively.
Cesarean Section: 1 g immediately after umbilical cord is clamped, then 1 g at 6 and 12 hours after first dose.
General: Lower doses are needed by renal-impaired clients.

Preparation: Supplied as a powder in 250-, 500-, and 1000-mg vials. Also available in 2- and 4-g/100-ml infusion containers and 2-g/200-ml infusion container. Reconstitute powder with 5 ml of sterile water for injection, bacteriostatic water for injection, 0.9% sodium chloride, or bacteriostatic sodium chloride for every 500 mg of drug.

Home Stability: Solution is stable for 10 hours in compatible infusion fluids or 24 hours if refrigerated.

Compatibilities: Compatible with solutions containing dextrose, saline, and KCl. Do not mix with any other antibiotic. Not compatible with total parenteral nutrition.

Administration:
Neonatal: Dilute to 50 mg/ml and administer by IV push over 3–5 minutes.
Pediatric: Dilute to 50–100 mg/ml and administer by IV push or IV Y-site over 3–5 minutes.
Adult: Dilute to 50–100 mg/ml and administer by IV push or IV Y-site over 3–5 minutes.
General: Solution may be infused over a longer period of time based on client condition.

Contraindications: Hypersensitivity to cephalosporins or penicillin derivatives. Individuals with a history of allergic problems are more susceptible to untoward reactions. Safe use in pregnancy has not been established. Use with caution in clients with renal impairment or history of GI disease.

Side Effects:
Primary: Hypersensitivity reactions such as skin rash, pruritus, anaphylaxis, urticaria, and febrile reactions. Superinfections, pain, and thrombosis of the IV site.
Secondary: Dizziness; vertigo; headache; fatigue; malaise; nausea; vomiting; anorexia; abdominal cramps; diarrhea; pseudomembranous colitis; neutropenia; leukopenia; pancytopenia; agranulocytopenia; thrombocytopenia; hypoprothrombinemia; hemolytic anemia; positive Coombs' test; increased SGOT, SGPT, alkaline phosphatase, BUN, serum creatinine, bilirubin; nephrotoxicity; oliguria; renal failure; decreased creatinine clearance.

Nursing Implications: Prior to and during therapy, culture and sensitivity tests should be completed.
Monitor for allergic reactions.
Monitor baseline and periodic renal function and prothrombin time. Assess for bleeding.
Monitor for superinfection. Assess for the onset of black, hairy tongue; oral lesions (stomati-

tis, glossitis); rectal or vaginal itching; vaginal discharge; loose, foul-smelling stools; unusual odor to urine.

Monitor infusion site hourly for signs of thrombophlebitis.

Observe clients closely for the first half-hour after initial dose for a wheal or redness at IV site indicating allergic reaction.

Report onset of diarrhea to the physician.

Monitor intake-output ratio. Report oliguria, hematuria, and changes in intake-output ratio. Caution clients on sodium-restricted diets.

Use glucose oxidase reagents to check urine glucose. False positive reactions can occur with Clinitest.

Generic Name: CHLORAMPHENICOL

Trade Name: CHLOROMYCETIN SODIUM SUCCINATE, MYCHEL-S

Classification: Antibiotic

Actions: Synthetic broad-spectrum antibiotic with bactericidal effect against gram-negative and gram-positive bacteria and most anaerobic microorganisms. Particularly effective against *Salmonella typhi* and other Salmonella species, *Streptococcus pneumoniae*, Neisseria, *Hemophilus influenzae*, Rocky Mountain spotted fever and other Rickettsia, Chlamydia, and Mycoplasma.

Indications: Only for serious infections such as acute infections caused by the Salmonella species, *Hemophilus influenzae* (meningeal), Rickettsia, lymphogranuloma-psittacosis group, and other gram-negative and gram-positive organisms causing bacteremia and meningitis. Also indicated in some cystic fibrosis regimens.

Dosage:
Neonatal:
Less Than 7 Days Old: 25 mg/kg/day every 12 hours.
Full-term Infant More Than 7 Days Old: 50 mg/kg/day every 12 hours.
Pediatric: 50–100 mg/kg/day every 6 hours.
Adult: 50–100 mg/kg/day every 6 hours.
General: Dosage should be reduced in clients with impaired hepatic or renal function.

Preparation: Supplied as a powder. Reconstitute with sterile water for injection or normal saline, 1 g with 10 ml of diluent for a final concentration of 100 mg/ml.

Home Stability: Use reconstituted drug within 24 hours.

Compatibilities: Compatible with solutions containing dextrose, saline, KCl, Ringer's, or lactated Ringer's. Do not mix with any other antibiotic. Not compatible with total parenteral nutrition.

Administration:
Neonatal: Inject slowly over 3–5 minutes into the IV tubing or site.

Pediatric: Inject slowly over 3–5 minutes into the IV tubing or site.
Adult: Further dilute with 50–100 ml of compatible solution and infuse over 15–30 minutes.

Contraindications: In the presence of less toxic yet effective drugs or in clients with a history of hypersensitivity or toxic reaction to the drug.

Side Effects:
Primary: Serious and potentially fatal blood dyscrasias, such as aplastic anemia, hypoplastic anemia, thrombocytopenia, and granulocytopenia, have occurred with short-term therapy. Aplastic anemia has resulted in leukemia. Other side effects include bone marrow depression and, in the presence of excessively high blood levels at any age, gray baby syndrome (cyanosis, abdominal distension, and cardiovascular collapse).
Secondary: Nausea, vomiting, glossitis and stomatitis, diarrhea or enterocolitis, headache, mild depression, mental confusion, delirium, optic and peripheral neuritis. Fever, macular and vesicular rashes, angioedema, urticaria, or anaphylaxis may occur with hypersensitivity.

Nursing Implications: Prior to initiation of therapy, bacterial culture and susceptibility tests are essential. Obtain baseline complete blood count, platelets, serum iron, and reticulocyte cell counts prior to therapy, at 48-hour intervals, and periodically during therapy.
Observe for signs of bone marrow depression. Notify physician if signs occur.
Observe for signs of gray baby syndrome. Notify physician if signs occur.
Assess for hypersensitivity reactions.
Monitor chloramphenicol blood levels closely (desired concentration 5–20 μg/ml).
Monitor vital signs every 4 hours. Closely assess intake and output.
Assess for signs of superinfection by susceptible organisms, stomatitis, glossitis with or without black tongue, anogenital irritation or itching, vaginal discharge, elevated temperature, diarrhea (enterocolitis), cough.
More frequent blood glucose monitoring may be indicated for clients receiving antidiabetic agents.

Generic Name: CHLOROTHIAZIDE SODIUM

Trade Name: DIURIL

Classification: Diuretic, antihypertensive

Actions: Affects the renal tubular mechanism of electrolyte reabsorption, causing excretion of sodium, chlorides, potassium, and water.

Indications: For treatment of edema associated with congestive heart failure, hepatic cirrhosis, corticosteroid and estrogen therapy, nephrotic syndrome, acute gomerulonephritis, and chronic renal failure.

Dosage:
Neonatal: Use in neonates is not recommended.
Pediatric: Use in children is not recommended.
Adult: 0.5–1.0 g 1–2 times a day.

Preparation: Dry white powder in 500-mg vials.

Home Stability: Not applicable.

Compatibilities: May infuse with dextrose or sodium chloride solutions.

Administration:
Neonatal: Not applicable.
Pediatric: Not applicable.
Adult: Add 18 ml of sterile water for injection to the 500-mg vial. Give slowly over 5 minutes.

Contraindications: Hypersensitivity to chlorothiazide sodium or sulfonamide drugs; anuria. Use with caution in clients with severe renal disease, impaired hepatic function, or progressive liver disease. Thiazides may potentiate the action of other antihypertensive drugs. Thiazides cross the placental barrier and are found in cord blood and breast milk; therefore, anticipated benefits must be weighed against possible hazards to the fetus.

Side Effects:
Primary: Volume depletion and dehydration, orthostatic hypotension, hyponatremia, hypochloremic alkalosis, hypokalemia, hyperglycemia.
Secondary: Aplastic anemia, agranulocytosis, weakness, dizziness, vertigo, muscle cramps, nausea, vomiting, transient blurred vision.

Nursing Implications: Assess for signs and symptoms of fluid and electrolyte imbalance, including tachycardia, hypotension, oliguria, dryness of mouth, thirst, weakness, lethargy, drowsiness, restlessness, muscle cramps, and fatigue.

Monitor intake and output, pulse, blood pressure, weight, and serum electrolytes frequently.

Assess for signs of hypokalemia (muscle weakness and cramping). Teach patients about potassium-rich foods (citrus fruits, tomatoes, bananas, dates, apricots). Be especially careful in patients receiving digitalis because of increased risk of digitalis toxicity.

Caution patient to change position slowly because of orthostatic hypotension.

Monitor BUN and creatinine for signs of deteriorating renal function.

Monitor blood glucose levels, especially in diabetics.

Monitor serum uric acid levels, especially in patients with a history of gout.

Administer in the morning to prevent nocturia.

Elderly patients are especially susceptible to excessive diuresis.

Generic Name: CHLORPHENIRAMINE MALEATE

Trade Name: CHLOR-PRO, CHLOR-TRIMETON

Classification: Antihistamine, antiemetic, anticholinergic, antiparkinsonism

Actions: Competes with histamine for cell receptor sites.

Indications: For relief of allergic reactions to blood or plasma; anaphylaxis; active treatment of motion sickness; parkinsonism.

Dosage:
Neonatal: 0.35 mg/kg/24 hours in divided doses every 6 hours.
Pediatric: 0.35 mg/kg/24 hours in divided doses every 6 hours.
Adult: 10 mg initially; may repeat as necessary but not to exceed 40 mg/24 hours.
For Anaphylactic Reactions: 20 mg initially.

Preparation: Supplied in 10-mg/ml vials.

Home Stability: Not applicable.

Compatibilities: May infuse with solutions containing dextrose, saline, or any combination thereof.

Administration:
Neonatal: Infuse over 1 minute at IV site undiluted.
Pediatric: Infuse over 1 minute at IV site undiluted.
Adult: Infuse over 1 minute at IV site undiluted.

Contraindications: Hypersensitivity, asthma, MAO inhibitor therapy, use in newborn or premature infants. Use with caution in narrow-angle glaucoma, peptic ulcer disease, prostatic hypertrophy, hypertension, and cardiac disease, as well as in the elderly. May have additive sedative effects with other central nervous system depressants.

Side Effects:
Primary: Drowsiness, nausea, dry mouth.
Secondary: Confusion, insomnia, headache, vertigo, palpitations, photosensitivity, diplopia, nasal stuffiness, vomiting, diarrhea, constipation, dysuria, urinary retention, urticaria.

Nursing Implications: Monitor vital signs frequently.
Assess for development of side effects, particularly in elderly or debilitated patients. Warn patients to avoid activities that require alertness until effects on central nervous system are determined. Cool drinks, ice chips, hard candy, or sugarless gum can relieve dry mouth. Encourage fluids to help prevent constipation.
Monitor intake and output for development of urinary retention.
Discontinuation of drug should be done slowly.

Generic Name: CHLORPROMAZINE

Trade Name: THORAZINE

Classification: Antipsychotic

Actions: Exact mechanism of action not completely understood, but agents in this classification block postsynaptic dopamine receptors in the brain. By inhibiting or altering dopamine release and increasing the firing rate of neuronal cells in the midbrain, the antipsychotic drugs suppress the clinical signs of schizophrenia. These medications may also depress the control of basic body functions such as metabolism, body temperature, level of consciousness, and hormonal balance.

Antipsychotic agents may be administered IM, IV, or orally; oral administration is used for maintenance therapy. Parenteral administration provides more active drug than oral doses. Drugs in this classification are widely distributed and stored in the tissues and may be eliminated in the urine for up to 6 months after therapy is discontinued.

Drugs in this family differ in the severity of their side effects. The major side effects are sedation, extrapyramidal effects, and orthostatic hypotension. It is possible to minimize these side effects by changing from one drug to another.

Indications: For treatment and management of psychotic disorders. May be used in treatment of severe nausea and vomiting.

Dosage:
Neonatal: Not recommended under 6 months of age.
Pediatric: 0.25 mg/pound of body weight IM every 6–8 hours.
Adult: 25–50 mg IM 3–4 times daily. Dose may vary depending on the condition under treatment.

Preparation: Injectable 12.5 mg/ml.

Compatibilities: Normal saline.

Administration:
Neonatal: Not recommended.
Pediatric: IM or by mouth.
Adult: IM or by mouth.
General: IV dose is not recommended except for severe hiccups, surgery, and tetanus. Drug *must* be diluted when given IV.

Contraindications: In patients who are comatose or experiencing central nervous system depression; in presence of blood dyscrasias, hepatic disease, coronary artery disease, or convulsive disorders.

Side Effects: All side effects listed have not been observed in use of this drug, but because of the similarities of the phenothiazines, they are listed for all drugs in this group.
Primary: Most common are the extrapyramidal reactions. These include but are not limited to aching and numbness in the limbs, motor restlessness, dystonia, tight feeling of throat, slurred speech, and ataxia. Other reactions include orthostatic hypotension, blurred vision and other ocular changes, dark urine, bradycardia, and dizziness.
Secondary: Jaundice, anemia, agranulocytosis, dermatitis, and pain at IM injection site.

Nursing Implications: Monitor vital signs and observe for hypotension or behavioral changes. Monitor level of consciousness. Ongoing assessments should include these observations on a daily basis.

Assess and observe for side effects. The development of extrapyramidal effects can be distressing; reassure client that they will subside.

Warn clients on home therapy that care should be used when activities require alertness or coordination. The drowsiness experienced should subside after a period of time.

Warn patients to avoid extended exposure to the sun. Also avoid getting drug on skin—it may cause contact dermatitis.

Dry mouth may be a side effect. Gum or candy may relieve the discomfort.

Generic Name: CIMETIDINE

Trade Name: TAGAMET

Classification: Gastrointestinal drug

Actions: Acts to decrease gastric acid secretion by inhibiting histamine action on gastric parietal cells. Inhibits gastric acid secretion stimulated during the day and night.

Indications: For treatment of gastric and duodenal ulcers over short period of time. May be prescribed for longer periods to prevent recurrence of an ulcer.

Dosage:

Neonatal and Pediatric:

Under 12 Years of Age: 20–40 mg/kg/day IV every 6 hours.

Over 12 Years of Age: 300 mg IV every 6 hours.

Adult: 300 mg every 6 hours. To increase dose, administer 300 mg at closer intervals, but do not exceed 2400 mg/day.

Preparation: Injectable 300 mg/2 ml.

Compatibilities: Compatible with 0.9% sodium chloride, 5% or 10% dextrose, lactated Ringer's, 5% sodium bicarbonate.

Administration:

Infusion: 300 mg diluted in 100 ml of IV fluid and infused over 15–20 minutes.

Injection: Dilute 300 mg to 20 ml with compatible solution and inject over at least 2 minutes.

There is a possibility of cardiac arrythmias and arrest after too rapid IV bolus administration.

Contraindications: None known.

Side Effects:

Primary: Mild and transient diarrhea, dizziness, urticaria, neutropenia.

Secondary: Hypersensitivity, rash, jaundice.

Nursing Implications: Monitor vital signs. Observe for signs of actively bleeding ulcer.

Rotate injection sites, because injection may cause temporary pain in the area.

Document response to drug therapy.

Generic Name: CISPLATIN

Trade Name: PLATINOL

Classification: Antineoplastic alkylating agent

Actions: Heavy metal compound that inhibits DNA precursors and causes cross-linking of DNA; also inhibits protein and RNA synthesis. Considered cell-cycle nonspecific.

Indications: Testicular, ovarian, bladder, cervical, and bone cancers, melanoma, lymphoma, and squamous cell cancer of the head and neck.

Dosage:
Neonatal: Not applicable.
Pediatric: 100–120 mg/m^2 IV every 3–4 weeks; 10–20 mg/m^2 IV every day for 5 days every 3–4 weeks; 80 mg/m^2 continuous drip for 24 hours; 20 mg/m^2 intra-arterially over 2 hours; 120 mg/m^2 intra-arterially over 45 hours; 90 mg/m^2 in 2 L dialysate intraperitoneally every 3 weeks (experimental).
Adult: See pediatric dosage.

Preparation: Available in 10-mg vials that should be mixed with at least 10 ml sterile water. It should be added to 250–500 ml of normal saline, D$_5$NS, or 0.3% saline for infusion since it is incompatible with D$_5$W alone.

Home Stability: Undiluted vials are stable for 2 years if refrigerated and protected from light or for 1 year if kept at room temperature.
The diluted drug is stable for 24 hours at room temperature and should be protected from light. If it is admixed with mannitol, it should be used in less than 24 hours.

Compatibilities: Only compatible with solutions that contain chloride and therefore should not be mixed with plain D$_5$W. Should not be infused through aluminum needles, since it reacts with this metal and loses its potency. Forms a precipitate with IVs containing bicarbonate. Concurrent administration of aminoglycosides increases the risk of renal failure. Loop diuretics increase the risk of ototoxicity. Cisplatin decreases the effects of phenytoin. As with most antineoplastic agents, it is advisable not to administer cisplatin with other admixture solutions.

Administration:
Neonatal: Not applicable.
Pediatric: Infuse IV at a minimum of 1 mg/minute. Slower infusions may decrease nausea and vomiting. Patients must be well hydrated to avoid nephrotoxicity. It is recommended that patients force fluids the day before therapy and receive prehydration of 1–2 L of IV solution 8–12 hours before administration and posthydration with 1–2 L of IV solution. Mannitol and/or Lasix are also recommended to promote diuresis. Antiemetics must be given to control nausea and vomiting and prevent dehydration. Intra-arterial infusions should include heparin, and aspirin should be given to decrease inflammatory-type reactions. The dwell time with intraperitoneal use should be 4 hours, and mannitol and sodium thiosulfate should also be given to decrease toxicity.
Adult: See pediatric administration.

Contraindications: Pregnancy. Cisplatin is usually not administered or the dose is considerably reduced if the patient's creatinine clearance is less than 60–70 mg/minute or if serum creatinine is greater than 1.5 mg/dl or if the patient has a hearing loss.

Side Effects:
Primary:
Nephrotoxicity: Decreased creatinine clearance, elevated serum creatinine and BUN leading to renal failure can occur. Hydration with KCl and diuresis with Lasix and mannitol can significantly minimize this toxicity. Electrolytes should be closely monitored.
Immunologic: Hypersensitivity and anaphylactoid reactions of increased heart rate, decreased blood pressure, facial swelling, and wheezing can occur and are fairly easily controlled by premedicating sensitive patients with Benadryl and/or treating symptoms with corticosteroids, antihistamines, or epinephrine.
Ototoxicity: Tinnitus and high-frequency hearing loss occur in about 30 percent of patients, especially children. Audiograms should be done periodically to assess the severity of this toxicity.

Neurotoxicity: Peripheral neuropathy with numbness and tingling.

Gastrointestinal: Severe nausea and vomiting within 1 hour and lasting 6–24 hours, anorexia.

Reproductive: May be teratogenic.

Secondary: Decreased WBC, platelets and RBCs 2 weeks after treatment; increased uric acid levels; opthalmologic toxicity; decreased magnesium and calcium resulting in tetany and seizures; liver toxicity; cardiac abnormalities. Risk of infertility and secondary malignancy is unknown.

Nursing Implications: Remember *not* to infuse cisplatin with plain D_5W or aluminum needles.

Maintain IV pre- and posthydration, and administer Lasix and mannitol as ordered.

Instruct patients to force fluids the day before treatment and to maintain fluid intake as best they can for at least a week after therapy. Patients should be told to report poor fluid intake from persistent nausea or vomiting to their physician.

Premedicate patients with antiemetics and administer regularly after cisplatin for 24–48 hours.

Monitor creatinine clearance, serum creatinine, electrolytes (magnesium, calcium, potassium, and phosphorus), and/or BUN closely.

Observe the patient frequently for hypersensitivity and anaphylactic reactions; monitor vital signs. A physician and emergency equipment and supplies should be immediately available.

Instruct patients and family members to report any noticeable decrease in the patient's ability to hear or problems with peripheral neuropathy.

Inform patient of the possibility of birth defects if pregnancy occurs while taking cisplatin.

Safe-handling precautions should continue for 9 days after a dose of cisplatin.

Generic Name: CLINDAMYCIN PHOSPHATE

Trade Name: CLEOCIN PHOSPHATE

Classification: Semisynthetic antibiotic

Actions: Semisynthetic antibiotic active against susceptible strains of anaerobic bacteria and gram-positive cocci such as Streptococcus, Pneumococcus, and Staphylococcus.

Indications: For treatment of the following serious infections when penicillin is contraindicated: respiratory tract infections (empyema, anaerobic pneumonitis), skin and soft tissue infections, septicemia, intra-abdominal infections (peritonitis or abscess), endometritis, nongonococcal tubo-ovarian abscess, pelvic cellulitis, vaginal cuff infections, and bone and joint infections (acute hematogenous osteomyelitis).

Dosage:
Neonatal: Not recommended for infants under 1 month of age.
Pediatric (over 1 Month of Age): 15–40 mg/kg in equally divided doses every 6–8 hours based on severity of infection. Maximum dosage: 300 mg/ 24 hours regardless of body weight.
Adult: 600–2700 mg/day in equally divided doses every 12, 8, or 6 hours. Maximum dosage: 4.8 g/day for life-threatening infections.

Preparation: Supplied as a liquid in 300-mg/2-ml ampules or 600-mg/4-ml ampules.

Compatibilities: Compatible with IV solutions containing sodium chloride, glucose, calcium, and potassium. Also compatible with the following antibiotics: cephalothin, kanamycin, gentamicin, penicillin, and carbenicillin. Do not administer with any other drug.

Administration:
Neonatal: Not applicable.
Pediatric: Do not administer via IV injection: cardiac arrest has been reported. Dilute and administer via intermittent infusion according to the following chart:

DOSE	DILUENT	TIME
300 mg	50 ml	10 minutes
600 mg	100 ml	20 minutes
900 mg	150 ml	30 minutes
1200 mg	200 ml	45 minutes

Maximum infusion is 1200 mg in a single 1-hour infusion.
Adult: See pediatric administration.

Contraindications: Hypersensitivity; in newborns; pregnancy; lactation.

Side Effects:
Primary: Pseudomembranous colitis, abdominal pain, allergic reactions, jaundice, nausea, thrombophlebitis, vomiting.
Secondary: Polyarthritis, abnormalities in hepatic function tests, transient leukopenia, eosinophilia, agranulocytosis, thrombocytopenia.

Nursing Implications: Prior to and during therapy, culture and sensitivity tests should be completed.

Monitor for hypersensitivity reactions: hypotension, facial edema, dyspnea, and restlessness may indicate pending anaphylactoid reaction. Contact physician if these symptoms should occur.

Monitor for symptoms of pseudomembranous colitis. Record frequency of bowel movements. Note if blood, pus, or mucus is present. Withhold drug if abdominal cramping or diarrhea occurs and contact physician.

Monitor baseline and periodic renal, hematologic, and hepatic functions.

Monitor for superinfection: fever, redness, soreness, pain, swelling, drainage, monilial rash in perineal area, change in cough, or diarrhea.

Monitor respiratory functions in clients receiving concurrent neuromuscular blocking agents. Clindamycin may potentiate their effects.

Assess IV site frequently for thrombophlebitis, and rotate device every 48–72 hours.

Generic Name: COLCHICINE

Trade Name: COLCHICINE

Actions: Exact mechanism of action in gout is unknown, but acts to decrease production of lactic acid by leukocytes, which decreases the depositing of uric acid. Also reduces inflammatory response to the deposited crystals and decreases phagocytosis. By interrupting this cycle, relieves the symptoms of acute gout attack. Although not an analgesic, pain relief is an effect of the drug.

Indications: For treatment of gout—relieves the pain in an acute attack and may prevent further attacks. IV use will give a rapid response.

Dosage:

Neonatal and Pediatric: Safety not established.
Adult: Initial dose: 0.5–2 mg every 6 hours until desired response obtained, not to exceed 4 mg in 24 hours. Patient may be transferred to oral therapy.

Preparation: Injectable 1 mg/2 ml.

Compatibilities: Compatible with nonbacteriostatic normal saline.

Administration:

Adult: Must be given IV; IM route will cause severe local irritation.

Contraindications: Hypersensitivity; serious gastrointestinal, hepatic, renal, or cardiac disorders; blood dyscrasias.

Side Effects:

Primary: Bone marrow depression and aplastic anemia, agranulocytosis or thrombocytopenia, peripheral neuritis, myopathy.
Secondary: Vomiting, diarrhea, abdominal pain and nausea. GI symptoms may occur with IV administration, and drug should be discontinued if symptoms occur.

Nursing Implications: Note appearance of joints and document patient discomfort.

Assess relief from symptoms and discomfort.

Observe closely for any GI symptoms—drug must be stopped if they develop to prevent overdose. Notify physician.

Encourage fluid intake, and measure urine output carefully. This will promote urate excretion.

Obtain appropriate lab work.

A dosage change may be necessary a few days before and after a minor surgical or dental procedure. Notify physician.

Generic Name: COLISTIMETHATE SODIUM

Trade Name: COLY-MYCIN M

Classification: Antibiotic

Actions: Polypeptide antibiotic with neuromuscular blocking action, bactericidal against gram-negative bacilli: *Pseudomonas aeruginosa, Enterobacter aerogenes, Escherichia coli,* and *Klebsiella pneumoniae.*

Indications: For treatment of acute and chronic infections, especially of the urinary tract, due to the organisms listed above.

Dosage:
Neonatal: 2.5–5.0 mg/kg/24 hours equally divided into 2–4 doses and administered every 6–12 hours.
Pediatric: See neonatal dosage.
Adult: 2.5–5.0 mg/kg/24 hours equally divided into 2–4 doses and administered every 6–12 hours.
General: Normal renal function is necessary for this dosage.

Preparation: Supplied as a powder; reconstitute with 2 ml of sterile water for injection. Swirl gently to prevent frothing.

Home Stability: Store reconstituted drug in refrigerator for 7 days. Discard solutions diluted for infusion after 24 hours.

Compatibilities: Compatible with IV solutions containing sodium chloride, 5% dextrose, lactated Ringer's, or 10% invert sugar. Do not administer with other medications.

Administration:
Neonatal: Administer initial dose over 3–5 minutes by IV push. Second dose may be administered in 1–2 hours at 5–6 mg/hour by continuous infusion. If renal function is impaired, reduce the infusion rate according to physician's directions.
Pediatric: See neonatal administration.
Adult: See neonatal administration.

Contraindications: Hypersensitivity to the drug or multiple allergens; pregnancy.

Side Effects:
Primary: Circumoral paresthesia, dizziness, formication of extremities, numbness of extremities, pruritus, slurring of speech, tingling of extremities, vertigo.
Overdose: Anaphylaxis, apnea, decreased urine output, elevated BUN, elevated serum creatinine, muscle weakness, renal insufficiency.

Nursing Implications: Monitor serum blood levels. Serum half-life is 2–3 hours. Do not exceed 5 mg/kg/day in clients with normal renal function.
Prior to and during therapy, culture and sensitivity tests should be completed.
Monitor for hypersensitivity reactions: hypotension, facial edema, dyspnea, and restlessness may indicate pending anaphylactoid reaction. Contact physician if these symptoms should occur.
Monitor baseline and periodic renal, hematologic, and hepatic functions.
Monitor urinary input-output ratio. Report to the physician any change in the ratio. Decreased dosage is indicated in the presence of renal impairment.
Monitor for superinfection: fever, redness, soreness, pain, swelling, drainage, monilial rash in perineal area, change in cough, diarrhea.
Monitor respiratory functions in clients receiving concurrent neuromuscular blocking agents. Colistimethate may potentiate their effects.

Generic Name: CONJUGATED ESTROGENS

Trade Name: PREMARIN INTRAVENOUS

Classification: Hormone

Actions: Produces an increase in circulating prothrombin and accelerator globulin and a decrease in the antithrombin activities of the blood.

Indications: Dysfunctional uterine bleeding as a result of hormonal imbalance.

Dosage:
Neonatal: Not applicable.
Pediatric: Not applicable.
Adult: 25 mg; may repeat in 6–12 hours if needed.

Preparation: Vial containing powder and ampule with diluent.

Home Stability: Not applicable.

Compatibilities: May infuse with dextrose or saline. Not compatible with lactated Ringer's, Ringer's, sodium lactate injection, or any solution with an acid pH.

Administration:
Neonatal: Not applicable.
Pediatric: Not applicable.
Adult: Dilute with diluent provided and give by IV push at a rate of 5 mg/minute.

Contraindications: Pregnancy, thrombophlebitis, thromboembolic disorders. Use with caution in patients with epilepsy, migraines, asthma, cardiac and renal disease.

Side Effects:
Primary: Nausea, vomiting, flushing.

Nursing Implications: Assess uterine bleeding before and after administration.
Obtain baseline vital signs and check frequently during therapy.
Refrigerate solution after reconstitution; do not use if discolored or if precipitate is present.
Estrogens may be carcinogenic.

Generic Name: CORTICOTROPIN

Trade Name: ACTHAR

Classification: Adrenocorticotropic hormone (ACTH)

Actions: Stimulates the adrenal cortex to produce cortisol, corticosterone, and aldosterone. Effect is measured by analysis of pre- and post-infusion cortisol levels.

Indications: For diagnostic testing of adrenocortical function *only*.

Dosage:
Neonatal and Pediatric: 2–5 u/100 ml over an 8-hour period. Infants and young children require larger doses per kilogram of body weight than adults or older children.
Adult: 10–25 u over an 8-hour period; also 25 u as a single injection or 40 u every 12 hours for 48 hours.

Preparation: Supplied in vials containing 25 or 40 u of lyophilized ACTH in the dry form and approximately 9 and 14 mg of hydrolyzed gelatin. It is a white, water-soluble powder.

Home Stability: Reconstituted solution may be refrigerated but must be used within 24 hours.

Compatibilities: May be reconstituted with sterile water or sodium chloride. Compatible with 5% dextrose and lactated Ringer's as well.

Administration:
Neonatal and Pediatric: 2–5 u diluted in 100 ml of 5% dextrose or 0.9% sodium chloride, infused over an 8-hour period.

Adult: 10–25 u diluted in 500 ml of 5% dextrose or 0.9% sodium chloride, infused over an 8-hour period. This administration method is preferred, but 25 u may be given by rapid direct IV injection, or 40 u may be given as a continuous infusion every 12 hours for 48 hours.

Contraindications: Scleroderma, osteoporosis, hypertension, congestive heart failure, peptic ulcer or a history of recent surgery, ocular herpes simplex, systemic fungal infections, sensitivity to proteins with a porcine origin.

Side Effects:
Primary: Hypersensitivity as evidenced by skin reactions, dizziness, nausea, vomiting, fever.
Secondary: In some instances, anaphylactic shock.

Nursing Implications: Observe patient closely for signs of hypersensitivity reaction.

Assure that pre- and post-cortisol levels are drawn at specified time, depending on the method of administration.

Cortisol levels may be drawn as frequently as every 15 minutes for 1 hour and every 30 minutes thereafter.

Pretest doses of cortisone, hydrocortisone, or spironolactone should not be given.

In normal patients, one 8-hour infusion is adequate for diagnosis. In patients with hypopituitarism or secondary adrenocortical insufficiency, one 8-hour infusion daily for 4–5 days may be necessary for diagnosis.

Generic Name: COSYNTROPIN

Trade Name: CORTROSYN

Classification: Adrenocorticotropic hormone (ACTH)

Actions: Synthetic subunit of ACTH with action similar to that of purified natural ACTH: it stimulates the adrenal cortex and produces secretion of cortisol (hydrocortisone), corticosterone, and aldosterone as well as several weakly androgenic substances.

Indications: For diagnostic use only, to screen patients thought to have adrenocortical insufficiency. If a patient is found to have adrenal insufficiency, further studies are necessary to determine if it is primary or secondary.

Dosage:
Neonatal: 0.125 mg in children 2 years or less.
Pediatric: 0.25–0.75 mg, highly individualized. A maximum response has been noted with the smallest dose.
Adult: 0.25–0.75 mg. A maximum response has been noted with the smallest dose.

Preparation: Supplied as a lyophilized white to off-white powder in vials containing 0.25 mg of cosyntropin and 10 mg of mannitol. Also supplied with an ampule of solvent.

Home Stability: Reconstituted cosyntropin should not be retained for use later.

Compatibilities: May be added to either saline or glucose solutions. Enzymes found in blood and plasma may inactivate it.

Administration:
Neonatal: Dilute in 2–5 ml of saline and give IV over a 2-minute period.
Pediatric: See neonatal administration.
Adult: Dilute in 2–5 ml of saline and give IV over a 2-minute period; 0.25 mg may be given as a continuous IV infusion at the rate of 40 μg/hour over a 6-hour period when a greater stimulus to the adrenal cortex is desired.

Contraindications: Previous adverse reaction.

Side Effects:
Primary: Hypersensitivity reaction (rare), including pruritus and flushing.

Nursing Implications: Not intended for therapeutic use.
Assure that a control blood sample for cortisol analysis is drawn before the cosyntropin is given.
A second blood sample should be drawn either 20 or 60 minutes after injection, depending on which normal cortisol values are being used for interpretation.
On the day of the test, patients should omit their pretest doses of cortisone, hydrocortisone, or spironolactone.
Observe the patient for evidence of an allergic response during and immediately after administration.
Cosyntropin is preferable to ACTH as a diagnostic agent to screen for adrenocortical insufficiency because it is less likely to cause allergic reactions.

Generic Name: CYANOCOBALAMIN (VITAMIN B₁₂)

Trade Name: BETALIN 12

Classification: Vitamin

Actions: Essential vitamin in maintaining health and normal metabolic functioning. Used by the body for growth, cell reproduction, and maturation of red blood cells. Although vitamins are necessary for normal growth and development, they do not serve as sources of energy. Vitamins must be obtained from sources outside the body. A dietary deficiency in vitamin B_{12} will result in development of pernicious anemia. If this has been present for 3 months or longer, permanent lesions of the spinal cord can occur.

Indications: For treatment of vitamin B_{12} deficiency, which results in pernicious anemia. Parenteral form is given when absorption is impaired because of gastrointestinal pathology.

Dosage: To treat pernicious anemia:
Neonatal: 1000 μg/IM daily for 11 days. Diet should be low in protein.
Pediatric: 1000–5000 μg in 100-μg doses over about 2 weeks. Maintenance for life is 60 μg/month.
Adult: 100–1000 μg daily for about 2 weeks. Monthly maintenance is 100–1000 μg for life. The required dose may be less for vitamin B_{12} deficiency.

Preparation: Injectable form available as 30 μg/ml, 100 μg/ml, 120 μg/ml, and 1000 μg/ml.

Home Stability: Protect solution from light.

Compatibilities: Do not mix solution with other IV solutions or medications.

Administration: IV administration is not recommended for any age because it may cause anaphylactic reactions. It should be used only when other routes are impossible.
Neonatal: IM
Pediatric: IM, SC, or by mouth.
Adult: IM or by mouth.

Contraindications: Known hypersensitivity. Use with caution in patients with cardiac, pulmonary, or hypertensive disease, Leber's disease, and gouty conditions.

Side Effects:
Primary: Anaphylaxis, peripheral vascular thrombosis, pain or burning at injection sites.
Secondary: Transient diarrhea, itching, urticaria.

Nursing Implications: Assess patient for nutritional status. Some signs and symptoms of pernicious anemia are ataxia, paresthesias, numbness, weakness in extremities, visual disturbances, depression, and loss of bowel and bladder control. Additional symptoms may include weight loss, glossitis, anorexia, bleeding gingiva, constipation, and diarrhea.

Test dose may be administered to assess for sensitivity.

Warn patient of possibility of pain at the injection site.

Monitor patient daily for improvement in physical symptoms. Also monitor lab work for response, such as hemoglobin, hematocrit, and reticulocyte count.

Because of the possibility of hypokalemia, serum potassium levels should be monitored.

Provide nutritional counseling as necessary to patient and family.

Generic Name: CYCLOPHOSPHAMIDE

Trade Name: CYTOXAN, NEOSAR

Classification: Antineoplastic alkylating agent

Actions: Inert until metabolized by the liver and the plasma. Its metabolites cause cell destruction by cross-linking DNA strands. It is cell-cycle nonspecific.

Indications: Non-Hodgkin's lymphoma; adult acute leukemia; Hodgkin's and Burkitt's lymphoma; breast, endometrial, and oat cell lung cancers; multiple myeloma; sarcomas; nephrotic syndrome; rheumatoid arthritis; various autoimmune diseases; graft versus host reactions in organ transplants; multiple sclerosis.

Dosage:
Neonatal: Not applicable.
Pediatric: 500–1500 mg/m^2 IV in one dose every 3–4 weeks or 60–120 mg/m^2 by mouth daily for 1–2 weeks. Doses vary greatly with various diseases and drug combinations.
For Multiple Sclerosis: 100–125 mg IV every 6° daily for 10–14 days.
Adult: See pediatric dosage.

Preparation: Supplied in 25- and 50-mg tablets as well as in the injectable form in the following concentrations:

  100 mg/10 ml—add 5 ml of sterile water without benzyl alcohol preservative.
  200 mg/20 ml—add 10 ml of sterile water without preservative.
  500 mg/30 ml–add 25 ml of sterile water without preservative.

Vigorous shaking and *slight* warming of the prepared vials helps dissolve the drug crystals completely, which is necessary before administration.

Home Stability: Both tablets and unopened vials should be stored at room temperature not greater than 90°F. The IV preparations are stable for 24 hours at room temperature or 6 days in the refrigerator, except for solutions prepared without paraben-preserved bacteriostatic water, which should be discarded after 24 hours.

Compatibilities: Because cyclophosphamide is inactive outside the body, other admixtures may be given with it. Allopurinol and thiazide diuretics may increase the bone marrow suppression of cyclophosphamide. Barbiturates and other drugs such as phenytoin and chloral hydrate may increase the toxicity of cyclophosphamide. It may increase the sedative effects of barbiturates. Phenobarbital decreases the half-life of cyclophosphamide. Corticosteroids may reduce its effects and increase its toxicity; both of these drugs need dose adjustments in adrenalectomized patients. Cyclophosphamide may increase the side effect of apnea with succinylcholine, the cardiotoxicity of anthracyclines, and perhaps the toxicity of halothane and nitrous oxide. Chloramphenicol decreases the effects of cyclophosphamide while chlorpromazine increases its effects. Cyclophosphamide decreases the effects of digoxin and warfarin.

Administration:
Neonatal: Not applicable.
Pediatric: When taken by mouth, cyclophosphamide should be given with meals, and some patients prefer it with cold foods such as ice cream. The total daily dose can be taken all at once or divided into smaller doses. By the IV route, cyclophosphamide can be infused at any rate. All forms of the drug should be administered as early in the day as possible, at least before 5:00 P.M., to facilitate emptying of the bladder while the patient is still awake and able to force fluids. If cyclophosphamide cannot be given early in the day, the patient should be awakened about every 2 hours during the night to void and drink fluids. Patients should always void at the first feeling of bladder fullness while on cyclophosphamide. If patients cannot maintain oral hydration, IV hydration is mandatory. High-doses given IV may require continuous bladder irrigation to prevent hemorrhagic cystitis. Mesna and/or Lasix may also be administered with higher doses to minimize cystitis and water retention. Mesna may be given IV or by mouth with fruit juice or cola at a dose of 60–90 percent of the cyclophosphamide dose or 800 mg/m^2. The first dose should be given IV, with 4 subsequent doses IV or by mouth every 3–4 hours.
Adult: See pediatric administration.

Contraindications: Pregnancy. Presence of an infection, especially varicella-zoster. Doses are usually reduced by half if creatinine clearance is below 25 ml/minute. Use with caution in patients with hepatic dysfunction.

Side Effects:

Primary:

Hematopoietic: Primarily decreased white blood cells and some decreased platelets in 1–2 weeks. T cells, particularly suppressor cells, appear to be most suppressed.

Nephrotoxicity: Hemorrhagic cystitis may occur up to several weeks after treatment without adequate hydration and prompt emptying of the bladder during drug administration. This side effect may be controlled by bladder instillations of 5–10 percent formalin or acetylcysteine irrigations or IV administration of Mesna. Prolonged therapy with cyclophosphamide may fibrose the bladder, making it smaller and causing frequency in urination. Also, seizures, decreased sodium, and inappropriate antidiuretic hormone syndrome (resulting in water retention) have occurred with higher doses of cyclophosphamide and increased fluid intake with some patients, especially children.

Cutaneous: Some hair loss, which is reversible, occurs in most patients, but only 35–50 percent of patients experience total alopecia, and some hair regrowth occurs even while treatment continues. Hyperpigmentation of the nails and skin and ridge formation of the nails occur.

Gastrointestinal: Anorexia and nausea may occur with oral and lower IV doses. Moderate vomiting usually only occurs with higher IV doses within 3–12 hours and can last 8–10 hours.

Reproductive: Infertility and teratogenesis are definite. Permanent sterility is possible.

Secondary: Pneumonitis, pulmonary fibrosis, a temporary oropharyngeal and tongue-burning sensation with IV push administration, urticaria, anaphylactoid reactions, cardiac toxicity especially with high doses that are given in less than 48 hours. Risk of secondary bladder carcinoma and leukemia is relatively high.

Nursing Implications: Monitor complete blood count.

Instruct patient and family to take infection precautions beginning 1 week after treatment and continue these for 2 weeks.

Instruct patient to force fluids, void as soon as the urge is felt, take the drug early in the day with meals, and report any blood in the urine to the physician immediately.

Awake the patient to void every 2–3 hours and to drink fluids if an IV dose of cyclophosphamide cannot be given before 5:00 P.M.

Hemastix all urine and observe for gross bleeding.

Instruct patient on the possibility of hair loss, skin rash that itches, and changes in the nailbeds.

Medicate with regularly scheduled antiemetics for nausea that occurs with oral intake of cyclophosphamide. Premedicate and continue antiemetics for 24 hours for high doses of cyclophosphamide given IV.

Inform patient of the probability of birth defects if pregnancy occurs while taking cyclophosphamide and the possibility of permanent sterility.

Safe-handling precautions should continue for 3 days after the last dose of cyclophosphamide.

Generic Name: CYTARABINE (ARA-C)

Trade Name: CYTOSAR-U

Classification: Antineoplastic antimetabolite

Actions: Inhibits DNA polymerase and competes with cellular enzymes during the S phase of the cell cycle to cause cell death. Thus it is cell-cycle specific at the S phase.

Indications: Acute and chronic myeloid leukemia.

Dosage:
Neonatal: Not applicable.
Pediatric:
Induction/Consolidation Therapy: 100–150 mg/m^2 continuous IV daily for 5–10 days or 2–3 g/m^2 IV over 1 hour every 12 hours daily for 8–12 days.
Maintenance Therapy: 70–100 mg/m^2 every 6° for 5 days or 20 mg/m^2 SC daily for 7–21 days; 5–70 mg/m^2 intrathecally up to 3 days/week.
Adult: Same as for pediatric dosage, except high-dose Ara-C is usually 2 g/m^2 or less to minimize severe neurotoxicity in patients over 60 years of age.

Preparation: Supplied in 100-mg and 500-mg vials that should be mixed with 5 ml and 10 ml respectively of the supplied diluent; 1–2 ml of sterile water, normal saline, or D_5W, can be used to make smaller volumes for SC use. Elliott's B solution is used for reconstituting intrathecal doses. Normal saline or D_5W can be used for administering continuous infusions.

Home Stability: Undiluted vials should be refrigerated and are stable for 2 years. Reconstituted drug is stable at room temperature for 48 hours but should not be used if cloudy or hazy.

Compatibilities: Ara-C increases the cytotoxicity of cyclophosphamide and BiCNU. Ara-C is incompatible with fluorouracil. As with most antineoplastic agents, it is not advisable to administer Ara-C with other admixture solutions.

Administration:
Neonatal: Not applicable.
Pediatric: Infuse by continuous IV for 24 hours or administer IV drip over about 1 hour for high doses. Give SC or IM doses by rotating sites to avoid tissue irritation.
Adult: See pediatric administration.

Contraindications: Pregnancy. Previously uncontrolled allergy to Ara-C evidenced by fever, muscle and joint pain, chest pain, rash, conjunctivitis, and malaise within 6–12 hours of administration. (Corticosteroids are used to prevent and treat this syndrome.) Neurotoxicity with previous high doses of Ara-C or methotrexate neurotoxicity (lower doses may be resumed after symptoms subside). Use with caution if patient has hepatic dysfunction. Ara-C decreases the effect of oral digoxin.

Side Effects:
Primary:
Hematopoietic: Decreased WBCs and platelets within 7 days and lasting for 1–3 weeks, with some anemia.
Gastrointestinal: Anorexia, moderate nausea and vomiting (especially with high doses), stomatitis, esophagitis, diarrhea, anal ulceration, abdominal pain, ileus, gastrointestinal bleeding, and electrolyte imbalance.
Neurotoxicity: Occurs primarily with high doses. Lethargy, change in level of consciousness, confusion, inability to move or use extremities correctly.
Ophthalmologic: Conjunctivitis often occurs with high-dose Ara-C unless prophylactic steroid eye drops are administered.
Reproductive: Teratogenetic; probably causes infertility.
Secondary: Flulike syndrome with fever, headache, and arthralgia; rash or freckling, especially with exposure to sunlight; reversible hepatic dysfunction; acute pancreatitis with previous asparaginase therapy; urinary retention; meningism, paresthesias, paraplegias, seizures (within 24 hours), headaches, vomiting, and fever have occurred with intrathecal use, especially with CNS irradiation; a very low risk of hypersensitivity reactions exists. The risk of secondary malignancy is low.

Nursing Implications: Instruct patient and family to take infection and bleeding precautions beginning 1 week after treatment starts and continue these for 1–3 weeks.

Emphasis should be placed on good oral hygiene with a soft-bristled toothbrush.

Monitor white blood cells and platelets and take precautions against infection and bleeding according to hospital routine and the Oncology Nursing Societies' guidelines.

Medicate as needed with antiemetics for nausea. High-dose Ara-C requires medication with antiemetics before each dose and as needed afterward. Assess all emesis for blood via a guaiac test.

Guaiac all stools and diarrhea and obtain an order for an antidiarrheal if necessary.

When administering high-dose Ara-C, a neurological assessment should be done before each dose to avoid undue neurotoxicity. This assessment should include the following: (1) Instruct the patient to follow your finger as you move it from one side to the other in front of the patient's face. If the eyes move rapidly in the corners, nystagmus is present. (2) Have the patient sign her or his name. (3) Check level of consciousness. If any of these checks are not within normal limits, the drug should be held until the physician sees the patient and determines if continued administration is safe.

Make sure the patient takes steroid eye drops regularly, and check for any eye irritation or changes in vision.

Inform patient of the possibility of birth defects if pregnancy occurs while taking Ara-C and that sterility is probable.

Safe-handling precautions should continue for 2 days after the last dose of Ara-C.

Generic Name: DACARBAZINE

Trade Name: DTIC

Classification: Antineoplastic, miscellaneous agent

Actions: Exact cytotoxic action unknown, but appears to be an alkylator and antimetabolite and also interferes with proteins and inhibits RNA and DNA synthesis. Although somewhat more active at the G_2 phase, it is considered cell-cycle nonspecific.

Indications: Melanoma, soft tissue sarcomas, and refractory Hodgkin's lymphoma.

Dosage:
Neonatal: Not applicable.
Pediatric:
IV: 2–4.5 mg/kg/day daily for 10 days or 150–300 mg/m^2 daily for 5–10 days or 650–1450 mg/m^2 in one dose.
Intra-arterial: 250 mg/m^2 daily for 5 days.
Adult: See pediatric dosage.

Preparation: Available in amber vials of 100 and 200 mg that must be reconstituted with at least 2 ml of sterile water, normal saline, or D_5W. The mixed drug is clear and colorless or pale yellow. A pink color indicates drug decomposition and solution should be discarded.

Home Stability: Intact vials should be refrigerated and are stable for 4 years. Dilutions of 10 mg/ml are stable for 8 hours at room temperature and 72 hours if refrigerated. Large dilutions into 250–500 ml of D_5W or normal saline are stable for 24 hours if protected from light. Loss of drug activity with exposure to light is significant, and side effects of nausea, vomiting, hepatotoxicity, and venous irritation may also be worsened with light exposure. Change in solution color from yellow to pink indicates drug decomposition.

Compatibilities: Dacarbazine forms an immediate precipitate with Solu Cortef. Dilantin and phenobarbital may induce the metabolism of dacarbazine. Dacarbazine has an additive effect when given with allopurinol and may increase the toxicities of azathioprine or 6-mercaptopurine. It also may increase the cardiotoxicity of doxorubicin. As with most antineoplastic agents, it is advisable not to administer dacarbazine with other admixture solutions.

Administration:
Neonatal: Not applicable.
Pediatric: Infuse in 250–500 ml of D_5W or normal saline over about 1 hour. Smaller volumes can be given by IV push, but pain along the IV site is common, especially with rapid administration. IV sites should be monitored closely to avoid extravasation, particularly with IV push concentrations, which can cause severe pain and necrosis.
Adult: Same as pediatric.

Contraindications: Pregnancy, previous allergy to dacarbazine.

Side Effects:
Primary:
Hematopoietic: Moderate decrease in WBC and platelets 21–25 days after administration. Anemia may also occur.
Gastrointestinal: Nausea and vomiting can be severe for 1–12 hours, especially during the first few days of treatment.
Pyrogenic: Flulike syndrome of fever, malaise, and myalgia may occur 7 days after treatment and persist for 1–3 weeks.
Reproductive: Teratogenic.
Secondary: Alopecia, facial flushing and paresthesias, metallic taste, and urticaria. Occurrence of an anaphylactic reaction is rare. Risk of infertility and secondary malignancy is unknown.

Nursing Implications: Monitor complete blood count.

Instruct patient and family on infection and bleeding precautions during the third and fourth week after treatment begins.

Premedicate with antiemetics and continue them for 12–16 hours afterward. Inform patient that nausea and vomiting lessens with each dose in a 5–10 day series.

Obtain an order for acetaminophen to decrease fever and flulike symptoms.

Establish and maintain good venous access,

checking for patency every 10–15 minutes during IV drip infusion and instructing the patient to report any sensations of burning or pain.

Inform patient of the possibility of birth defects if pregnancy occurs while taking dacarbazine.

Safe-handling precautions should continue for 2 days after the last dose of dacarbazine.

Generic Name: DACTINOMYCIN/ACTINOMYCIN D

Trade Name: COSMEGEN

Classification: Antineoplastic antibiotic

Actions: Inhibits DNA-dependent RNA synthesis, especially messenger RNA. Although it has some increased activity in the G_1 phase, it is considered cell-cycle nonspecific.

Indications: Choriocarcinoma, Wilms' tumor, Kaposi's sarcoma, Ewing's sarcoma, rhabdomyosarcoma, melanoma, testicular tumors, childhood acute lymphocytic leukemia, and organ transplantation.

Dosage:
Neonatal (under 12 Months): Not recommended.
Pediatric (over 12 Months): 15 μg/kg/day IV or 450 μg (500 μg limit) m²/day IV for 5 days repeated every 2–8 weeks or 2 mg/m² IV every 3–4 weeks.
For Isolated Limb or Pelvic Perfusion: 30–50 μg/kg.
Adult: 500 μg/m² IV daily for 5 days or 2 mg weekly for 3 weeks.

Preparation: Available in 500-μg vials that require 1.1 ml of preservative-free sterile water for a concentration of 500 μg/ml.

Home Stability: Unopened vials should be stored at room temperature. Although the mixed drug can be stored at room temperature for 2–5 months, it should be discarded after 24 hours, since it has no preservative in it.

Compatibilities: Should not be given with live virus vaccines. Not compatible with preservatives in bacteriostatic diluents. As with most antineoplastic agents, it is not advisable to administer dactinomycin with other admixture solutions.

Administration:
Neonatal: Not applicable.
Pediatric (over 12 Months): Administer by slow IV push into the side arm of a free-flowing IV, checking patency every 2–3 minutes to avoid extravasation of this severe vesicant.
Adult: See pediatric administration.
General: Do not administer this drug through final cellulose filters.

Contraindications: Pregnancy; bone marrow depression or presence of viral infection, especially chickenpox or herpes zoster. Use with caution within 2 months after radiation therapy near the liver.

Side Effects:
Primary:
Hematopoietic: Decreased WBCs and platelets with some decrease in RBCs, usually occurring in 7–10 days and not beyond 3 weeks.
Gastrointestinal: Severe nausea and vomiting begins within a few hours and lasts 4–20 hours. Mucositis, esophagitis, proctitis, and diarrhea also occur in about 30 percent of patients, and discontinuing the drug should be considered.
Cutaneous: Reversible alopecia, acnelike skin changes, erythema, hyperpigmentation, and radiation "recall" on previously irradiated skin that develops as skin irritation and can even necrose. Extravasation causes immediate pain and swelling that can result in necrotic ulcers.
Reproductive: Teratogenic.
Secondary: Decreased serum calcium; hepatic and renal toxicity; fatigue and malaise. Risk of infertility is unknown. Risk of secondary malignancy is increased with radiation therapy.

Nursing Implications: Monitor complete blood count.
Instruct patient and family on infection and bleeding precautions during the second to fourth weeks after treatment.
Premedicate with antiemetics and continue them for 24 hours afterward.
Emphasize good oral hygiene with a soft-bristled toothbrush.
Guaiac all diarrhea and obtain an order for an antidiarrheal if necessary.
Inform patient of the possibility of hair loss and skin changes, especially at previous radiation therapy sites.
Establish and maintain good venous access, checking for patency every 2–3 minutes during IV push administration and instructing the patient to report any sensations of burning or pain.
Monitor liver and renal function studies.
Inform patient of the possibility of birth defects if pregnancy occurs while taking dactinomycin.
Continue safe-handling precautions for 8 days after the last dose of dactinomycin.

Generic Name: DANTROLENE SODIUM

Trade Name: DANTRIUM

Classification: Skeletal muscle relaxant

Actions: Acts directly on skeletal muscle to reduce muscle tension. Interference with intracellular calcium movement produces relaxation. Has no effect on smooth or cardiac muscle. Also used to treat malignant hyperthermia and is the only drug that has been found successful in treatment. In this case it also acts by interfering with calcium release in muscle fiber.

Indications: Oral route used to treat muscle spasms resulting from spinal cord injury, stroke, multiple sclerosis, or cerebral palsy. IV route used in treatment of malignant hyperthermia. Oral dose may be administered several days preoperatively as prophylaxis for patients with this condition.

Dosage:
Muscle Spasticity:
Pediatric: 0.5 mg/kg 2 times daily increasing to 3 times daily on the fourth day. Can increase up to 3 mg/kg (in increments of 0.5 mg/kg) 2–4 times daily as needed.
Adult: 25 mg once a day, increasing up to 100 mg (in 25-mg increments) 2–4 times daily.
Malignant Hyperthermia:
All Ages: Begin with 1 mg/kg and continue (up to 10 mg/kg) until symptoms subside. This can be repeated if the symptoms reappear. There should be continuous administration until the symptoms subside.

Preparation: Vials containing lyophilized mixture of dantrolene, mannitol, and sodium hydroxide to make a pH of 9.5. This is reconstituted with 60 ml sterile water (without bacteriostatic agent). Give within 6 hours of reconstitution.

Administration: Continuous infusion as reconstituted above.
Malignant Hyperthermia: Done by anesthesiologist. Discontinue anesthesia. Given by continuous rapid IV administration.

Contraindications: By mouth (for spasticity): Active hepatic disease and when spasticity necessary to maintain an upright posture. Safety not established in women with childbearing potential, nursing mothers, and children under 5 years.

Side Effects:
Primary: Muscle weakness, dizziness, drowsiness, fatigue, headache, tachycardia, blurred vision, severe diarrhea.
Secondary: Confusion, blood pressure changes, excessive tearing, abnormal hair growth.

Nursing Implications: Baseline assessment of muscular spasticity prior to beginning of therapy.
Maintain a safe environment until the patient's response to the drug is known. Warn patients at home of drug actions and reactions.
Monitor for signs of hepatic damage. Obtain hepatic function tests.
Monitor for signs of malignant hyperthermia—they most commonly occur during surgery to several hours after. Symptoms include skeletal muscle rigidity, sudden tachycardia, increased temperature, rapid respiration, hypotension, and acidosis. Inform the physician immediately if any symptoms are noted.
Avoid extravasation, which can cause severe tissue damage.
Monitor patient carefully during IV administration.

Generic Name: DAUNORUBICIN HYDROCHLORIDE

Trade Name: CERUBIDINE

Classification: Antineoplastic antibiotic

Actions: Binds to the DNA molecule and thus interferes with RNA and DNA synthesis. Intermediate doses affect late S and G_2 phases, while higher doses affect all phases, making this drug cell-cycle nonspecific.

Indications: Acute myeloid and lymphatic leukemias; lymphomas; solid tumors in children, including Wilms' tumor, rhabdomyosarcoma, neuroblastoma, and Ewing's sarcoma.

Dosage:
Neonatal: Not applicable.
Pediatric: 1 mg/kg IV daily for 5 days or 30–60 mg/m² IV daily for 3 days.
Adult: See pediatric dosage.
Maximum Cumulative Dose: 500–600 mg/m² in adults, 300 mg/m² in children over 2, 10 mg/kg in children less than 2 or with a body surface area less than 0.5 m² to prevent irreversible cardiotoxicity.

Preparation: Supplied in 20-mg glass vials, which can be reconstituted with 5–10 ml of D_5W, normal saline, or sterile water.

Home Stability: Unopened vials may be stored at room temperature for 2 years if kept from direct sunlight. The reconstituted solution is stable for 24 hours at room temperature and 36 hours in the refrigerator.

Compatibilities: Not compatible with heparin or dexamethasone. Appears to decrease the cellular uptake of methotrexate, thereby reducing methotrexate's effectiveness, when given just before or along with methotrexate. As with most antineoplastic agents, it is advisable not to administer daunorubicin with other admixture solutions.

Administration:
Neonatal: Not applicable.
Pediatric: Administer by slow IV push into the side arm of a free-flowing IV, checking patency every 2–3 minutes to avoid extravasation of this vesicant.
Adult: See pediatric administration.

Contraindications: Congestive heart failure or other heart disease. Consider lower cumulative doses for patients with previous chest irradiation. Use with caution in children. Hepatic dysfunction with a bilirubin of more than 1.5 mg/100 ml requires a dose reduction of daunorubicin by 50 percent. Renal dysfunction with a serum creatinine of more than 3 mg/dl also requires a dose reduction of 50 percent.

Side Effects:
Primary:
Hematopoietic: Decreased white blood cells with a nadir between the first and second week. Platelets may decrease somewhat.
Cardiac Toxicity: EKG abnormalities initially, developing into irreversible congestive heart failure from cardiomyopathy.
Gastrointestinal: Moderate nausea and vomiting.
Cutaneous: Tissue destruction and ulceration if extravasated; radiation "recall" on previously irradiated skin that develops as skin irritation and can necrose; complete alopecia that is reversible; hyperpigmentation or skin rash; loosening of the nails.
Nephrotoxicity: Urine will be red in color for several days after treatment. Increased serum uric acid with rapid tumor lysis.
Reproductive: Teratogenetic.
Secondary: Stomatitis, diarrhea, hepatic and renal toxicity. Risk of infertility or secondary malignancy is unknown.

Nursing Implications: Monitor complete blood count.

Instruct patient and family on infection precautions to be taken between first and second week after administration.

Monitor patient closely for early signs of congestive heart failure. Remind the physician to obtain and compare periodic systolic time interval ratios.

Record cumulative dose with administration of each new dose.

Premedicate with antiemetics and continue them for 24 hours.

Inform the patient of the possibility of complete hair loss that is reversible and of skin changes at previous radiation therapy sites.

Establish and maintain good venous access, checking for patency every 2–3 minutes during IV push administration and instructing the patient to report any sensations of burning or pain.

Inform patient that urine will be red for several days after receiving the drug.

Inform patient of the possibility of birth defects if pregnancy occurs while taking daunorubicin.

Safe-handling precautions should continue for 21 days after the last dose of daunorubicin.

Generic Name: DEFEROXAMINE MESYLATE

Trade Name: DESFERAL

Classification: Heavy metal antagonist

Actions: Highly specific agent used in treatment of iron intoxication. It is an iron-chelating agent that binds with the ferric ions. The resultant compound is water soluble and easily excreted in the urine. Most excretion of iron occurs at the beginning of therapy and will turn the urine a reddish-brown.

Indications: Treatment of acute iron intoxication. May be used in addition to gastric lavage, control of shock, and correction of acidosis.

Dosage:

Neonatal and Pediatric: Initial dose 20 mg/kg, followed by 10 mg/kg every 4 hours for 8 hours. Further doses, depending on clinical symptoms, of 10 mg/kg every 4–12 hours. Maximum 6 g/day.

Adult: Initial dose of 1 g followed by 0.5 g every 4 hours for 8 hours. Further doses, depending on clinical symptoms, of 0.5 g every 4–12 hours. Maximum dose 6 g/day.

General: The above doses are for acute intoxication. Doses for chronic overload are slightly less.

Preparation: Injection 500 mg/vial.

Compatibilities: Compatible with sterile water, saline, glucose in water, or Ringer's.

Administration: IM is the preferred route for all patients except those in shock. IV infusion should not exceed 15 mg/kg/hour. It is also possible to administer SC or by mini-infusion pump.

Contraindications: Severe renal impairment, anuria.

Side Effects:

Primary: Pain at injection site, urticaria, hypotension, allergic reactions with long-term therapy, blurred vision, diarrhea.

Secondary: Rash, tachycardia, abdominal discomfort.

Nursing Implications: Obtain complete history of ingestion—product, amount ingested, time of ingestion.

Do a complete assessment to determine clinical signs of intoxication: lethargy, bloody diarrhea, abdominal pain, restlessness, and hematemesis. Shock may develop.

Monitor vital signs and intake and output closely.

Have emergency equipment and medications available in case of shock and arrest.

Generic Name: DESLANOSIDE INJECTION

Trade Name: CEDILANID-D

Classification: Cardiac glycoside

Actions: Increases the force of myocardial contraction, increases the refractory period of the atrioventricular node, and to a lesser degree affects the sinoatrial node and conduction system via the parasympathetic and sympathetic nervous system.

Indications: Congestive heart failure, especially low-output failure; atrial fibrillation; atrial flutter; paroxysmal atrial tachycardia.

Dosage:

Neonatal (under 2 Weeks): Digitalizing dose is 0.022 mg/kg; give in divided doses every 3–4 hours.

Pediatric: Digitalizing dose for children 2 weeks–3 years of age is 0.025 mg/kg; for children 3 years and over, 0.022 mg/kg. Give in divided doses every 3–4 hours or in single dose if necessary.

Adult: Digitalization obtained within 12 hours by giving 1.6 mg either as single injection or divided into 2 doses. Maintenance therapy accomplished by oral preparations within 12 hours.

Preparation: 2-ml ampules containing 0.4 mg deslanoside (0.2 mg/ml).

Home Stability: Not applicable.

Compatibilities: Compatible with solutions containing dextrose, saline.

Administration:

Neonatal (under 2 Weeks): May give undiluted at a rate of 0.2 mg/minute.

Pediatric (over 2 Weeks): May give undiluted or diluted in 10 ml of sodium chloride injection at a rate of 0.2 mg/minute.

Adult: May give undiluted or diluted in 10 ml of sodium chloride injection at a rate of 0.2 mg/minute.

General: Onset of action is within 5 minutes, with a peak effect 2–4 hours after IV administration. Therapeutic action persists for 2–5 days.

Contraindications: Digitalis toxicity, hypersensitivity, ventricular fibrillation, ventricular tachycardia. Use with caution in the elderly, in patients with acute myocardial infarction, severe pulmonary disease, advanced heart failure, hypothyroidism, and renal insufficiency. Also use with caution in conjunction with drugs that may cause hypokalemia (amphotericin B, carbenicillin, ticarcillin, corticosteroids, and diuretics) or hypercalcemia and hypomagnesemia (parenteral calcium, thiazides). Usefulness in patients with Stokes-Adams attacks, chronic constrictive pericarditis, or idiopathic hypertrophic subaortic stenosis is doubtful. Quinidine and verapamil may cause an increase in serum digitalis concentration. Concomitant use of deslanoside and sympathomimetics increases the risk of cardiac arrhythmias. Beta-adrenergic blockers or calcium channel blockers together with deslanoside may cause complete heart block.

Side Effects (Toxic): Anorexia, nausea, vomiting, diarrhea, headache, weakness, agitation, apathy, yellow-green halos around visual images, blurred vision, ST depression, PR prolongation, premature ventricular contractions, paroxysmal and nonparoxysmal nodal rhythms, atrioventricular dissociation, paroxysmal atrial tachycardia with block, severe bradycardia, atrioventricular blocks leading to complete heart block.

Nursing Implications: Dosage is highly individualized and must be adjusted to patient's clinical condition.

Obtain baseline data on heart rate and rhythm, blood pressure, and electrolytes before giving first dose.

Continuous cardiac monitoring is required during IV digitalization and essential if digitalis toxicity is suspected. Record and report to physician any significant changes (sudden increase or decrease in rate, irregular beats, and particularly regularization of a previously irregular rhythm). Obtain a blood pressure reading and a 12-lead EKG with these changes.

Hold if apical pulse is less than 60 beats/minute; notify physician.

Assess heart tones, jugular venous distension, peripheral edema, lung sounds, dyspnea, pulse quality, and color, temperature, and capillary refill of extremities every 4 hours and as needed to ascertain effectiveness of treatment.

Monitor serum potassium levels; hypokalemia makes the myocardium more sensitive to digitalis and tends to reduce the positive inotropic effect.

Monitor serum calcium levels; calcium affects contractility and excitability of the heart in a manner similar to digitalis.

Monitor serum magnesium levels; hypomagnesemia predisposes patients to digitalis toxicity.

Question patients about use of cardiac glycosides within the previous 2–3 weeks before administering a loading dose.

Assess for signs and symptoms of digitalis toxicity.

Take apical-radial pulse for a full minute. Report any significant pulse deficit to the physician.

**Generic Name: DEXAMETHASONE
SODIUM PHOSPHATE**

Trade Name: DECADRON

Classification: Corticosteroid

Actions: Members of this family have many and varied effects because they influence almost every cell in the body. Some of these actions are accelerated protein metabolism that results in muscle weakness and wasting, suppression of immune response and impaired wound healing, redistribution of fat, and increased formation of adipose tissue. Blood glucose levels increase because it is utilized less. This causes an increase in the release of insulin. Steroids suppress the body's immune response by affecting histamine release and inhibit the chain of events that leads to the inflammatory response. Finally, they have an effect on the reabsorption and distribution of some electrolytes and other elements necessary for normal body function. Any patient who has been on long-term therapy should have steroids withdrawn slowly to prevent development of acute adrenal insufficiency.

Indications: Treatment of many disorders including (but not limited to) inflammatory, endocrine, collagen, dermatologic, rheumatic, allergic, respiratory, hematologic, and gastrointestinal diseases and diseases of the nervous system.

Dosage: Highly variable depending on disease or condition; ranges from 0.75–9.0 mg/day by mouth.

Preparation: Injectable 4, 10, and 24 mg/ml.

Administration: IM, IV, and by mouth.

Contraindications: Hypersensitivity, systemic fungal infections. The smallest dose for the shortest period of time should be used because of the chance of side effects. May stunt growth in children. Do not give immunizations during therapy. Use with caution in patients with congestive heart failure, hypertension, osteoporosis, or active infections. May aggravate diabetes mellitus, Cushing's syndrome, and optic nerve damage.

Side Effects: Many effects are dependent on dose or length of therapy. The following side effects are related to the drug itself.
Primary: Fluid and electrolyte disturbances, osteoporosis, long bone fracture, central nervous system effects, increased incidence of infections, impaired wound healing, ocular effects, endocrine effects.
Secondary: Abrupt withdrawal may lead to withdrawal syndrome or adrenal insufficiency.

Nursing Implications: Obtain baseline information on height, weight, vital signs, physical assessment, and laboratory results.

Check drug label carefully—some solutions should not be administered IV, only IM.

Any patient who has been on long-term therapy *must* have dose tapered. Observe for clinical symptoms of withdrawal.

Continuing assessment includes weight, vital signs, and laboratory follow-up. Assess for side effects.

The patient at home should be instructed to avoid contact with any person having an active infection because of decreased resistance.

Dietary adjustments may be necessary for diabetic patients. Any patient on long-term therapy may need to increase protein intake.

Monitor patient for improvement in condition under therapy. Document observations.

Additional patient teaching may include diarrhea and tarry stools; avoiding exposure to infection; reporting any possible infections and unhealed cuts; having eyes examined periodically along with routine laboratory tests.

Generic Name: DEXPANTHENOL

Trade Name: ILOPAN

Classification: Water-soluble B complex vitamin.

Actions: Exact mechanism of action unknown but used after abdominal surgery to decrease incidence of paralytic ileus. Also minimizes postoperative abdominal distension and helps in return of intestinal motility.

Indications: Postoperative use to minimize chance of paralytic ileus after abdominal surgery and help speed return of intestinal motility.

Dosage:
Pediatric and Adult: 250 mg or 500 mg IM. Repeat again in 2 hours, then every 6 hours until chance of ileus has passed.
Adynamic Ileus: 500 mg IM in dosing intervals as above.

Preparation: Injectable 250 mg/ml.

Administration: IM; when given IV, must be *slowly* infused—rate varies.

Contraindications: Hemophilia. Do not give within 1 hour of succinylcholine.

Side Effects:
Primary: Itching, tingling, generalized dermatitis, urticaria, slight decrease in blood pressure.
Secondary: Colic, vomiting, diarrhea.

Nursing Implications: Assess abdomen by palpation and auscultation for rigidity and bowel sounds. Document observations.
Ongoing assessment: note presence or absence of bowel sounds, distension, passage of flatus or stool, and intake and output.
Record all observations.

Generic Name: DEXTRAN, HIGH MOLECULAR WEIGHT

Trade Name: DEXTRAN 75, DEXTRAN 70, GENTRAN 75, MACRODEX

Classification: Volume expander

Actions: Provides hemodynamically significant plasma volume expansion by approximating colloidal properties of human albumin.

Indications: Treatment of shock or impending shock.

Dosage:
Neonatal: Not applicable.
Pediatric: Variable, not to exceed 20 ml/kg/day.
Adult: Variable, not to exceed 20 ml/kg/day.

Preparation: 6% solution in 500-ml bottles of normal saline or 5% solution of dextrose in water.

Home Stability: Not applicable.

Compatibilities: May infuse with saline or dextrose.

Administration:
Neonatal: Not applicable.
Pediatric: Not applicable.
Adult: Give first 500 ml at a rate of 20–40 ml/minute. If additional doses are needed, reduce flow to lowest rate possible to maintain hemodynamic status desired.

Contraindications: Congestive heart failure, sensitivity to dextran, lactation and pregnancy, severe renal disease, thrombocytopenia, severe bleeding disorders, marked hemostatic defects (thrombocytopenia, hypofibrinogenemia, etc). Use with caution in heart disease, renal shutdown, and pulmonary edema.

Side Effects:
Primary: Overhydration, fever, joint pain, nausea, wheezing.
Secondary: Bleeding, dehydration, hypotension, tightness of chest, urticaria, vomiting; severe anaphylaxis and death may occur.

Nursing Implications: Monitor fluid indicators diligently. Obtain baseline pulse, blood pressure, central venous pressure, pulmonary arteriole wedge pressure, pulmonary artery pressure, and urinary output. Check every 5–15 minutes during and after infusion until stable. Slow or discontinue infusion rate if a rapid rise in pressures occurs or if anuria or oliguria develops.

Assess for signs of circulatory overload: dyspnea, wheezing, rales, ronchi, change in blood pressure during therapy.

Monitor electrolytes and hematocrit for possible dehydration, overhydration, and blood loss.

Monitor serum blood glucose levels.

May reduce coagulability of the circulating blood; assess for onset of bleeding. Have type and cross-match drawn before infusion begins. Monitor hemoglobin, hematocrit, and serum protein evaluations.

Crystallization can occur at low temperatures; submerge in warm water and dissolve all crystals before infusion.

Generic Name: DEXTRAN 40, LOW MOLECULAR WEIGHT

Trade Name: GENTRAN 40, LMD 10%, RHEOMACRODEX

Classification: Volume expander

Actions: Increases plasma volume by mobilizing water from body tissues and holding it in the vascular space.

Indications: Adjunctive therapy in shock; prophylaxis during surgical procedures that have a high incidence of venous thrombosis and pulmonary embolism.

Dosage:
Neonatal: Not applicable.
Pediatric: Not applicable.
Adult: 20 ml/kg total during first day; 10 ml/kg during next 4 days; then discontinue therapy. For prophylaxis: 10 mg/kg on day of surgery; 500 ml daily for 2–3 days; then 500 ml every 2–3 days for up to 2 weeks.

Preparation: 10% solution in 500-ml bottles.

Home Stability: Not applicable.

Compatibilities: May infuse with saline or dextrose.

Administration:
Neonatal: Not applicable.
Pediatric: Not applicable.
Adult: Give first 500 ml over 15–30 minutes. Infuse subsequent doses over 8–24 hours.

Contraindications: Congestive heart failure, hypofibrinogenemia, sensitivity to dextran, lactation and pregnancy, severe renal disease, thrombocytopenia. Use with caution in heart disease, renal shutdown, and pulmonary edema.

Side Effects:
Primary: Overhydration, fever, joint pain, nausea, wheezing.
Secondary: Bleeding, dehydration, hypotension, tightness of chest, urticaria, vomiting. Severe anaphylaxis and death may occur.

Nursing Implications: Monitor fluid indicators diligently. Obtain baseline pulse, blood pressure, central venous pressure, pulmonary arteriole wedge pressure, pulmonary artery pressure, and urinary output. Check every 5–15 minutes during and after infusion until stable. Slow or discontinue infusion rate if a rapid rise in pressures occurs or if anuria or oliguria develops.

Assess for signs of circulatory overload: dyspnea, wheezing, rales, change in blood pressure during therapy.

Monitor electrolytes and hematocrit for possible dehydration, overhydration, and blood loss.

Monitor serum blood glucose levels.

May reduce coagulability of the circulating blood; assess for onset of bleeding. Have type and cross-match drawn before infusion begins.

Crystallization can occur at low temperatures; submerge in warm water and dissolve all crystals before infusion.

Generic Name: DEXTROSE

Trade Name: DEXTROSE

Classification: Dextrose

Actions: Supplies calories and energy for patients unable to take carbohydrates orally. Also minimizes glyconeogenesis. Provides calories for protein synthesis, metabolism, and prevention of fatty acid deficiency.

Indications: Hypoglycemia, inability to absorb enteral carbohydrates.

Dosage: Highly variable, depending on patient's age, weight, nutritional status, and fluid balance. Many parenteral forms are available.

Preparation: Infusion: 2.5%, 5%, 10%, 20%, 50%.

Administration: Infuse over several hours. Higher concentrations are administered through a central venous catheter. In some cases, 25% dextrose may be administered at 1 ml/minute. Too rapid administration can cause hyperglycemia and a fluid shift.

Contraindications: Intracranial or intraspinal hemorrhage, hyperglycemia, diabetic coma.

Side Effects:
Primary: Must be diluted to 25% or less to avoid sclerosing and thrombi, osmotic diuresis, and dehydration.
Secondary: Hyperglycemia, fluid and electrolyte imbalance.

Nursing Implications: Continuous infusion should be controlled with an infusion pump to insure accurate and safe administration. Monitor closely.
Never stop infusion suddenly—wean to a lower concentration or rate before stopping.
Monitor peripheral IV site for extravasation.
Monitor intake and output.
Monitor lab results as required.

Generic Name: DIAZEPAM

Trade Name: VALIUM

Classification: Benzodiazepine with antianxiety and sedative effects, Schedule IV controlled substance.

Actions: Acts to reduce anxiety by depressing the central nervous system at the subcortical level. The resultant effects are anticonvulsive, hypnotic, sedative antianxiety, and skeletal muscle relaxant. Will not stop abnormal activity from the focus of a seizure but will stop the spread of activity. Especially useful in treating status epilepticus.

Indications: Treatment of anxiety or short-term relief of anxiety symptoms. Used before some procedures to decrease anxiety and decrease patient's memory of the procedure. Also indicated for treatment of status epilepticus. After termination of seizure activity, maintenance anticonvulsant therapy should be begun.

Dosage:
Neonatal: 0.1–0.3 mg/kg; may be repeated every 3–5 minutes. Maximum dose: 5 mg.
Pediatric: 0.1–0.3 mg/kg; may be repeated every 3–5 minutes. Maximum dose: 10–15 mg.
Adult: 5–10 mg IV initially, maximum dose 30 mg in 1 hour; more may be administered depending on patient's response.

Preparation: Injectable form available as 5 mg/ml in 2-ml ampules and syringes, also 10-ml vials.

Compatibilities: Because of its propylene glycol diluent, Valium is not compatible with any other medication or IV solution.

Administration:
Neonatal: Slow IV bolus over 3 minutes, no faster than 5 mg/minute.

Pediatric: See neonatal administration.
Adult: Absorption of IM dose is variable. IV administration provides more reliable absorption. Rate should not exceed 5 mg/minute. Do not dilute.

Contraindications: Known hypersensitivity to benzodiazepines, acute alcohol intoxication, shock, coma, acute narrow-angle glaucoma, psychosis.

Side Effects:
Primary: Sedation, drowsiness. If given too rapidly by IV bolus may cause hypotension, respiratory depression, bradycardia, or cardiac arrest.
Secondary: Phlebitis at injection site, constipation, nausea.

Nursing Implications: Avoid too rapid IV administration. Monitor patient for hypotension and respiratory depression during administration.

Use with caution when administering with narcotic analgesics. May be necessary to decrease dosage.

Emergency equipment should be readily available in case of respiratory arrest.

Warn patient that drowsiness may occur. Assist with ambulation where appropriate.

After long-term therapy, dosage should be decreased gradually to prevent withdrawal symptoms.

This drug should be given by direct IV bolus. Infusion should be avoided because of the chance for precipitation with incompatible IV solutions and the chance the drug will be absorbed by the IV tubing.

Smoking will decrease the effectiveness of drug therapy. When possible encourage patient to stop smoking.

Generic Name: DIAZOXIDE

Trade Name: HYPERSTAT

Classification: Antihypertensive

Actions: Relaxes smooth muscle in the peripheral arterioles to lower peripheral resistance.

Indications: Severe nonmalignant and malignant hypertension.

Dosage:
Neonatal: Not applicable.
Pediatric: 1–3 mg/kg.
Adult: 1–5 mg/kg, not to exceed 150 mg per injection.

Preparation: 20-ml ampules containing 300 mg of diazoxide.

Home Stability: Not recommended for home use.

Compatibilities: Do not dilute. Diazoxide is to be administered undiluted rapidly for maximum effect.

Administration:
Neonatal: Not applicable.
Pediatric: Give calculated dose, undiluted, by IV push in less than 30 seconds through a peripheral vein, dosage not to exceed 150 mg per injection. May repeat in 5–15 minutes if needed. Repeat every 4–24 hours as needed for maintenance of blood pressure.
Adult: See pediatric administration.

Contraindications: Treatment of compensatory hypertension such as that with aortic coarctation or arteriovenous shunt. Hypersensitivity to diazoxide, thiazides, or sulfonamide-derived drugs. Use with caution in patients with impaired cerebral or cardiac circulation, diabetes, or uremia. Actions may be potentiated if used concurrently with other antihypertensives or thiazide diuretics. Do not administer within 6 hours of hydralazine, reserpine, alphaprodein, methyldopa, beta-blockers, prazosin, minoxidil, nitrates, or other papaverinelike compounds.

Side Effects:
Primary: Hypotension, orthostatic hypotension, nausea, vomiting, dizziness, weakness, headache, hyperglycemia, sodium and water retention.

Nursing Implications: Continuous blood pressure monitoring is preferred; if not possible, obtain baseline blood pressure and check every 3–5 minutes during administration of bolus and until pressure is stabilized. Hourly checks should then be continued.

Continuous cardiac monitoring is needed; observe for ischemic changes and arrhythmias.

Assess heart tones, jugular venous distension, peripheral edema, lung sounds, dyspnea, and capillary refill every 4 hours and as needed to ascertain effectiveness of the treatment.

Monitor fluid status via hourly urine outputs, intake, and daily weights.

Monitor electrolytes, particularly sodium.

Monitor glucose levels carefully; assess for signs of hyperglycemia or hyperosmolar nonketotic coma.

Monitor uric acid levels for increases.

Keep patient supine for 1 hour after administration, then observe for and teach patient about orthostatic hypotension.

Generic Name: DIETHYLSTILBESTROL DIPHOSPHATE

Trade Name: STILPHOSTROL

Classification: Synthetic estrogen

Actions: Potent, long-lasting, nonsteroidal estrogen. In male clients with androgenic hormone–dependent conditions such as metastatic carcinoma of the prostate, estrogens counter the androgenic influence by competing for receptor sites.

Indications: Palliative treatment of inoperable cancer of the prostate or treatment of breast carcinoma.

Dosage:
Neonatal: Not applicable.
Pediatric: Not applicable.
Adult: Initial dose: 0.5 g/24 hours, followed by 1 g daily for 5 days. Maintenance dose: 250–500 mg 1–2 times weekly.

Preparation: Supplied in 5-ml ampules containing 250 mg of drug.

Home Stability: Not applicable.

Compatibilities: Compatible with 0.9% sodium chloride or 5% dextrose in water. Do not mix with any other medication or IV solution.

Administration:
Neonatal: Not applicable.
Pediatric: Not applicable.
Adult: Dilute 0.5 g in 300 ml of 0.9% normal saline or 5% dextrose in water and administer at a rate of 1–2 ml/minute during the first 10–15 minutes; continue the infusion at a rate that will administer the remaining dose over 1 hour.

Contraindications: Known hypersensitivity, marked liver function, thrombophlebitis, thromboembolic disorders, cerebral thrombosis or embolism, or a past history of any of these disorders. Use with caution in clients with a history of renal insufficiency or metabolic bone diseases associated with hypercalcemia.

Warnings: Large doses of estrogen have been shown to increase the risk of nonfatal myocardial infarction, pulmonary embolism, and thrombophlebitis in men.
Discontinue the drug if there is sudden onset of proptosis, diplopia, or migraine, or if assessment reveals papilledema or retinal vascular lesions.

Side Effects:
Primary: A statistically significant association has been shown between use of estrogen-containing drugs and thrombophlebitis, pulmonary embolism, and cerebral thrombosis. An association also exists for retinal thrombosis and optic neuritis. Headache, malaise, nervousness, fatigue, depression, anxiety, dizziness, hypersensitivity reactions including anaphylaxis, rash, salt and water retention, edema, rise in blood urea nitrogen, hypercalcemia.
Secondary: Anorexia, nausea, vomiting, diarrhea, cholestatic jaundice, abdominal cramps, breast engorgement (male and female) and tenderness, loss of libido, acne, purpura, hair loss, erythema nodosum, itching, hemorrhagic eruption, erythema multiforme, sterile abscesses.

Nursing Implications: Assess for thrombophlebitis: pain, swelling, positive Homans' sign in the legs.
Assess for cerebral thrombosis: change in mental status, weakness and numbness of the face or extremities, seizures.
Assess for pulmonary embolism: sudden dyspnea, chest pain.
Assess for coronary thrombosis: chest pain, diaphoresis, decrease in blood pressure.
Assess clients susceptible to congestive heart failure for increase in weight, peripheral edema, increase in respiratory or heart rate, dyspnea or orthopnea, rales, and distended jugular veins.
Assess intake-output ratio. Report oliguria and changes in the intake-output ratio.
Instruct clients to take contraceptive measures.
Assess IV site frequently for signs of thrombophlebitis and for sterile abscess.
Assess baseline and periodic renal, hepatic, and hematologic functions, especially calcium and phosphorus levels; estrogen influences the metabolism of calcium and phosphorus.

Generic Name: DIGOXIN

Trade Name: LANOXIN, DIGOXIN INJECTION, DIGOXIN IN TUBEX

Classification: Cardiac glycoside

Actions: Increases the force of myocardial contraction, increases the refractory period of the atrioventricular node, and to a lesser degree affects the sinoatrial node and conduction system via the parasympathetic and sympathetic nervous system.

Indications: Congestive heart failure, especially low-output failure; atrial fibrillation; atrial flutter; and paroxysmal atrial tachycardia.

Dosage:

Neonatal and Pediatric: Digitalizing dose should be given in several portions, half the total given as the first dose followed by additional fractions at 4–8-hour intervals.

AGE	DIGITALIZING DOSE (μg/kg)
Preterm	15–25
Full term	20–30
1–24 months	30–50
2–5 years	25–35
5–10 years	15–30
Over 10 years	8–12

Daily maintenance dose for preterm infants is 20–30 percent of the loading dose; for other pediatric clients, 25–35 percent of the loading dose.

Adult: Loading dose of 400–600 μg followed at 4–8-hour intervals by additional doses of 100–300 μg. Usual total is 600–1000 μg.

General: These dosage guidelines are based on average patient response. Clinical response should be carefully assessed before each additional dose.

Preparation: Lanoxin: 500 μg in 2 ml, 100 μg in 1 ml (pediatric).

Home Stability: Not applicable.

Compatibilities: Compatible with solutions containing dextrose, saline.

Administration:

Pediatric: Dilute dosage in 5–10 ml and give slowly over 5 minutes.

Adult: See pediatric administration.

Contraindications: Digitalis toxicity, hypersensitivity, ventricular fibrillation, ventricular tachycardia. Use with caution in the elderly and in patients with acute myocardial infarction, severe pulmonary disease, advanced heart failure, hypothyroidism, and renal insufficiency. Also use cautiously in conjunction with drugs having potential for causing hypokalemia (amphotericin B, carbenicillin, ticarcillin, corticosteroids, and diuretics) and hypercalcemia and hypomagnesemia (parenteral calcium, thiazides). Usefulness in patients with Stokes-Adams attacks, chronic constrictive pericarditis, or idiopathic hypertrophic subaortic stenosis is doubtful. Quinidine and verapamil may cause an increase in serum digitalis concentration. Concomitant use of digoxin and sympathomimetics increases the risk of cardiac arrhythmias. Beta-adrenergic blockers or calcium channel blockers together with digoxin may cause complete heart block.

Side Effects (Toxic): Anorexia, nausea, vomiting, diarrhea, headache, weakness, agitation, apathy, yellow-green halos around visual images, blurred vision, ST depression, PR prolongation, premature ventricular contractions, paroxysmal and nonparoxysmal nodal rhythms, atrioventricular dissociation, paroxysmal atrial tachycardia with block, severe bradycardia, and atrioventricular blocks leading to complete heart block.

Nursing Implications: Dosage is highly individualized and must be adjusted to patient's clinical condition.

Obtain baseline data on heart rate and rhythm, blood pressure, and electrolytes before giving first dose.

Continuous cardiac monitoring is required during IV digitalization and essential if digitalis toxicity is suspected. Record and report to physician any significant changes (sudden increase or decrease in rate, irregular beats, and particularly regularization of a previously irregular rhythm). Obtain a blood pressure reading and a 12-lead EKG with these changes.

Hold if apical pulse is less than 60 beats/minute; notify physician.

Assess heart tones, jugular venous distension, peripheral edema, lung sounds, dyspnea, pulse quality, and the color, temperature, and capillary refill of extremities every 4 hours and as needed to ascertain the effectiveness of treatment.

Monitor serum potassium levels; hypokalemia causes the myocardium to be more sensitive to digitalis and tends to reduce the positive inotropic effect.

Monitor serum calcium levels; calcium affects contractility and excitability of the heart in a manner similar to that of digitalis.

Monitor serum magnesium levels; hypomagnesemia predisposes patients to digitalis toxicity.

Question patients about use of cardiac glycosides within the previous 2–3 weeks before administering a loading dose.

Assess for signs and symptoms of digitalis toxicity.

Take apical-radial pulse for a full minute. Report any significant pulse deficit to the physician.

Generic Name: DIGOXIN IMMUNE FAB

Trade Name: DIGIBIND

Classification: Digoxin binding agent

Actions: Promotes a rapid release of digoxin from binding sites in the heart by binding the digoxin to itself, thus rendering the digoxin inactive.

Indications: Digoxin (or digitoxin) intoxication.

Dosage:
Neonatal: Not applicable.
Pediatric: Calculated based on amount of digoxin in the body.
Adult: See pediatric dosage.
Duration of Therapy: Short-term therapy only.

Preparation: Each 5-ml vial contains 40 mg of purified digoxin antibody fragments.

Home Stability: Not applicable.

Compatibilities: Dissolve with sterile water for injection and dilute with normal saline. Do not infuse with other medications.

Administration:
Neonatal: Not applicable.
Pediatric: Dissolve with 4 ml of sterile water for injection; may dilute further with 36 ml of normal saline to achieve a concentration of 1 mg/ml. Small doses may be administered with a tuberculin syringe. Infuse over 30 minutes through a 0.22-micron filter.
Adult: Dissolve with 4 ml of sterile water for injection; may dilute further with normal saline. Infuse over 30 minutes through a 0.22-micron fil-

ter. If cardiac arrest is imminent, digoxin immune Fab can be given as a bolus injection.

Contraindications: None known, but use with caution in pregnancy and lactation and in patients who have had previous therapy with digoxin immune Fab.

Side Effects:
Primary: Reappearance of heart failure, rapid ventricular response to atrial fibrillation, hypokalemia.
Secondary: Possible allergic reaction, especially in those allergic to sheep proteins and those who have received digoxin immune Fab in the past.

Nursing Implications: Total serum digoxin levels will be inaccurate following administration of the drug. It causes such a great release of digoxin from the heart and tissues that, typically, total serum digoxin is 10–20-fold higher than pretreatment. However, essentially all of it is bound to digoxin immune Fab and therefore inactive.

Monitor cardiac rhythm continuously until the drug is eliminated from the body. This occurs within a few days, longer for patients with renal failure.

Monitor serum potassium levels carefully, especially over the first several hours after administration. When the effect of digitalis is reversed by digoxin immune Fab, potassium shifts back into the cells, and serum hypokalemia can result.

Improvement in signs and symptoms of digitalis intoxication usually begins within one-half hour or less.

Assess frequently for signs of congestive heart failure.

Digoxin therapy cannot be reinstated until digoxin immune Fab is eliminated from the body, which can take several days.

Generic Name: DIHYDROERGOTAMINE MESYLATE

Trade Name: DHE 45

Classification: Adrenergic blocking agent (vaso-constrictor)

Actions: Alpha-adrenergic blocking agent with a direct effect on peripheral and cranial blood vessels.

Indications: Prevention or abortion of vascular headaches.

Dosage:
Neonatal: Not applicable.
Pediatric: Not applicable.
Adult: 1 mg; may repeat after 1 hour. Total daily dosage not to exceed 2 mg; total weekly dosage not to exceed 6 mg.

Preparation: 1 mg in 1-ml ampules.

Home Stability: Not applicable.

Compatibilities: May infuse with dextrose, saline, or dextrose in saline.

Administration:
Neonatal: Not applicable.
Pediatric: Not applicable.
Adult: May give undiluted over 1 minute.

Contraindications: Hypersensitivity, peripheral and occlusive vascular disease, coronary artery disease, hypertension, hepatic or renal dysfunction, sepsis, pregnancy. Use cautiously with beta-blockers because of possible excessive vasoconstriction.

Side Effects:
Primary: Numbness and tingling in fingers and toes, transient tachycardia or bradycardia, precordial distress and pain, increased arterial pressure.
Secondary: Nausea, vomiting, itching, weakness in legs, muscle pain in extremities, localized edema.

Nursing Implications: Most effective when used to prevent migraine or soon after onset. Provide quiet, dark, low-stimulus environment and assist patient in relaxation. After migraine, explore stress factors and possible stress-reduction techniques with patient.

Use smallest dose that achieves desired effect.

Avoid prolonged administration; do not exceed dosage recommendations.

Instruct patient to report tingling, numbness, or feelings of cold in extremities; severe vasoconstriction may result in tissue damage. Provide careful skin care, avoid shearing forces, keep linens off of feet and toes, and protect skin from possible damage.

Generic Name: DIMENHYDRINATE

Trade Name: DRAMAMINE

Classification: Antiemetic

Actions: Exact mechanism of action unknown, but effects are antihistaminic, antiemetic, central nervous system depressant, and anticholinergic.

Indications: Treatment of symptoms of motion sickness including nausea, vomiting, and vertigo.

Dosage:
Neonatal and Pediatric: IV doses not established. IM: 1.25 mg/kg 4 times a day. Maximum dose: 300 mg/day.
Adult: IV and IM: 50 mg qid.

Preparation: Injectable 50 mg/ml.

Compatibilities: Compatible with normal saline.

Administration:
Neonatal and Pediatric: IM, rotate sites.

Adult: IM, IV: Mix in 10 normal saline; administer over not less than 2 minutes.

Contraindications: Hypersensitivity to dimenhydrinate or diphenhydramine. Use with caution in patients with narrow-angle glaucoma, myasthenia gravis, or cardiovascular disease.

Side Effects:
Primary: Drowsiness, mydriasis, dry mouth, urinary retention, tachycardia, hypotension.
Secondary: Dry respiratory passages, blurred vision, dizziness.

Nursing Implications: Obtain history of nausea and vomiting. Assess for signs for dehydration and obtain ordered laboratory work.

Observe patient for side effects during and after administration—hypotension, drowsiness, etc. Assist with ambulation as necessary. Patient may need to remain flat for a period of time.

Warn patient to use caution in doing tasks that require alertness.

Observe for any other symptoms. This drug can mask signs of toxicity or disease.

Generic Name: DIPHENHYDRAMINE HYDROCHLORIDE

Trade Name: **ALLERDRYL 50, BENADRYL**

Classification: Antihistamine

Actions: Competes with histamine for cell receptor sites.

Indications: Allergic reactions to blood or plasma, anaphylaxis, active treatment of motion sickness.

Dosage:
Neonatal: Not applicable.
Pediatric: 5 mg/kg/24 hours or 150 mg/m^2/24 hours divided into 4 doses. Maximum daily dosage: 300 mg.
Adult: 10–50 mg, 100 mg if needed. Maximum daily dosage: 400 mg.

Preparation: 10- and 30-ml vials containing 10 mg/ml.

Home Stability: Not applicable.

Compatibilities: May infuse with solutions containing dextrose, saline, or any combination thereof.

Administration:
Neonatal: Not applicable.
Pediatric: Dilute and infuse at a rate of 25 mg/minute.
Adult: See pediatric administration.

Contraindications: Hypersensitivity, asthma, MAO inhibitor therapy, use in newborn or premature infants. Use with caution in patients with narrow-angle glaucoma, peptic ulcer disease, prostatic hypertrophy, hypertension, and cardiac disease, as well as in the elderly. May have additive sedative effects with other central nervous system depressants.

Side Effects:
Primary: Drowsiness, nausea, dry mouth.
Secondary: Confusion, insomnia, headache, vertigo, palpitations, photosensitivity, diplopia, nasal stuffiness, vomiting, diarrhea, constipation, dysuria, urinary retention, urticaria.

Nursing Implications: Monitor vital signs frequently.
Assess for development of side effects, particularly in elderly or debilitated patients. Warn patients to avoid activities that require alertness until effects on the central nervous system are determined. Cool drinks, ice chips, hard candy, and sugarless gum can relieve dry mouth. Encourage fluids to help prevent constipation.
Monitor intake and output for development of urinary retention.
Discontinuation of drug should be done slowly.

Generic Name: DIPHTHERIA ANTITOXIN

Trade Name: GENERIC ONLY

Classification: Antitoxin

Actions: Neutralizes toxins produced by *Corynebacterium diphtheriae.*

Indications: Treatment of diphtheria.

Dosage:
All Ages:
Pharyngeal or Laryngeal Disease (48 Hours): 20,000–40,000 u.
Nasopharyngeal Lesions: 40,000–60,000 u.
Extensive Disease or Neck Swelling: 80,000–120,000 u.

Preparation: Injectable: 10,000- and 20,000-u vials.

Administration: IM or slow IV infusion. Any person with clinical symptoms should receive antitoxin immediately. All contacts of unimmunized persons with disease should receive prophylactic treatment.

Side Effects:
Primary: Anaphylaxis, serum sickness, skin rash, fever.
Secondary: Local pain or urticaria.

Nursing Implications: Allergy history is imperative before administration of horse serum.

Health history should include symptoms and history of exposure to diphtheria.

Monitor vital signs and assess for any signs of an upper respiratory obstruction.

Have supportive equipment and medications available because of the risk of anaphylactic reactions. Monitor closely during infusion.

Generic Name: DOBUTAMINE HYDROCHLORIDE

Trade Name: DOBUTREX

Classification: Adrenergic

Actions: Stimulation of the cardiac beta receptors produces an inotropic effect with comparatively mild chronotropic, hypertensive, arrhythmic, and vasodilative effects.

Indications: Short-term therapy for adults with cardiac decompensation due to depressed contractility.

Dosage:
Neonatal: Not applicable.
Pediatric: Not applicable.
Adult: Rate of infusion usually 2.5–10 $\mu g/kg/$ minute. Rarely, infusion rates up to 40 $\mu g/kg/$ minute have been required.

Preparation: White powder in vials equivalent to 250 mg of dobutamine.

Home Stability: Not applicable.

Compatibilities: Compatible in dextrose, saline, or sodium lactate solutions. Do not infuse with calcium gluconate, potassium phosphate, or in alkaline solutions. May infuse through the same tubing as dopamine, lidocaine, and potassium chloride.

Administration:
Neonatal: Not applicable.
Pediatric: Not applicable.
Adult: For continuous infusion only. Must be diluted in at least 50 ml prior to administration. Onset of action is within 1–2 minutes, but peak effects may not be seen for up to 10 minutes. Plasma half-life is 2 minutes.

Contraindications: Hypersensitivity, idiopathic hypertrophic subaortic stenosis. Additive effect when used with nitroprusside. Beta-blockers may make dobutamine ineffective.

Side Effects:
Primary: Increased heart rate, blood pressure, ventricular ectopy.
Secondary: Nausea, headache, anginal pain, nonspecific chest pain, palpitations, shortness of breath.

Nursing Implications: Record baseline heart rate and rhythm, blood pressure, quality of pulses, and color, temperature, and capillary refill of extremities before beginning infusion.

Continuous cardiac monitoring is essential during treatment. Report arrhythmias or changes in heart rate to physician.

Monitor blood pressure every 5 minutes during titration until stabilized, then every 15 minutes.

Monitoring of hemodynamic parameters is beneficial in assessing patient's response to therapy. Therapeutic effects should result in an increase in cardiac output and a decrease in pulmonary arteriole wedge pressure.

Assess heart tones, jugular venous distension, peripheral edema, lung sounds, dyspnea, pulse quality, and color, temperature, and capillary refill of extremities every 4 hours and as needed.

Fluid status should be monitored via hourly urine outputs, intake, daily weights, pulmonary arteriole wedge pressure, and central venous pressure.

Titrate according to physician's guidelines, avoiding an excessive blood pressure response, which can cause acute pulmonary edema, arrhythmias, and cardiac arrest.

Discontinue drug slowly, monitoring vital signs every 5 minutes until drug is stopped and blood pressure is stabilized.

Infuse via largest vein possible and assess IV site frequently for signs of infiltration or blanching along course of infused vein.

Infuse via automatic infusion pump.

Oxidation of dobutamine can cause pink discoloration of the solution, but there is no loss of potency if used within 24 hours of reconstitution.

Generic Name: DOPAMINE HYDROCHLORIDE

Trade Name: DOPASTAT, INTROPIN

Classification: Catecholamine

Actions: Exerts a positive inotropic effect on the myocardium, resulting in increased cardiac output. Can cause increased resistance in peripheral vascular beds and concomitant decreases in mesenteric and vascular beds that offset each other, resulting in static or decreased systemic vascular resistance.

Indications: Low cardiac output and hypotension related to myocardial infarction, trauma, endotoxic septicemia, open heart surgery, renal failure, chronic cardiac decompensation.

Dosage:
Neonatal: Not applicable.
Pediatric: Safety and efficacy in children has not been established.
Adult: 2–5 μg/kg/minute titrating in 5–10-μg increments every 10–30 minutes. Average dose is 20 μg/kg/minute, but doses up to 50 μg/kg/minute have been required in some instances to obtain the desired hemodynamic and/or renal response.

Preparation: 5-ml ampules (40 and 80 mg/ml), 10-ml jets (40 mg/ml), and 5-ml vials and jets (40, 80, and 160 mg/ml).

Home Stability: Not applicable.

Compatibilities: May infuse with saline, 5% dextrose in water, 5% dextrose in saline or half normal saline, 5% dextrose in lactated Ringer's, sodium lactate, and lactated Ringer's. Do not infuse with alkaline solutions.

Administration:
Neonatal: Not applicable.
Pediatric: Not applicable.
Adult: Continuous infusion only.

Contraindications: Uncorrected tachyarrhythmias, ventricular fibrillation, pheochromocy-toma. Use with caution in patients with occlusive vascular disease, cold injuries, diabetic endarteritis, arterial embolism and in pregnancy. Use cautiously with MAO inhibitors, cyclopropane, or halogenated hydrocarbon anesthetics.

Side Effects:
Primary: Necrosis and tissue sloughing with extravasation, hypotension, tachycardia.
Secondary: Angina, ectopy, headaches, nausea, vomiting, piloerection.

Nursing Implications: Record baseline heart rate and rhythm, blood pressure, quality of pulses, and color, temperature, and capillary refill of extremities before beginning infusion.

Continuous cardiac monitoring is essential during treatment. Report arrhythmias or changes in heart rate to physician.

Monitor blood pressure every 5 minutes during titration until stabilized, then every 15 minutes.

Monitoring of hemodynamic parameters is beneficial in assessing patient's response to therapy. Therapeutic effects should result in an increase in cardiac output and a decrease in pulmonary arteriole wedge pressure.

Assess heart tones, jugular venous distension, peripheral edema, lung sounds, dyspnea, pulse quality, and color, temperature, and capillary refill of extremities every 4 hours and as needed.

Monitor urinary output hourly. Report inadequate outputs to physician.

Infuse via automatic infusion pump.

Titrate according to physician's guidelines, avoiding an excessive blood pressure response, which can cause acute pulmonary edema, arrhythmias, and cardiac arrest.

Discontinue drug slowly, monitoring vital signs every 5 minutes until drug is stopped and blood pressure is stabilized.

Infuse via largest vein possible and assess IV site frequently for signs of infiltration or blanching along course of infused vein. If extravasation occurs, infiltrate site with 5–10 mg phentolamine within 12 hours.

Generic Name: DOXAPRAM HYDROCHLORIDE

Trade Name: DOPRAM

Classification: Respiratory stimulant

Actions: Acts on peripheral carotid chemoreceptors to stimulate respiration. When dosage level is increased, the central receptors are stimulated along with other parts of the brain and spinal cord. Respiratory depression due to opiates is antagonized. After administration, effect is seen within 20–40 seconds; duration of action is about 5–12 minutes.

Indications: Treatment of respiratory depression due to anesthesia, drug-induced central nervous system depression, and patients with chronic pulmonary disease in an acute hypercapnic state.

Dosage: Highly variable depending on condition under treatment. May be given as single dose, repeated doses, or infusion of varying strengths. Continual assessment and supportive treatment are necessary during administration. Not recommended for children under 12.

Preparation: 20 mg/ml injectable.

Compatibilities: Compatible with 5% or 10% dextrose in normal saline or water.

Administration: See Dosage.

Contraindications: Any convulsive state, impaired respiratory mechanism (muscle paresis, flail chest, pneumothorax, airway obstruction), cerebrovascular accident, hypertension, hypersensitivity, head injury, pulmonary disease (pulmonary embolism), bronchial asthma, neuromuscular disorders causing respiratory failure, pulmonary fibrosis or other restrictive disease, coronary artery disease, frank uncompensated heart failure. Use with caution in patients with cerebral edema, any cardiac arrhythmia, and in pregnancy. Dopram by itself may not stimulate breathing enough in drug-induced respiratory depression.

Side Effects:

Primary: Headache, dizziness, apprehension, seizures, disorientation, pupillary dilation, chest pain, arrhythmias, cough, dyspnea.

Secondary: Sneezing, nausea, vomiting, diarrhea, urinary retention or incontinence.

Nursing Implications: Obtain accurate history of respiratory depression, especially if drug-induced.

Monitor vital signs closely, also laboratory results (blood gases).

Maintain patent airway. Have emergency equipment available.

Assess level of consciousness and nature of respirations. Document effectiveness of therapy.

Generic Name: DOXORUBICIN HYDROCHLORIDE

Trade Name: ADRIAMYCIN

Classification: Antineoplastic antibiotic

Actions: Interferes with nucleic acid synthesis by binding with DNA and preventing DNA-directed RNA and DNA transcription. Although most active in the S phase, considered cell-cycle nonspecific since it has some activity during all phases.

Indications: Sarcomas, carcinomas, melanomas, leukemias, lymphomas, neuroblastomas.

Dosage:
Neonatal: Not applicable.
Pediatric: IV: 60–90 mg/m^2 every 3 weeks or 20–30 mg/m^2 3 times every 3 weeks or 30 mg/m^2 every week or 60–90 mg/m^2 by IV drip over 10–96 hours every 3–4 weeks.
   Intra-arterially: 25 mg/m^2 every day for 3 days.
   Intraperitoneally or into the bladder: 30–60 mg/m^2 in 150 ml of normal saline every month.
Adult: See pediatric dosage.

Preparation: A red powder, available in 10- and 50-mg vials, which can be mixed with sterile water and D$_5$W or normal saline for IV push administration.

Home Stability: Unopened vials are stable for 2 years if protected from light and stored at room temperature. In solution, doxorubicin is stable for 24 hours at room temperature and 48 hours in the refrigerator. It should be protected from light if not used within 8 hours.

Compatibilities: Not compatible with aminophylline, dexamethasone, keflin, fluorouracil, diazepam, heparin, and hydrocortisone, and the same final filter should not be used with these drugs. Necrotizing colitis has occurred with Ara-C. Barbiturates increase the plasma clearance of doxorubicin. Mercaptopurine increases doxorubicin hepatotoxicity. Doxorubicin decreases the effectiveness of oral digoxin. Compatible with dacarbazine and has been mixed with it in liter solutions and infused over 24 hours for 4 days. However, as with most antineoplastic agents, it is usually advisable not to administer doxorubicin with other admixture solutions.

Administration:
Neonatal: Not applicable.
Pediatric: Administer by slow IV push into the side arm of a free-flowing IV, checking for patency every 2–3 minutes to avoid extravasation of this severe vesicant. This drug should not be given by IV drip through a peripheral IV.
Adult: See pediatric administration.

Contraindications: Allergy to lincomycin, bone marrow depression, poor liver function (dose reductions required for serum bilirubin greater than 1.2), congestive heart failure. Watch for cardiotoxicity in patients with hypertension, coronary artery disease, angina, and previous myocardial infarction. To prevent irreversible cardiotoxicity, cumulative doses should not exceed 550 mg/m^2 with doxorubicin or daunorubicin or 450 mg/m^2 with cyclophosphamide or mitomycin or previous radiation therapy to the chest. Concurrent administration of vitamin E or N-acetylcysteine or weekly or continuous drip administration of doxorubicin may decrease cardiotoxicity. Dose reductions should also be considered if other anthracyclines have been given. Single doses of more than 150 mg should be double-checked.

Side Effects:
Primary:
Hematopoietic: Decreased white blood cells after 7–14 days, with recovery in 1–3 weeks.
Cutaneous: Extensive tissue damage if extravasated; radiation "recall" on previously irradiated areas of the skin, the esophagus, and the lung; complete and often sudden hair loss that is reversible.
Cardiac Toxicity: Pericarditis, myocarditis, EKG changes, hypotension, and usually irreversible cardiomyopathy.
Gastrointestinal: Moderate nausea and vomiting, stomatitis, esophagitis, and diarrhea. Ascites and adhesions occur with intraperitoneal administration.
Nephrotoxicity: Urine will be red for 24–48 hours after administration. Bladder instillations may cause urgency, local irritation, and cystitis.

Increased uric acid levels occur with rapid tumor lysis.

Reproductive: Teratogenic and probably causes infertility.

Secondary: Decreased platelets and RBCs, hyperpigmentation of the skin, nailbed changes, conjunctivitis, and excessive tearing and facial flushing if the drug is administered too fast. Hives and/or red streaking may appear along the vein where the drug is being administered. This necessitates slowing administration, increasing flushing of the vein, and applying heat along with elevation of the arm to increase venous flow. Hypersensitivity reactions are infrequent. Risk of secondary malignancy is unknown.

Nursing Implications: Monitor CBC.

Instruct patient and family on infection precautions during the second and fourth weeks after treatment.

Establish and maintain good venous access, checking for patency every 2–3 minutes during IV push administration and instructing the patient to report any sensations of burning or pain. Do not give by continuous infusion through a peripheral vein. Consult a plastic surgeon immediately if extravasation is suspected, since the drug remains active for 10 days or more and may continue to cause tissue damage (ulcerations to the bone have occurred) unless surgically removed.

Inform the patient of probable complete hair loss, which may occur all at once. Reassure patient that condition is reversible.

Inform the patient of possible skin changes at previous radiation therapy sites. Also, the patient may have esophageal discomfort and difficulty swallowing if this area has been previously irradiated.

Inform patient of expected red discoloration of urine.

Monitor uric acid levels and prepare to administer allopurinol.

Observe closely for signs of cardiac changes, especially congestive heart failure.

Record cumulative dose with administration of each new dose.

Remind physician to obtain and compare periodic systolic time interval ratios.

Premedicate with antiemetics and continue them for 24 hours afterward.

Emphasize good oral hygiene with a soft-bristled toothbrush.

Obtain an order for an antidiarrheal if necessary.

Inform patient of possibility of birth defects if pregnancy occurs while taking doxorubicin and of probable sterility.

Safe-handling precautions should continue for 10 days after the last dose of doxorubicin.

Generic Name: DOXYCYCLINE HYCLATE

Trade Name: VIBRAMYCIN

Classification: Antibiotic (tetracycline)

Actions: Broad-spectrum antibiotic with bactericidal action against Rickettsia, *Mycoplasma pneumoniae,* agents of psittacosis and ornithosis, agents of lymphogranuloma venereum and relapsing fever, and infections caused by the following gram-negative organisms: *Hemophilus ducreyi, Pasteurella pestis* and *tularensis, Bartonella bacilliformis,* Bacteroides, *Vibrio comma* and *fetus,* Brucella. When bacteriologic testing indicates susceptibility, doxycycline hyclate is an alternate drug of choice for the following organisms: *Escherichia coli, Enterobacter aerogenes,* Shigella, Mima, Herellea, *H. influenza,* Klebsiella, Streptococcus, *Diplococcus pneumoniae,* and *Staphylococcus aureus.* When penicillin is contraindicated, doxycycline hyclate is indicated in the treatment of *Neisseria gonnorrhoeae, Treponema pallidum,* Clostridium, *Bacillus anthracis, Fusobacterium fusiforme,* and Antinomyces.

Indications: For action against the above-stated organisms when sensitivity testing shows susceptibility.

Dosage:
Neonatal: Not recommended.
Pediatric:
8 Years and over Weighing 45 kg or Less: Initial 2 doses: 4.4 mg/kg/day in divided doses every 12 hours with subsequent dosage of 2.2 mg/kg/day given once daily or in 2 equally divided doses.
8 Years and over Weighing 45 kg or More: Initial dose: 200 mg/day in divided doses every 12–24 hours with subsequent dosage of 100–200 mg/day given once daily or in 2 equally divided doses depending on the severity of the causative organism.
Adult: Initial dose: 200 mg/day in divided doses every 12–24 hours with subsequent dosage of 100–200 mg/day given once daily or in 2 equally divided doses depending on the severity of the causative organism. Continued administration for at least 24–48 hours after symptoms and fever have subsided. In the treatment of primary and secondary syphilis, recommended dosage is 300 mg/day for at least 10 days. Studies indicate that use of recommended doses does not lead to excessive accumulation in those with renal impairment.

Preparation: Supplied as a powder. Reconstitute with sterile water for injection: add 10 ml of diluent to a 100-mg vial and 20 ml to a 200-mg vial.

Home Stability: Protect the solution from direct sunlight. Infuse within 12 hours of preparation. Darkening solution indicates deterioration of the medication. If lactated Ringer's or 5% dextrose with lactated Ringer's is used, infuse within 6 hours of preparation. Discontinue the solution.

Compatibilities: Compatible with solutions containing dextrose, saline, Ringer's, or lactated Ringer's. Do not administer with total parenteral nutrition or any other medication. Infusion must be completed within 6 hours when administered with lactated Ringer's.

Administration:
Neonatal: Not recommended.
Pediatric: Further dilute the drug to a concentration of 0.5 mg/ml and infuse over 1–4 hours. Administer via infusion pump.
Adult: Further dilute the drug to a concentration of 0.5 mg/ml and infuse over 1–4 hours or administer via continuous infusion over 12 hours at a concentration of 0.1–0.4 mg/ml. Protect the solution from direct sunlight. Administer via infusion pump.

Contraindications: Hypersensitivity to the drug. Not recommended in pregnancy or lactation. Use of this drug during the years of tooth development can cause permanent discoloration of the teeth and enamel hypoplasia. Do not use tetracyclines in this age group or in pregnancy unless other drugs are ineffective or contraindicated.

Side Effects:
Primary: Hypersensitivity reactions including anaphylaxis, liver damage, photosensitivity, systemic moniliasis, thrombophlebitis, renal toxicity including a rise in BUN.

Secondary: Anorexia, nausea, vomiting, diarrhea, glossitis, dysphagia, enterocolitis, *Candida albicans* overgrowth in the perineal area (Monilia) and mouth (thrush), hemolytic anemia, thrombocytopenia. In infants: bulging fontanels, papilledema, which usually disappears with discontinuation of the drug.

Nursing Implications: Prior to and during therapy, culture and sensitivity tests should be completed.

Monitor for allergic reactions.

Monitor baseline and periodic renal, hepatic, and hematologic functions.

Monitor for superinfection. Assess for the onset of black, hairy tongue; oral lesions (stomatitis, glossitis); rectal or vaginal itching; vaginal discharge; loose, foul-smelling stools; unusual odor to urine.

Monitor infusion site for signs of thrombophlebitis.

Clients on anticoagulants may require lower doses of those drugs while on doxycycline hyclate.

Monitor intake-output ratios. Notify physician of gastrointestinal disturbance or changes in renal status.

Notify physician of signs of increasing intracranial pressure.

Generic Name: DROPERIDOL

Trade Name: INAPSINE

Classification: Neuroleptic agent

Actions: Used only preoperatively during induction and maintenance of anesthesia. Produces marked sedation and antiemetic effect. May also potentiate other central nervous system depressants. May cause hypotension and decrease peripheral vascular resistance. Acts within 3–10 minutes with full effect in 30 minutes. Has duration of 2–4 hours.

Indications: To produce tranquilization and decrease occurrence of nausea and vomiting during surgical procedures. Also used as adjunct in maintaining anesthesia.

Dosage: Individualized based on patient's age, weight, health status, and other variables. The following are guidelines only.
Neonatal: Not applicable.
Pediatric (2–12 Years): 1–1.5 mg/20–25 pounds.
Adult: 2.5–10 mg IM or IV.

Preparation: Injectable 2.5 mg/ml.

Home Stability: Not appropriate for home use.

Administration: IV or IM only.

Contraindications: Intolerance or hypersensitivity.

Side Effects:
Primary: Hypotension, tachycardia, extrapyramidal effects. Hypertension is possible if administered with narcotic analgesics.
Secondary: Postoperative drowsiness, dizziness, chills and shivering.

Nursing Implications: Monitor vital signs closely.

Assess patient when administering premedication dose for signs of adverse reactions. Take vital signs before administration. Hold if respirations are depressed.

Have supportive equipment available for use: oxygen, suction equipment, etc.

Give medication 30–60 minutes before the procedure to allow for full effect.

Generic Name: EDETATE CALCIUM DISODIUM (EDTA)

Trade Name: CALCIUM DISODIUM VERSENATE

Classification: Heavy metal antagonist

Actions: Treatment of acute and chronic lead poisoning. The calcium is easily displaced by the ions of lead to form stable complexes that can be excreted in the urine. Excretion of lead usually begins about 1 hour after parenteral administration and reaches a peak after 24–48 hours. Oral administration should be avoided because it may enhance lead absorption.

Indications: Lead poisoning and lead encephalopathy.

Dosage:
Neonatal and Pediatric: 30–50 mg/kg/day in divided doses for 3–5 days. Rest for 2 days, then repeat. It is not unusual for children to require 2 courses of therapy. Maximum dose is 70 mg/kg/day.
Adult: 1 g in 250–500 ml of D_5W or 0.9% normal saline infused over 1–2 hours daily or every 12 hours for 3–5 days. Repeat after 2 days if indicated.

Preparation: Injectable form available as 200 mg/ml in 5-ml ampules.

Compatibilities: Compatible with D_5W or 0.9% normal saline. Not compatible with $D_{10}W$, Ringer's, lactated Ringer's, protein hydrolysates, or 10% invert sugar.

Administration:
Neonatal and Pediatric: Deep IM route is preferred. IV infusion over 2 hours if patient is symptomatic; 6–8 hours is preferred.

Adult: Infusion over 1–2 hours. May give every 12 hours in divided doses. Physician should order infusion and rate.

Contraindications: Severe renal disease and anuria. IV form is contraindicated in lead encephalopathy because of increased intracranial pressure.

Side Effects:
Primary: Rapid IV administration can cause increased intracranial pressure. Less often, IV doses may cause nausea, vomiting, headache, hypotension, and inverted T waves on EKG. Nephrotoxicity can lead to renal tubular necrosis.
Secondary: Fever, chills, thrombophlebitis, histaminelike reactions.

Nursing Implications: Assessment of patient's environment to identify sources of lead.

Physical assessment should be done to document symptoms of lead poisoning. They may include abdominal pain, tarry stools, metallic taste, diarrhea, anorexia with weight loss, sensory disturbances, ataxia, convulsions, and coma.

Obtain baseline data on urine output. Initiate measurement of intake and output.

If giving dosage IM rotate sites. Procaine may be added to dose to decrease discomfort.

Monitor patient as follows: infusion rate every 15 minutes, vital signs at least every 4 hours, urine output, CNS symptoms, and relief of other symptoms of lead poisoning.

Once the source of lead is determined, education of the family may be necessary to prevent further ingestion.

Monitor lead levels.

Generic Name: EDROPHONIUM CHLORIDE

Trade Name: TENSILON

Classification: Cholinergic

Actions: Drugs in this classification act to facilitate transmission of impulses across the myoneural junction and inhibit destruction of acetylcholine. They have a variety of onsets and durations of action.

Indications: This family of drugs is indicated in the diagnosis and treatment of myasthenia gravis. Edrophonium can also be used specifically when a curare antagonist is needed. The duration of action is very short.

Dosage: Varies greatly depending on condition under treatment and age of patient, with range from 0.5–10 mg IV.

Preparation: Injectable 10 mg/ml.

Administration:

All Ages: IV is recommended route although it may be administered IM.

Contraindications: Hypersensitivity, obstructions (mechanical intestinal and urinary), bradycardia, hypotension. Use with caution in patients with bronchial asthma or cardiac dysrhythmias. Atropine and epinephrine should be available in case of hypersensitivity reaction. Do not use neostigmine bromide or pyridostigmine bromide in patients with urinary tract infections or a history of hypersensitivity to bromides.

Side Effects: The following side effects may occur but have not been observed with each agent.

Primary: Ocular changes; convulsions; dysphonia; dysphagia; respiratory changes including increased secretions, paralysis, and laryngospasm; arrhythmias, gastrointestinal disturbances, muscle weakness.

Secondary: Urinary frequency and incontinence, thrombophlebitis with IV use.

Nursing Implications: Complete assessment of patient, including symptoms observed.

Emergency equipment should be readily available in case of hypersensitivity reaction.

Observe myasthenic patient for any exacerbation of symptoms.

If drug is being administered as curare antagonist, observe patient for return of muscle movement.

If patient has myasthenia gravis, determine if in a crisis or in a cholinergic crisis. Because symptoms are so similar, it may be necessary to do an edrophonium test.

Monitor vital signs closely.

Patient teaching should include spacing activities to avoid fatigue, signs of drug overdosage or underdosage, and need for follow-up care and close medical supervision.

Generic Name: EPHEDRINE SULFATE

Trade Name: BRONKAID, MARAX, PAZO, THEOFEDRAL

Classification: Cerebral stimulant

Actions: Alkaloid sympathomimetic that has a positive inotropic action resulting in a stronger myocardial contraction as well as an elevated heart rate and blood pressure. Vasoconstricts the arterioles, relaxes the smooth muscle of the bronchi, and dilates the pupils. Increases the metabolic and respiratory rate.

Indications: Pressor agent during spinal anesthesia, Stokes-Adams syndrome, and narcotic, barbiturate, and alcoholic poisoning.

Dosage:
Neonatal: Not applicable.
Pediatric: 3 mg/kg/day divided into 4–6 doses.
Adult: 25–50 mg repeated every 3–4 hours as needed, not to exceed 150 mg/day.

Home Stability: Not applicable.

Compatibilities: May infuse with dextrose or saline solutions. Not compatible with alkaline solutions.

Administration:
Neonatal: Not applicable.
Pediatric: 10 mg/minute, undiluted.
Adult: 10 mg/minute, undiluted.

Contraindications: Hypersensitivity, labor and delivery if maternal blood pressure exceeds 130/80 mmHg, overdose of phenothiazines. Use with caution in patients with heart disease, angina, diabetes, hyperthyroidism, and prostatic hypertrophy. Hypertensive crisis may occur in conjunction with MAO inhibitors. May cause cardiac arrhythmias with digitalis; may cause severe hypertension with ergonovine or oxytocin, hypotension and bradycardia with hydantoins. Potentiated by tricyclic antidepressants and urinary alkalizers.

Side Effects:
Primary: Cardiac arrhythmias, nausea, nervousness, palpitation, precordial pain, sweating, tachycardia.
Secondary: Anorexia, headache, insomnia, painful urination, urinary retention, vertigo, vomiting. With higher doses, confusion, delirium, euphoria, and hallucinations may occur.

Nursing Implications: Assess pulse rate and rhythm, blood pressure, and respiratory rate and pattern before infusion and every 5 minutes during therapy until stable.
Assess IV site for patency; can cause necrosis at site.
Assess neurological status during therapy.

Generic Name: EPINEPHRINE HYDROCHLORIDE

Trade Name: ADRENALIN

Classification: Adrenergic

Actions: Most potent alpha receptor agent also possessing beta receptor action; imitates all actions of the sympathetic nervous system except those on the arteries of the face and sweat glands.

Indications: For restoration of cardiac rhythm in cardiac arrest.

Dosage:
Neonatal: Not applicable.
Pediatric: 10 μg/kg.
Adult: 0.5–1.0 mg IV, may follow with a continuous infusion of 1–4 μg/minute.

Preparation: Sterile clear liquid in concentrations of 1:100 (1 mg = 1 ml) and 1:10,000 (1 mg = 10 ml).

Home Stability: Not applicable.

Compatibilities: May infuse with solutions containing 5% dextrose in water, saline, or any combination of the two. Do not mix with alkaline solutions.

Administration:
Neonatal: Not applicable.
Pediatric: Give by IV push, diluting 1 mg in 10 ml. Give before sodium bicarbonate.
Adult: See pediatric administration.

Contraindications: Narrow-angle (congestive) glaucoma, shock, cardiac dilatation, coronary insufficiency, organic brain damage, during general anesthesia with halogenated hydrocarbons or cyclopropane, and during labor. Use with extreme caution in patients with long-standing bronchial asthma and emphysema associated with degenerative heart disease. Use with caution in the elderly and patients with hyperthyroidism, angina, hypertension, psychoneurosis, or diabetes. Concurrent use with digitalis, mercurial diuretics, or propranolol is not recommended. Tricyclic antidepressants may potentiate actions.

Side Effects:
Primary: Tachycardia, ventricular fibrillation, cerebrovascular accident, nervousness, headache, hyperglycemia, pallor.
Secondary: Hypertension, widened pulse pressure, angina, pulmonary edema, dyspnea, cerebral hemorrhage, disorientation, agitation.

Nursing Implications: Continuous cardiac monitoring is essential; record rhythm and rate before administration and with any changes thereafter.

Resuscitation efforts must be continued until cardiac rhythm is achieved. External cardiac massage is vital after epinephrine administration so that the drug can be circulated.

After restoration of rhythm, continue frequent checks of heart rhythm, rate, quality of pulses, and blood pressure. Notify physician of any changes.

Generic Name: ERGONOVINE MALEATE

Trade Name: ERGOTRATE MALEATE

Classification: Oxytocic

Actions: Increases the strength, duration, and frequency of uterine contractions and decreases uterine bleeding by directly stimulating the smooth muscle of the uterus and vasoconstricting the uterine vessels.

Indications: For prevention or control of postpartum or postabortal hemorrhage. Investigationally indicated for the diagnosis of Prinzmetal's angina.

Dosage:
Adult: 0.2 mg IV for emergency use only. For severe uterine bleeding, may require a repeated dose every 2–4 hours.
Investigational Dosage: 0.05 mg–0.2 mg IV during coronary arteriography to provoke spontaneous coronary arterial spasms responsible for Prinzmetal's angina.

Compatibilities: Do not mix with other medications.

Administration:
Adult: Administer at IV site via stopcock or T-connector undiluted. IV route is reserved for lifesaving measures; administer over a period of at least 60 seconds.

Contraindications: Hypersensitivity, pregnancy, induction of labor, cases of threatened spontaneous abortion.

Side Effects:
Primary: Hypertensive or cardiovascular accidents in the presence of regional anesthesia (caudal or spinal) and with ephedrine, epinephrine, methoxamine, and other vasopressors.
Secondary: Nausea, vomiting, diarrhea, hypersensitivity, ergotism, elevation of blood pressure, headache.

Nursing Implications: Assess blood pressure prior to administration and every 3–5 minutes after administration. Notify physician of any changes in vital signs.
Assess uterine response every 15 minutes after administration. Notify physician of change in uterine response (severe cramping or atony).
Assess client's calcium level; uterine response may be poor in calcium-deficient clients. Administer a calcium supplement if ordered.
Assess for signs of ergotism, although rare. They include pale, cold, or numb fingers and toes, nausea, vomiting, diarrhea, headache, and muscle pain or weakness. Notify physician.

Generic Name: ERYTHROMYCIN LACTOBIONATE
ERYTHROMYCIN GLUCEPTATE

Trade name: GENERIC ONLY
ILOTYCIN GLUCEPTATE

Classification: Antibiotic

Actions: Bacteriostatic antibiotic against Group A beta-hemolytic streptococcus, alpha-hemolytic streptococcus, *Staphylococcus aureus,* *Streptococcus pneumoniae, Mycoplasma pneumoniae, Hemophilus influenzae, Corynebacterium diphtheriae, Listeria monocytogenes,* and *Neisseria gonorrhoeae.*

Indications: When penicillin is contraindicated, to treat susceptible strains of infections caused by staphylococci, pneumococci, and streptococci, gonorrhea, syphilis, Legionnaires' disease, and active diphtheria in conjunction with antitoxin and for prophylaxis against endocarditis preoperatively in clients with a history of rheumatic fever or congenital heart disease.

Dosage:
Neonatal: 30–50 mg/kg/24 hours administered every 6 hours.
Pediatric: 15–20 mg/kg/24 hours divided into even doses and administered every 6 hours or by continuous infusion. Maximum dosage: 4 g/ 24 hours.
Adult: See pediatric dosage and the following.
Acute Pelvic Inflammatory Disease Caused by *N. gonorrhoeae:* 500 mg every 6 hours for 3 days followed by 250 mg of oral erythromycin every 6 hours for 7 days.
Legionnaires' Disease: 1–4 g/day in divided doses. Optimal doses have not been established.
General: Reduced dosage is indicated in the presence of hepatic impairment.

Preparation: Supplied as a powder in the following vial sizes: 250 mg, 500 mg, and 1000 mg. Reconstitute with sterile water for injection only. Do not use bacteriostatic water for injection. Dilute as follows:

VIAL SIZE	DILUENT	CONCENTRATION
250 mg	10 ml	25 mg/ml
500 mg	10 ml	50 mg/ml
1000 mg	20 ml	50 mg/ml

Home Stability: After reconstitution, store in refrigerator. Erythromycin lactobionate is stable for 14 days refrigerated and 24 hours at room temperature. Erythromycin gluceptate is stable for 7 days refrigerated.

Compatibilities:
Erythromycin Gluceptate: Compatible with 5% dextrose in water or normal saline if administered within 4 hours. When adding erythromycin gluceptate to a volume of solution that must be infused over more than 4 hours, buffer the solution to a pH of 7 using a sodium bicarbonate 4% solution.
Erythromycin Lactobionate: When added to 5% dextrose in water, 5% dextrose in lactated Ringer's, 5% dextrose in normal saline, Normosol-M in 5% dextrose in water, or Normosol-R in 5% dextrose in water, buffering compounds must first be added to the solution. When infusing with normal saline, lactated Ringer's, or Normosol-R without 5% dextrose, buffering is not indicated. Once diluted, use within 8 hours.
General: Do not mix with other medications or total parenteral nutrition.

Administration:
Neonatal: Further dilute solution to a concentration of 1000 mg in 100 ml of solution and infuse solution over 20–60 minutes. Slow infusion if pain at IV site develops.
Pediatric: See neonatal administration.
Adult: Further dilute solution to a concentration of 1000 mg in 100 ml of solution and infuse solution over 20–60 minutes or via continuous infusion over 4 hours. Continuous infusion is the method of choice. Slow infusion if pain at IV site develops.

Contraindications: Hypersensitivity to the drug. Safety in pregnancy and lactation has not been established; the drug does cross the placental barrier and is excreted in breast milk.

Side Effects:
Primary: Hypersensitivity reactions including anaphylaxis.
Secondary: Venous irritation, reversible hearing loss (with 4 g or more per day), and altered liver function tests.

Nursing Implications: Prior to and during therapy, culture and sensitivity tests should be completed.

Monitor for hypersensitivity reactions.

Monitor baseline and periodic renal and hepatic functions.

Monitor for superinfection: fever, redness, soreness, pain, swelling, drainage, monilial rash in perineal area, change in cough, diarrhea.

Monitor digoxin and theophylline levels. Concurrent administration with erythromycin will potentiate these levels.

Generic Name: ESMOLOL HYDROCHLORIDE

Trade Name: BREVIBLOC

Classification: Antiarrhythmic, beta-blocking agent

Actions: Inhibits the beta-1 receptors located chiefly in cardiac muscle, causing a decrease in heart rate.

Indications: Supraventricular tachycardia; specifically atrial fibrillation and atrial flutter.

Dosage:
Neonatal: Not applicable.
Pediatric: Not applicable.
Adult: Initial loading dose of 500 μg/kg/minute over 1 minute followed by maintenance infusion of 50 μg/kg/minute. If desired effect is not achieved after 4 minutes of the maintenance dose, the loading dose may be repeated and the maintenance infusion increased by 50 μg/kg/minute. Maintenance doses over 200 μg/kg/minute are not recommended.

Duration of Therapy: For short-term therapy only.

Preparation: 2.5 mg/ampule.

Home Stability: Not applicable.

Compatibilities: Compatible with solutions of dextrose, normal saline, Ringer's, lactated Ringer's, and any combination of the above. Compatible with potassium chloride (40 mEq/l) in 5% dextrose. Not compatible with sodium bicarbonate.

Administration:
Neonatal: Not applicable.
Pediatric: Not applicable.
Adult: Dilute two 2.5-mg ampules in 500 ml or diluent and administer as a loading dose or maintenance infusion. Do not administer undiluted.

Contraindications: Sinus bradycardia, heart block greater than first degree, overt heart failure, cardiogenic shock. Use with caution in patients with hypotension, cardiac failure, bronchospastic disease, diabetes, and hypoglycemia.

Side Effects:
Primary: Hypotension and infusion-site phlebitis.
Secondary: Somnolence, dizziness, confusion, agitation, wheezing, dyspnea, nausea.

Nursing Implications: Patient should be on continuous cardiac monitoring during therapy.

Keep patient supine during therapy.

Monitor heart rate, rhythm, and blood pressure every minute during loading doses and titration. Following stabilization on maintenance dose, monitor vital signs every 5 minutes.

Breath sounds should be assessed every 4–5 minutes during therapy, as well as other indicators of congestive heart failure.

Infuse via infusion pump.

Titration is based on heart rate response. Once the drug is discontinued, the effects are reversed within 10–20 minutes. Oral agents, if desired, should be introduced during esmolol therapy with reduction of the esmolol dosage by one-half. Esmolol can be discontinued if the heart rate is stabilized 1 hour after the second dose of the oral agent.

Generic Name: ETHACRYNATE SODIUM

Trade Name: EDECRIN SODIUM

Classification: Diuretic

Actions: Acts on the ascending limb of the loop of Henle and on the proximal and distal tubules, inhibiting the reabsorption of sodium to a greater extent than most diuretic agents.

Indications: Treatment of edema associated with congestive heart failure, pulmonary edema, cirrhosis of the liver, and renal disease including nephrotic syndrome; short-term management of ascites.

Dosage:
Neonatal: Not recommended.
Pediatric: Not recommended.
Adult: 0.5–1.0 mg/kg. Normal dose for average-sized adult is 50 mg. Usually only one IV dose is needed.

Preparation: Vials of dry white powder containing 50 mg of ethacrynic acid.

Home Stability: Not applicable.

Compatibilities: May infuse with dextrose or sodium chloride solutions or any combination of the two.

Administration:
Neonatal: Not applicable.
Pediatric: Not applicable.
Adult: Add 50 ml of 5% dextrose injection or sodium chloride to the vial; do not use if resulting solution is hazy or opalescent. Give slowly through the tubing of a running injection over a period of several minutes.

Contraindications: Hypersensitivity, anuria. Use with caution in patients with electrolyte imbalance, advanced cirrhosis of the liver. Avoid giving concurrently with drugs known to have ototoxic effects. May potentiate effects of warfarin. Additive effect when used with other diuretics.

Side Effects:
Primary: Volume depletion; dehydration; muscle cramps; orthostatic hypotension; paresthesia; thirst; anorexia; sudden onset of watery, profuse diarrhea; deafness; tinnitus; vertigo; sense of fullness in the ears; hyponatremia; hypochloremic alkalosis; hypokalemia.
Secondary: Skin rash, headache, fever, chills, hematuria, blurred vision, fatigue, apprehension, confusion.

Nursing Implications: Potential for volume and electrolyte depletion leading to profound water loss, dehydration, reduction in blood volume, and circulatory collapse. Therefore monitor intake and output, serum electrolytes, blood pressure, and pulse rate frequently.

Assess for signs of hypokalemia (muscle weakness and cramping). Teach patients about potassium-rich foods (citrus fruits, tomatoes, bananas, dates, apricots). Be especially careful with patients receiving digitalis because of the risk of digitalis toxicity.

Caution patient to change position slowly because of orthostatic hypotension.

Monitor BUN and creatinine for signs of deteriorating renal function.

Administer in the morning to prevent nocturia.

Elderly patients are especially susceptible to excessive diuresis.

Generic Name: ETOPOSIDE/VP-16

Trade Name: VEPESID

Classification: Antineoplastic plant alkaloid

Actions: Inhibits cells from entering mitosis and disrupts cell division at metaphase if they have already entered mitosis. Also depresses DNA, RNA, and protein synthesis to some extent, especially at the G_2 and S phases, and is therefore considered cell-cycle nonspecific.

Indications: Nonlymphocytic leukemias, oat cell lung cancer, lymphosarcoma, Hodgkin's lymphoma, reticulum cell sarcoma, breast and germinal cell cancers, especially testicular cancer.

Dosage:
Neonatal: Not applicable.
Pediatric: Safe use in children has not been determined.
Adult: 125–140 mg/m^2 IV 3 times a week every 5 weeks or 200–250 mg/m^2 IV every week or 50–60 mg/m^2 IV daily for 5 days every 2–4 weeks or 100–130 mg/m^2 by mouth daily for 5 days every 3 weeks or 300–400 mg daily for 5 days every 9 days.

Preparation: Supplied in 100-mg/5-ml ampules and in various oral preparations. Must be diluted in at least 1 ml of normal saline for each milligram of drug.

Home Stability: Unopened ampules are stable for 3 years at room temperature if protected from light. Must be diluted with at least 1 ml of normal saline per each milligram, but this solution is only stable for 30 minutes. A dilution of 5 ml of normal saline per milligram of drug is stable for 6 hours. Cloudy solutions should be discarded.

Compatibilities: Not compatible with D$_5$W. As with most antineoplastic agents, it is advisable not to administer this drug with other admixture solutions.

Administration:
Neonatal: Not applicable.
Pediatric: Not applicable.
Adult: Infuse over 30–60 minutes to avoid se-

vere drop in blood pressure. Do not administer by intraperitoneal, intrapleural, or intrathecal routes.

Contraindications: Previous allergy to the drug.

Side Effects:
Primary:
Hematopoietic: Decreased WBC count and some decrease in platelets about 16 days after treatment with recovery in 4–6 days.
Gastrointestinal: Mild nausea, vomiting, abdominal cramps, anorexia, and diarrhea, primarily with oral preparations.
Cutaneous: Alopecia, phlebitis along the venipuncture site, and possible reactivated redness of previously irradiated skin.
Immunologic: Allergic reactions with fever, chills, shortness of breath, bronchospasm, wheezing, decreased blood pressure, and anaphylaxis. (Treat with antihistamines, pressors, volume expanders, and epinephrine.)
Reproductive: Teratogenic.
Secondary: Headache, fever, fatigue, bradycardia, hypertension, decreased blood pressure if given over less than 30 minutes, aftertaste, stomatitis, peripheral neuropathy, and paresthesias. Risk of infertility is unknown. Secondary malignancy is possible.

Nursing Implications: Monitor complete blood count.

Instruct patient and family on infection precautions during the third week after treatment.

Administer antiemetics if needed.

Inform patient of possible hair loss that is reversible and skin reactions at previous radiation therapy sites.

Instruct patient to report any discomfort along the venipuncture site.

Take baseline blood pressure and check blood pressure halfway through drug administration or if the patient complains of dizziness or lightheadedness. Take blood pressure again at the completion of drug administration.

Observe closely for signs of allergic reactions.

Inform patient of the possibility of birth defects if pregnancy occurs while taking VP-16.

Safe-handling precautions should continue for 3 days after the last dose of VP-16.

Generic Name: FACTOR IX COMPLEX (HUMAN)

Trade Name: KONYNE, PROFILNINE, PROPLEX, PROPLEX SX

Classification: Coagulant

Actions: Made up of human coagulation factors II, VII, IX, and X. These respond in the body as the patient's own factors would.

Indications: Deficiency of one or more of the specific coagulation factors in Factor IX complex.

Dosage:
Neonatal: Highly individualized, depending on the deficiency of the patient.
Pediatric: See neonatal dosage.
Adult: See neonatal dosage.

Preparation: 50 u of dry powder; diluent is usually provided.

Home Stability: Not applicable.

Compatibilities: Infuse with saline.

Administration:
Neonatal: Completely individualized, not to exceed 10 ml/minute. Decrease rate of administration if side effects develop. Dilute 50 u in 2 ml of sterile water.
Pediatric: Completely individualized, not to exceed 10 ml/minute. Decrease rate of administration if side effects develop. Dilute 50 u in 1–2 ml of sterile water.
Adult: See pediatric administration.

Contraindications: Liver disease with suspicion of intravascular coagulation or fibrinolysis. Use with extreme caution in newborns, infants, and patients with liver disease.

Side Effects:
Primary: Chills, fever, flushing, headache, tingling.
Secondary: Anaphylaxis, disseminated intravascular coagulation, hepatitis, postoperative thrombosis.

Nursing Implications: Assess patient carefully for signs of anaphylactic reaction and side effects.

Obtain baseline coagulation factor levels and monitor during and after administration. Guard against overdosage.

Assess for signs of postoperative thrombosis or disseminated intravascular coagulation.

Store powder at 2–8°C.

Generic Name: 5-FLUOROURACIL (5FU)

Trade Name: FLUOROURACIL/ADRUCIL

Classification: Antineoplastic antimetabolite

Actions: Acts as a false metabolite to inhibit formation of an essential component of DNA synthesis. RNA synthesis is affected somewhat. Considered cell-cycle specific at the S phase.

Indications: Breast cancer, adenocarcinoma of the gastrointestinal tract, basal cell carcinoma, malignant dermatoses.

Dosage:
Neonatal: Not applicable.
Pediatric: 400–600 mg/m^2 by IV push or continuous drip daily for 4 days as a loading dose, then once a week or 200–250 mg/m^2 IV every other day for 4 days every 4 weeks or 500–600 mg/m^2 by IV push or continuous drip every week or 1100 mg/m^2 by continuous drip over 24 hours. One example of an intra-arterial dose is 20–30 mg/kg daily for 4 days, then 15 mg/kg daily for 17 days. Intrapericardial doses range from 500–1000 mg. Intrapleural doses can be 2–3 g. Intraperitoneal doses range from 130 μcg/l–1 g/l × 8, with 4 hours for each dwell time, every 2 weeks. Topical applications of 5% (25 g) cream applied twice daily for 2–4 weeks.
Adult: See pediatric dosage.

Preparation: Supplied as a clear yellowish fluid in ampules of 500 mg/10 ml and as a 25-g 5% cream.

Home Stability: Ampules should be protected from light and stored at room temperature. If a precipitate is visible from storage or cooler temperatures, shake the ampules vigorously and/or place them in warm water until clear. If mixed with D$_5$W or normal saline, the solution should be used within 24 hours.

Compatibilities: Not compatible with diazepam, doxorubicin, Ara-C, methotrexate, or any acid admixtures such as penicillin, tetracycline, multivitamins, etc. May be more effective when given with methotrexate if fluorouracil is given second. Thymidine may increase fluorouracil toxicity. Thiazide diuretics increase bone marrow depression caused by fluorouracil. Cimetidine increases the effects of fluorouracil. As with most antineoplastic agents, it is advisable not to administer fluorouracil with other admixture solutions.

Administration:
Neonatal: Not applicable.
Pediatric and Adult: IV push through the side arm of a free-flowing IV is preferred to direct IV push. If the latter is done, the vein should be flushed before and after with 5–10 ml of normal saline. Place a porous gauze dressing over the area where the topical cream (Efudex) is applied.
Adult: See pediatric administration.

Contraindications: Previous allergy to drug, inadequate liver or renal function, intrathecal administration. Use with caution in patients with possible serious infections, bone marrow suppression, poor nutrition, history of high-dose pelvic radiation, previous alkylating agent therapy, or extensive bone marrow metastasis.

Side Effects:
Primary:
Hematopoietic: Decreased WBCs and platelets with a nadir of 7–14 days (lessened with intra-arterial use).
Gastrointestinal: Mild nausea and vomiting, esophagitis, diarrhea, proctitis, gastrointestinal bleeding. Stomatitis, preceded by a sore mouth and tongue, is a sign of early severe toxicity, and the drug should be stopped.
Cutaneous: Hair loss that may be reversible while therapy continues; changes in finger- and toenails (cracking and loss); hyperpigmentation of the skin, especially along vein sites with exposure to the sun; dry skin; skin rashes (ulceration and necrosis are expected with topical application, and healing requires 1–2 months).
Secondary: Headache, visual disturbances, conjunctivitis, excessive tearing, cerebellar ataxia, somnolence, muscle incoordination, decreased blood pressure, cardiotoxicity, possible need for increased doses of cortisone for patients with an adrenalectomy. Risk of hypersensitivity reaction, infertility, or secondary malignancy is low. Risk of teratogenesis is unknown.

Nursing Implications: Monitor complete blood count.

Instruct patient and family on infection and bleeding precautions during the second week after treatment.

Medicate with antiemetics as needed.

Instruct patient to check mouth daily and report any sores or discomfort to the physician.

Guaiac all stools and emesis.

Inform patient of possible hair loss and nail changes.

Encourage patient to avoid direct sunlight and wear sunscreens, especially when receiving topical treatments. Inform patient that the latter will progress from redness and ulceration to necrosis over a 2–4 week period, with healing requiring 1–2 months.

Continue safe-handling precautions for 1 day after the last dose of drug.

Generic Name: FOLIC ACID

Trade Name: FOLACIN

Classification: Vitamin

Actions: Water-soluble vitamin (B_9) essential for humans to maintain health. Thought to be important for nucleoprotein synthesis and to maintain erythropoiesis. Encourages formation of red and white blood cells and platelets in some megaloblastic anemias. Essential for blood cell formation.

Indications: Treatment of anemia due to nutritional deficiency.

Dosage:
Neonatal: 0.1 mg/day.
Pediatric:
Under 4: 0.3 mg/day.
Over 4: 0.4 mg/day.
Adult: 0.4 mg/day.

Preparation: Injectable form available in 5 and 10 mg/ml.

Home Stability: Protect solution from light.

Administration:
All Ages: IM, IV, or SC. Give parenterally only if the disease is severe or if gastrointestinal absorption is impaired.

Contraindications: Aplastic, normocytic, or refractory anemia. Because it may mask the symptoms of pernicious anemia, it is also not recommended in the treatment of any undiagnosed anemia.

Side Effects:
Primary: Allergic reactions including pruritus, rash, erythema.
Secondary: Malaise, allergic bronchospasms.

Nursing Implications: Assess patient for nutritional status. Signs and symptoms of deficiency include shortness of breath, fatigue, slight jaundice pallor, and fainting.

Nutritional counseling may be needed to assist patient in maintaining a well-balanced diet.

Assess patient for improvement in physical status related to vitamin deficiency.

Generic Name: FUROSEMIDE

Trade Name: LASIX

Classification: Diuretic

Actions: Inhibits reabsorption of sodium in the loop of Henle as well as in the proximal and distal tubules.

Indications: Treatment of edema associated with congestive heart failure, hepatic and renal disease, including nephrotic syndrome.

Dosage:
Neonatal: Initial dose is 1 mg/kg. Dosage may be increased by 1 mg/kg no sooner than 2 hours after the previous dose until the desired diuretic effect has been obtained. Doses greater than 6 mg/kg are not recommended.
Pediatric: See neonatal dosage.
Adult:
For Edema: Initial dose is 20–40 mg. Dosage may be increased in 20-mg increments no sooner than 2 hours after the previous dose until the desired diuretic effect has been obtained.
For Acute Pulmonary Edema: Initial dose is 40 mg. If this dose does not achieve satisfactory response within 1 hour, the dose may be increased to 80 mg.

Preparation: 2-, 4-, and 10-ml ampules; 2-ml Tubex; 2-, 4-, and 10-ml jets. Concentration is 10 mg/ml.

Home Stability: Not applicable.

Compatibilities: May infuse with solutions containing saline, dextrose, and lactated Ringer's.

Administration:
Neonatal: Give over 1–2 minutes.
Pediatric: Give over 1–2 minutes.
Adult: Give over 1–2 minutes. Doses over 80 mg should be administered as a controlled infusion at a rate not exceeding 4 mg/minute.

Contraindications: Hypersensitivity, anuria, increasing azotemia and oliguria. Do not use in cases of hepatic coma or severe electrolyte disturbances until the condition is improved or corrected. Contraindicated in women of childbearing potential and nursing mothers. Should not be used concomitantly with cephaloridine due to enhancement of nephrotoxicity. May increase ototoxic potential of aminoglycosides. May potentiate effects of antihypertensive medications. Patient sensitive to sulfonamides may show allergic reactions to furosemide.

Side Effects:
Primary: Volume depletion and dehydration, orthostatic hypotension, hyponatremia; hypochloremic alkalosis, hypokalemia, hyperglycemia.
Secondary: Weakness, dizziness, vertigo, muscle cramps, nausea, vomiting, transient blurred vision, tinnitus, hearing loss.

Nursing Implications: Potential for volume and electrolyte depletion leading to profound water loss, dehydration, reduction in blood volume, and circulatory collapse. Therefore monitor intake and output, serum electrolytes, blood pressure, and pulse rate frequently.

Assess for signs of hypokalemia (muscle weakness and cramping). Teach patients about potassium-rich foods (citrus fruits, tomatoes, bananas, dates, apricots). Be especially careful in patients receiving digitalis because of increased risk of digitalis toxicity.

Caution patient to change position slowly because of orthostatic hypotension.

Monitor BUN and creatinine for signs of deteriorating renal function.

Monitor serum uric acid levels, especially in patients with a history of gout.

Administer in the morning to prevent nocturia.

Elderly patients are especially susceptible to excessive diuresis.

Generic Name: GALLAMINE TRIETHIODIDE

Trade Name: FLAXEDIL

Classification: Neuromuscular blocker

Actions: Competes at receptor site with acetylcholine to block impulses for skeletal muscle movement, producing paralysis. Causes a histaminelike action. Like other neuromuscular blockers, it produces no effect on pain perception.

Indications: When skeletal muscle relaxation is required and in management of ventilated patients.

Dosage:
All Ages (Guideline Only): 1 mg/kg; repeat dose of 0.5–1.0 mg/kg.

Preparation: Injectable 20 mg/ml.

Administration:
All Ages: Slow IV push over 30–90 seconds.

Contraindications: Myasthenia gravis, hypersensitivity, sensitivity to iodine, impaired renal function, and when tachycardia is hazardous.

Side Effects:
Primary: Tachycardia, prolonged dose-related effects.
Secondary: Increased secretions.

Nursing Implications: Before administration, intubation and supportive equipment must be available.

Monitor patient for recovery from anesthesia. Observe for a return of muscle movement and swallow and gag reflexes. This drug is usually administered by an anesthesiologist.

Maintain a patent airway.

This drug does not provide sedative effects.

Generic Name: GENTAMICIN SULFATE

Trade Name: APOGEN, BRISTAGEN GARAMYCIN, JENAMICIN, U-GENICIN

Classification: Antibiotic (aminoglycoside)

Actions: Semisynthetic aminoglycoside derivative from *Micromonospora purpurea* with neuromuscular blocking action. Inhibits protein synthesis in bacterial cell and is bactericidal. Effective against a wide variety of gram-negative bacilli: *Escherichia coli,* Enterobacter, *Klebsiella pneumoniae,* and most strains of *Pseudomonas aeruginosa,* Proteus, Serratia, *Providencia stuartii,* Citrobacter, Salmonella, and Shigella. Also effective against Staphylococcus, including pencillin- and methicillin-resistant strains.

Indications: Bacteremia and septicemia, including neonatal sepsis; serious infections such as those of the urinary or respiratory tract, bones, joints, and central nervous system, including meningitis; burns and postoperative infections.

Dosage:
Neonatal:

Premature or Full-term Neonates 1 Week of Age or Less: 5 mg/kg/day divided into 2 equal doses every 12 hours.
Over 1 Week: 7.5 mg/kg/day divided into equal doses every 8 hours.
Pediatric: 6.0–7.5 mg/kg/day divided into equal doses every 8 hours.
Adult: Usual dose: 3–5 mg/kg/day divided into equal doses every 8 hours. Dosage is based on ideal body weight.
General: Dosage is highly individualized and should be based on therapeutic drug monitoring.
Trough serum level: $< 2\ \mu g/ml$.
Peak serum level: 4–10 $\mu g/ml$.

Duration of Therapy: 7–10 days.

Preparation: Supplied as a colorless solution, which does not require refrigeration, in 10- and 40-mg/ml vials.

Home Stability: Stable at room temperature as prepared by manufacturer for at least 2 years.

Compatibilities: Compatible with solutions containing dextrose, saline, KCl, Ringer's, or lactated Ringer's. Compatible with the following drugs: aminophylline, dopamine, multivitamin solution, and vitamin B complex with C. Compatible with total parenteral nutrition.

Administration:
Neonatal: Infuse over 1–2 hours. Administer at appropriate IV site based on infusion rate. Dilution should be based on fluid volume needs.
Pediatric: Infuse over 30–60 minutes. Administer at appropriate IV site based on infusion rate. Dilution should be based on fluid volume needs.
Adult: Dilute in 50–200 ml (1 mg/ml) IV solution and administer over 30–120 minutes.

Contraindications: Known gentamicin sensitivity. Use with caution in clients with impaired renal function, eighth cranial nerve impairment, dehydration, fever, myasthenia gravis, parkinsonism, hypocalcemia. Do not administer concurrently with penicillins. If concurrent administration is prescribed, administer the drugs 2 hours apart. The neuromuscular blockade effects are enhanced with combined administration of the following drugs: decamethonium, ether, succinylcholine, tubocurarine, and related anesthetics. Cephalosporins may potentiate the nephrotoxic effects of gentamicin. Concurrent administration of other aminoglycosides, ethacrynic acid, and furosemide may enhance the ototoxic effects.

Side Effects:
Primary:
Nephrotoxicity: Proteinurea, presence of red and white blood cells in the urine; granular casts; azotemia; oliguria; urinary frequency; frank hematuria; increase in BUN and serum creatinine; decrease in creatinine clearance and specific gravity; renal damage and failure.
Ototoxicity: Auditory: high-frequency hearing loss; complete hearing loss (occasionally permanent); tinnitus; fullness, ringing, or buzzing in ears. Vestibular: dizziness, vertigo; ataxia; nausea, vomiting; nystagmus.
Neurotoxicity: Drowsiness, headache, unsteady gait, weakness, clumsiness, paresthesias, tremors, muscle twitching and weakness, convulsions,

neuromuscular blockade with respiratory depression.

Secondary: Nausea, vomiting, stomatitis, skin rash, urticaria, pruritus, generalized burning sensation, drug fever, arthralgia, eosinophilia, anemia, leukopenia, granulocytopenia, thrombocytopenia, unusual thirst, difficulty breathing, superinfections, peripheral neuritis.

Nursing Implications: Monitor serum blood levels initially and throughout therapy.

Document the *exact* time of medication administration for determination of blood levels.

Assess renal function prior to initial administration via baseline BUN, creatinine and creatinine clearance, specific gravity, and urine analysis.

Monitor renal function throughout therapy via assessment of BUN, creatinine and creatinine clearance, specific gravity, urine analysis, and strict intake and output.

Encourage hydration of client to reduce chemical irritation of renal tubles.

Assess eighth cranial (vestibulocochlear) nerve function prior to initial administration and throughout therapy and upon discharge via audiometric tests and assessment of vestibular disturbance.

Monitor for overgrowth infection as evidenced by diarrhea, anogenital itching, vaginal discharge, stomatitis, or glossitis.

Antidote: Peritoneal dialysis or hemodialysis will assist in removing the drug from the bloodstream.

Generic Name: GLUCAGON

Trade Name: Generic only

Classification: Hormone

Actions: Produced in the pancreatic islets and acts to stimulate glycogenolysis in the liver. Blood glucose is raised by the breakdown of glycogen to glucose and the inhibition of glycogen synthesis. Maximum effects are seen 20–30 minutes after parenteral administration. Effect produced only if liver glycogen is available. Effect is brief, and administration of carbohydrates is necessary to replenish stores in the liver.

Indications: To counteract hypoglycemia of insulin shock and severe hypoglycemia in diabetic patients.

Dosage:
Neonatal: 0.3 mg/kg in a single dose, IV, IM, or SC.
Pediatric: 0.025 g/kg in a single dose, IV, IM, or SC. May repeat in 20 minutes.
Adult: 0.5–1 mg IV, IM, or SC. May repeat within 20 minutes for 2 doses.

Preparation: Powdered injectable form: 1- and 10-mg vials.

Compatibilities: Compatible with dextrose and water solutions.

Administration: IM, IV, or SC. IV will give fastest response. It may also be necessary to administer IV glucose along with glucagon.

Contraindications: Hypersensitivity (glucagon is a protein). Avoid use in patients with hyperinsulinism.

Side Effects:
Primary: Nausea and vomiting, hypersensitivity.

Nursing Implications: Observe for signs of hypoglycemia. Obtain glucose level.
First response is normally observed in 5–20 minutes. Note when and what type of response is observed.
Remain with patient to give supportive treatment. Document events leading up to reaction (i.e., oral intake, insulin administration, dose, urine output).

Generic Name: GLYCOPYRROLATE

Trade Name: ROBINUL

Classification: Cholinergic blocking agent

Actions: Inhibits the neurotransmission of impulses in the parasympathetic nervous system at the junction between postganglionic nerve endings and effector organs by inhibiting the effects of acetylcholine.

Indications: Intraoperatively for bradyarrhythmias, reversal of neuromuscular blockade, and peptic ulcer disease.

Dosage:
Neonatal: Not applicable.
Pediatric:
Intraoperatively: 0.002 mg/lb, not to exceed 0.1 mg in a single dose every 2–3 minutes.
Reversal of Neuromuscular Blockade: 0.2 mg for each 1.0 mg neostigmine or 5 mg pyridostigmine.
Adult:
Intraoperatively: 0.1 mg every 2–3 minutes.
Reversal of Neuromuscular Blockade: 0.2 mg for each 1.0 mg neostigmine or 5 mg pyridostigmine.
Peptic Ulcer Disease: 0.1–0.2 mg every 4 hours, given a total of 3–4 times daily.

Preparation: 1-, 2-, 5-, and 20-ml vials containing 0. 2 mg/ml.

Home Stability: Not applicable.

Compatibilities: May infuse with normal saline or 5% or 10% dextrose in water. May mix in same syringe with neostigmine or pyridostigmine.

Administration:
Neonatal: Not applicable.
Pediatric: May give undiluted at a rate of 0. 2 mg over 1–2 minutes.
Adult: See pediatric administration.

Contraindications: Hypersensitivity, narrow-angle glaucoma, prostatic hypertrophy, gastrointestinal obstructive disease, paralytic ileus, intestinal atony, unstable cardiovascular status in acute hemorrhage, toxic megacolon. Use with caution in asthma, coronary artery disease, congestive heart failure, cardiac arrhythmias, hypertension, hyperthyroidism, autonomic neuropathy, hepatic or renal disease, ulcerative colitis, or hiatal hernia.

Side Effects:
Primary: Constipation, dry mouth, dilated pupils, blurred vision.
Secondary: Tachycardia, paradoxical bradycardia, palpitations, disorientation, irritability, incoherence, headache, sedation, muscular weakness, photophobia, vomiting, nausea, epigastric distress, urinary hesitancy or retention, flushing, dryness, rash, bronchial plugging, fever.

Nursing Implications: Monitor vital signs frequently.
Assess for development of side effects, particularly in elderly or debilitated patients. Warn patients to avoid activities that require alertness until effects on the central nervous system are determined. Intermittent constipation, distension, and abdominal pain may indicate onset of paralytic ileus. Cool drinks, ice chips, hard candy, or sugarless gum can relieve dry mouth. Encourage fluids to help prevent constipation.
Monitor intake and output for development of urinary retention.
Discontinuation of drug should be done slowly.

Generic Name: GONADORELIN HYDROCHLORIDE

Trade Name: FACTREL

Classification: Synthetic luteinizing hormone-releasing hormone (diagnostic agent)

Actions: Chemical structure and composition identical to natural hormone, which has gonadotropin-releasing effects upon the anterior pituitary.

Indications: Recommended for diagnostic use only to evaluate response and functional capacity of gonadotropes of the anterior pituitary, in patients with suspected gonadotropin deficiency or in patients who have had a pituitary tumor removed. Not useful in differentiating pituitary disorders from hypothalamic disorders.

Dosage:
Pediatric: 2.5 μg/kg. Maximum dosage: 200 μg.
Adult: 100 μg as a single dose. Maximum dosage: 200 μg.

Preparation: Supplied as a white powder in vials containing 100 or 500 μg gonadorelin hydrochloride and 100 mg lactose. A sterile diluent of alcohol and water is supplied.

Home Stability: Factrel is hygroscopic and thus moisture-sensitive. It is stable at room temperature. The solution should be prepared immediately before use.

Compatibilities: Compatible with dextrose and saline solutions.

Administration:
Pediatric: As a bolus over 15–30 seconds.
Adult: As a bolus over 15–30 seconds.

Contraindications: Hypersensitivity to the drug or any of the components.

Side Effects:
Primary: Headaches, flushing, abdominal pain, light-headedness, nausea.
Secondary: Hypersensitivity reactions consisting of urticaria, tachycardia, and bronchospasm are rare. High doses given repetitively may cause luteolysis and inhibition of spermatogenesis.

Nursing Implications: The following drugs affect the secretion of gonadotropins from the pituitary and thus should be discontinued during testing: androgens, estrogens, progestins, glucocorticoids, spironolactone, levodopa, oral contraceptives, digoxin, phenothiazines, and dopamine antagonists.

Plasma luteinizing hormone levels should be drawn at 15 minutes before and immediately before administration of gonadorelin hydrochloride and at 15, 30, 45, 60, 90, and 120 minutes after administration.

The patient should fast overnight.

This diagnostic test can be done in conjunction with L-arginine, glucagon, and TRH stimulations but not with levodopa stimulation, because levodopa is a neurotransmitter.

Generic Name: HEMIN

Trade Name: PANHEMATIN

Classification: Enzyme inhibitor, blood derivative

Actions: Exact mechanism of action not understood, but probably acts to repress synthesis of porphyrin precursors, because it blocks one enzyme essential to the porphyrin/heme biosynthetic pathway. Used to treat patients in acute episodes of hepatic porphyrias. Not curative but does help eliminate symptoms.

Indications: Treatment of acute episodes of intermittent porphyrias.

Dosage: IV: 1–4 mg/kg/day over 10–15 minutes for 3–14 days. If treating a severe case, repeat dose *no sooner than* every 12 hours. Maximum dosage is 6 mg/kg/24 hours.
General: Safe use in pregnancy, nursing women, and children has not been established.

Preparation: Sterile, lyophilized black powder in single-dose vials. Reconstitute with sterile water for injection, USP.

Administration: Reconstitute immediately before use. Shake for 2–3 minutes after adding diluent. See Dosage for rate of administration. Each milliliter of hemin contains 7 mg of hemin. A filter *must* be used—0.45 micron or smaller—to prevent administration of particulate matter.

Contraindications: Known hypersensitivity, use in porphyria cutanea tarda.

Side Effects:
Primary: Phlebitis when administered through small arm veins, coagulopathy, reversible renal shutdown.
Secondary: Decreased hematocrit.

Nursing Implications: Before administration, patient should have a complete evaluation and diagosis of acute porphyria. Usual criteria include
   1. Clinical symptoms
   2. Positive Watson-Schwartz or Hoesch test
In addition, alternative therapy with glucose should be attempted before administration of this drug.
   Administer drug through a large vein or central venous catheter with a 0.45-micron or smaller filter.
   Assess patient's initial symptoms and document observations. Possible symptoms are depression, anxiety, insomnia, disorientation, psychoses, dark urine, abdominal pain, and seizures.
   Monitor intake and output.

Generic Name: HEPARIN SODIUM

Trade Name: HEPARIN LOCK FLUSH, HEP-LOCK, HEPRINAR, LIPO-HEPIN, LIQUAEMIN SODIUM, PANHEPARIN, PANHEPARIN LOK

Classification: Anticoagulant

Actions: Inhibits the conversion of prothrombin to thrombin and fibrinogen to fibrin. Adhesiveness of platelets is reduced.

Indications: Prevention of thrombi and emboli, treatment of disseminated intravascular coagulation, and to maintain patency of heparin lock needle.

Dosage:
Neonatal: Titrate according to clotting times.
Pediatric: For anticoagulation, titrate to obtain coagulation 2–3 times the control.
Adult:
For Anticoagulation: Titrate to obtain coagulation 2–3 times the control, usually 20,000–40,000 u/24 hours.
To Maintain Patency of Heparin Lock: 10–100 u diluted in 0.5–1.0 ml of normal saline every 8–12 hours.

Preparation: Clear fluid in single or multidose vials or individual Tubex-type syringes.

Home Stability: Not applicable.

Compatibilities: May infuse with sodium chloride, dextrose, or Ringer's.

Administration:
Neonatal: May be given diluted or undiluted and by direct IV.
Pediatric: See neonatal administration.
Adult: See neonatal administration.

Contraindications: Active bleeding, blood dyscrasias, history of bleeding, hypersensitivity, liver disease, recent surgery, subacute bacterial endocarditis. Use with caution in pregnancy. Potentiated by chloramphenicol and salicylates. Inhibited by antihistamines, barbiturates, digitalis, calcium disodium edetate, hyaluronidase, hydroxyzine, penicillin, and phenothiazines. Potentiates oral anticoagulants, phenytoin, and thyroxine.

Side Effects:
Primary: Bruising, prolonged coagulation times, epistaxis, hematuria, and other bleeding.
Secondary: Allergic reaction, alopecia.

Nursing Implications: Obtain baseline partial thromboplastin time and check periodically during and after anticoagulation treatment until levels return to normal.

Assess hourly for signs of bleeding during and after anticoagulation treatment until coagulation studies return to normal.

Apply pressure to all puncture sites for 5–30 minutes, depending on site, to prevent bleeding.

Read label carefully; many different concentrations are available.

Protamine sulfate is a heparin antagonist and is indicated in overdose or heparin reversal.

Generic Name: HETASTARCH

Trade Name: HESPAN

Classification: Replacement solution

Actions: Plasma volume expander with colloidal properties like those of human albumin. It will expand plasma volume and improve hemodynamic status for approximately 24–36 hours.

Indications: Treatment of hypovolemic shock due to hemorrhage, burns, surgery, and other traumas. Because Hespan is not a substitute for blood or plasma it should be used as an adjunct in treatment of shock.

Dosage: Varies with the volume of blood lost.

Preparation: Injectable: 6% Hespan in 0.9% sodium chloride.

Compatibilities: This drug should be infused alone. Do not mix with medications or IV additives.

Administration: Rate of infusion depends on volume of blood lost and patient's condition. An infusion pump is suggested to insure controlled rate.

Contraindications: Severe bleeding disorders; congestive, cardiac, or renal failure; oliguria and anuria.

Side Effects:
Primary: Vomiting, fever, chills, headaches, peripheral edema, anaphylactic reactions.
Secondary: Urticaria, periorbital edema.

Nursing Implications: Monitor vital signs frequently. Assess for signs of hemorrhage. The administration of large volumes may alter bleeding times. Monitor lab values.

Measure and record intake and output. Also monitor for signs of fluid overload.

Generic Name: HISTAMINE PHOSPHATE

Trade Name: HISTAMINE PHOSPHATE

Classification: Histamine

Actions: Acts on the vascular system, smooth muscle, and exocrine glands and increases volume and acidity of gastric juice.

Indications: Diagnostic test for pheochromocytoma.

Dosage:
Neonatal: Not applicable.
Pediatric: Not applicable.
Adult: 0.01 mg, followed in 5 minutes by 0.05 mg if no response to initial dose.

Preparation: 1-ml ampules containing 0.1 mg.

Home Stability: Not applicable.

Compatibilities: May infuse with 5% dextrose or saline solution.

Administration:
Neonatal: Not applicable.
Pediatric: Not applicable.
Adult: Give undiluted by IV push following the test protocol (see Nursing Implications).

Contraindications: Severe hypertension and in the elderly. Use with caution in patients with severe asthma or severe allergic conditions.

Side Effects:
Primary: Flushing, dizziness, headache, bronchial constriction, dyspnea, visual disturbances, faintness, syncope, urticaria, palpitations, hypertension, hypotension, tachycardia, nervousness, abdominal cramps.
Secondary: Diarrhea, vomiting, metallic taste, local or generalized allergic manifestations, convulsions, vasomotor collapse, shock.

Nursing Implications: Withhold antihypertensives, sympathomimetics, sedatives, and narcotics for at least 24 (preferably 72) hours before test. Patient does not fast. Perform test only on patients with resting blood pressures less than 150/110. Keep epinephrine and phentolamine on hand to treat severe hypotension or severe hypertension.

To perform the test: Patient is supine with an IV of 5% dextrose or saline infusing at keep-open rate. Record blood pressure until stabilized, then collect a 2-hour urine for catecholamine assay. After this is completed, administer histamine by IV push and begin a second 2-hour urine for catecholamine assay. Record blood pressure, pulse, and respirations every 30 seconds for 15 minutes. If no response is observed after 5 minutes, administer 0.05 mg of histamine by IV push. Expected response to the test is headache, flushing, and a drop in blood pressure followed by an increase within 2 minutes. A positive result is shown by an increase in blood pressure 60/40 mmHg above the baseline and greater than that with the cold pressor test, or an increase in blood pressure 20/10 mmHg greater than with the cold pressor test. Explain procedure to patient, including sensations that may be experienced. Offer support during the test.

Treat overdose with epinephrine and antihistamines. Treat anaphylaxis and resuscitate as necessary.

Generic Name: HYDRALAZINE HYDROCHLORIDE

Trade Name: APRESOLINE

Classification: Antihypertensive

Actions: Relaxes smooth muscle in the peripheral arterioles to lower peripheral resistance.

Indications: Severe essential hypertension; reduction of afterload in severe congestive heart failure.

Dosage:
Neonatal: Not applicable.
Pediatric: 1.7–3.5 mg/kg daily or 50–100 mg/m² daily in 4–6 divided doses.
Adult: 20–40 mg with a maximum daily dose of 300–400 mg.

Preparation: 20 mg in 1-ml ampule.

Home Stability: Home use is not recommended.

Compatibilities: May infuse with solutions containing dextrose, saline, or combinations of dextrose and saline.

Administration:
Neonatal: Not applicable.
Pediatric: May give undiluted at a rate of 10 mg/minute.
Adult: See pediatric administration.

Contraindications: Hypersensitivity, coronary artery disease, mitral valvular rheumatic heart disease. Use with caution in patients with renal disease and concurrently with MAO inhibitors. Potentiated by concurrent use of other antihypertensives, especially diazoxide.

Side Effects:
Primary: Angina, tachycardia, palpitations, hypotension, nausea, vomiting, diarrhea, anorexia, lupus erythematosus-like syndrome, weight gain.
Secondary: Peripheral neuritis, dizziness, arrhythmias, orthostatic hypotension, rash.

Nursing Implications: Continuous blood pressure monitoring is preferred; if not possible, obtain baseline blood pressure and then check every 3–5 minutes until pressure is stabilized. Hourly checks should then be continued.

Continuous cardiac monitoring is needed; observe for ischemic changes and arrhythmias.

Assess heart tones, jugular venous distension, peripheral edema, lung sounds, dyspnea, and capillary refill every 4 hours and as needed.

Monitor fluid status via hourly urine outputs, intake, and daily weights.

Monitor electrolytes, particularly sodium.

Assess for signs of lupus erythematosus-like syndrome (sore throat, fever, muscle and joint aches, skin rash). Notify physician if these develop.

Monitor complete blood count, lupus erythematosus cell preparation, and antinuclear antibody titer determinations before and periodically during therapy.

Generic Name: HYDROCORTISONE PHOSPHATE

Trade Name: CORTEF

Classification: Corticosteroid

Actions: The members of this family have many and varied effects because they influence almost every cell in the body. Some of these actions are accelerated protein metabolism, which results in muscle weakness and wasting, suppression of immune response and impaired wound healing, redistribution of fat, and increased formation of adipose tissue. Blood glucose levels also increase because it is utilized less, and this causes an increase in the release of insulin. Steroids suppress the body's immune response by affecting histamine release and inhibit the chain of events that leads to the inflammatory response. Finally, they have an effect on the reabsorption and distribution of some electrolytes and other elements necessary for normal body function.

Any patient who has been on long-term therapy should have steroids withdrawn slowly to prevent development of acute adrenal insufficiency.

Indications: Steroids are indicated in the treatment of many disorders, including (but not limited to) inflammatory, endocrine, collagen, dermatologic, rheumatic, allergic, respiratory, hematologic, and gastrointestinal diseases and disorders of the central nervous system.

Dosage: Highly variable depending on the disease or condition under treatment. This form of corticosteroid is not for IV use. Administer part of the total dose IM.

Preparation: 25 and 50 mg/ml.

Administration: See Dosage.

Contraindications: Hypersensitivity, systemic fungal infections. The smallest dose for the shortest period of time should be used because of the chance of side effects. May stunt growth in children. Do not give immunizations during therapy. Use with caution in patients with active infections, congestive heart failure, hypertension, osteoporosis. May aggravate diabetes mellitus, Cushing's syndrome, and optic nerve damage.

Side Effects: Many effects are dependent on dose or length of therapy. The following side effects are related to the drug itself.
Primary: Fluid and electrolyte disturbances, osteoporosis, long bone fractures, effects on the central nervous system, increased incidence of infections, impaired wound healing, ocular effects, endocrine effects.
Secondary: Abrupt withdrawal may lead to withdrawal syndrome or adrenal insufficiency.

Nursing Implications: Obtain baseline information—height, weight, vital signs, physical assessment, and laboratory results.

Any patient who has been on long-term therapy *must* have dose tapered. Observe for clinical symptoms of withdrawal.

Continuing assessment includes weight, vital signs, and laboratory follow-up. Assess for side effects. Because of decreased resistance, patient at home should be instructed to avoid contact with any person who has an active infection.

Dietary adjustments may be necessary for diabetic patients. Patients on long-term therapy may need to increase protein intake.

Monitor patient for improvement in condition under therapy. Document observations.

Additional patient teaching may include telling the patient to expect diarrhea, tarry stools; report any infections or unhealed cuts. Eye examinations should be done periodically as well as routine laboratory tests.

Generic Name: HYDROMORPHONE HYDROCHLORIDE

Trade Name: DILAUDID

Classification: Narcotic analgesic

Actions: Drugs in this class act to relieve moderate to severe pain and provide preoperative sedation. A patient's perception of pain is altered by preventing or changing the transmission of painful stimuli along the sensory pathways in the central nervous system. These pathways are specific to the perception and emotional response of the patient to pain. In addition, these drugs suppress the respiratory and cough centers of the brain and have an antiperistaltic effect on the smooth muscle of the intestine. Because of their actions, narcotics can produce physical and psychological dependence. When used to treat severe pain, as in terminal illness, these medications should be given around the clock to maximize the relief of pain as well as the anxiety produced by the pain.

Indications: Management of moderate to severe pain owing to a diversity of causes. Should not be used in cases of mild pain or pain that can be relieved by non-narcotic analgesics.

Dosage:
Neonatal: Safety for use in infants and children has not been established.
Pediatric: See neonatal dosage.
Adult: 2 mg IM, SC, or IV every 4–6 hours. For severe pain: 3–4 mg every 4–6 hours as needed.

Preparation: Injectable form available in 1, 2, or 4 mg/ml.

Home Stability: Medication should be stored at 59–86°F and protected from light.

Compatibilities: When administered by direct IV push over 2–3 minutes, this medication does not mix with other solutions.

Administration:
Neonatal: Safety not established.
Pediatric: Safety not established.
Adult: Must be given IV over 3–5 minutes.

Contraindications: Known sensitivity to narcotic analgesics, use during delivery of a premature infant, use in patients taking monoamine oxidase inhibitors or those who have taken them within 14 days. Use with caution in patients with head injuries, increased intracranial pressure, shock, central nervous system and respiratory depression, chronic obstructive pulmonary disease and when administering to patients receiving other narcotic analgesics.

Side Effects:
Primary: Respiratory depression and apnea during IV administration, hypersensitivity reaction, hypotension, bradycardia, nausea, vomiting, dizziness, sedation, sweating.
Secondary: Physical dependence. Constipation can occur because of effect on smooth muscle of bowel. Urinary retention, pain at injection site, and phlebitis are possible after IV administration.

Nursing Implications: Because of the chance for respiratory depression, a narcotic antagonist should be available for rapid administration, especially if the route of choice is IV. Naloxone is the antagonist most often used.

Monitor vital signs frequently: for IV dose, every 5–10 minutes; for SC dose, every 15–30 minutes.

Supportive equipment should be readily available in case of cardiac or respiratory arrest. A patent airway should be maintained.

Monitor infants when the drug is used during labor and delivery.

Monitor intake and output when this drug is given repeatedly because it may cause urinary retention.

To augment the use of narcotic analgesics, give before severe pain occurs. Nursing actions also include emotional support and patient comfort measures. Because of depression of respiratory centers, postoperative use in management of pain should include patient's turning, coughing, and deep breathing to prevent pulmonary complications.

Patients should be warned to avoid activities that require alertness.

Assist patient with ambulation. This medication may cause orthostatic hypotension.

Generic Name: HYOSCYAMINE SULFATE

Trade Name: LEVSIN

Classification: Anticholinergic

Actions: Blocks actions of acetylcholine on vagus nerve, thus decreasing gastrointestinal motility and inhibiting gastric acid secretions.

Indications: Treatment of gastrointestinal tract disorders due to spasms; adjunctive therapy for peptic ulcers; preanesthetic agent to control secretions; intraoperative therapy for bradycardia; reversal of neuromuscular blockade.

Dosage:
Neonatal: Not applicable.
Pediatric: Not applicable.
Adult: 0.25–0.5 mg every 4 hours for a total of 3-4 doses daily.
Preanesthetic: 5 μg/kg 30–60 minutes before anesthesia.
Intraoperative Bradycardia: 0.125 mg; repeat as needed.
Reversal of Neuromuscular Blockade: 0.2 mg for each milligram neostigmine or the equivalent dose of physostigmine or pyridostigmine.

Preparation: 0.5 mg in 1-ml ampules.

Home Stability: Not applicable.

Compatibilities: May infuse with 5% dextrose in water.

Administration:
Neonatal: Not applicable.
Pediatric: Not applicable.
Adult: May give undiluted over at least 1 minute.

Contraindications: Hypersensitivity, narrow-angle glaucoma, obstructive uropathy, obstructive disease of gastrointestinal tract, severe ulcerative colitis, myasthenia gravis, paralytic ileus, intestinal atony, unstable cardiovascular status in acute hemorrhage, toxic megacolon. Use with caution in patients with autonomic neuropathy, hyperthyroidism, coronary artery disease, cardiac arrhythmias, congestive heart failure, hypertension, hiatal hernia associated with reflux esophagitis, hepatic or renal disease, ulcerative colitis, or in patients over 40 years of age.

Side Effects:
Primary: Confusion or excitement in elderly patients, palpitations, blurred vision, dry mouth, constipation, paralytic ileus, urinary hesitancy and retention.
Secondary: Headache, insomnia, drowsiness, dizziness, nervousness, weakness, tachycardia, mydriasis, increased ocular tension, cycloplegia, photophobia, dysphagia, heartburn, loss of taste, nausea, vomiting, impotence, urticaria, decreased sweating or anhidrosis, fever, allergic reactions.

Nursing Implications: Monitor vital signs frequently.

Assess for development of side effects, particularly in elderly or debilitated patients. Warn patients to avoid activities that require alertness until effects on the central nervous system are determined. Intermittent constipation, distension, and abdominal pain may indicate onset of paralytic ileus. Cool drinks, ice chips, hard candy, or sugarless gum can relieve dry mouth. Encourage fluids to help prevent constipation.

Monitor intake and output for development of urinary retention.

Discontinuation of drug should be done slowly.

Generic Name: IMMUNE GLOBULIN

Trade Name: GAMIMUNE

Classification: Immune serum

Actions: IV administration of this serum provides antibodies for immediate use by the body.

Indications: Immunodeficiency syndrome.

Dosage:

All ages: 100/mg/kg once a month by IV infusion. If necessary, dose may be increased to 200 mg/kg. It is also possible to repeat the dosage on a more frequent basis.

Preparation: Injectable, 5% solution in 50- and 100-ml vials.

Administration: Rate of infusion: 0.01–0.02 ml/kg/minute for the first 30 minutes. If no difficulties occur, rate can be increased to 0.02–0.04 ml/kg/minute. Slow rate if side effects occur.

Contraindications: Hypersensitivity to immune serum globulin.

Side Effects:

Primary: Low-grade fever, urticaria, anaphylaxis, chills, abdominal cramps, anxiety, headache.

Secondary: Back pain, dizziness, malaise, rash.

Nursing Implications: Obtain as complete an allergy history as possible.

Have supportive equipment and medications available in case of allergic reaction.

Monitor patient closely during infusion.

Generic Name: INSULIN IV

Trade Name: REGULAR INSULIN, ACTRAPID INSULIN

Classification: Insulins

Actions: Exact mechanism unknown but enhances transmembrane transport of glucose into most body cells. Also inhibits fatty acid mobilization, promotes conversion of glucose to glycogen, stimulates protein production, restores efficient sugar and fat utilization in the diabetic, and induces potassium movement into the liver and adipose and muscle tissues.

Indications: To replace or supplement endogenous insulin in diabetic patients. As an intravenous infusion to treat diabetic ketoacidosis or coma.

A patient may be placed on a continuous infusion of insulin when not in diabetic ketoacidosis or coma, when it is necessary to determine the number of units of insulin the patient requires over a 24-hour period to maintain blood sugar in the desired range.

Given IV to produce hypoglycemia, insulin stimulates growth hormone production. This helps to evaluate pituitary growth hormone reserve in patients with known or suspected growth hormone deficiency.

Added to solutions of dextrose to treat severe hyperkalemia, insulin facilitates intracellular shift of potassium.

Dosage:
Neonatal:
Treatment of Diabetic Ketoacidosis: 0.1 u/kg/hour.
Pediatric:
Treatment of Diabetic Ketoacidosis: 0.1 u/kg/hour. The same dosage may be given as a bolus before continuous infusion is started.
Test for Growth Hormone Secretion: 0.075 u/kg.
Adult:
Treatment of Diabetic Ketoacidosis: 0.33 u/kg. IV bolus may or may not be given, followed by 7–10 u/hour by continuous infusion.
Test for Growth Hormone Secretion: 0.05–0.1 u/kg.

Preparation: Clear and colorless liquid in a multidose vial. It should not be used if even slightly colored or cloudy.

Home Stability: Once used, the vial should be refrigerated but not frozen. Check label carefully for expiration date. Keep away from heat and sunlight. Insulin prepared for continuous infusion should be made fresh every 8 hours.

Compatibilities: Usually diluted with 0.9% sodium chloride. Compatible with dextrose solutions, KCl, KPO_4 (potassium phosphate), and cimetidine. Recommended dilution: 30 u of regular insulin per 150 ml of 0.9% sodium chloride. This provides 1 u/5 ml of insulin.

Administration:
Neonatal:
Treatment of Diabetic Ketoacidosis: Continuous infusion until blood sugar drops to 250 mg%; then SC insulin may be used.
Pediatric:
Treatment of Diabetic Ketoacidosis: IV bolus may or may not be given, followed by a continuous infusion until blood sugar drops to 250 mg%; then SC insulin may begin.
Test for Growth Hormone Secretion: Rapid IV injection.
Adult:
Treatment of Diabetic Ketoacidosis: IV bolus may or may not be given, followed by a continuous infusion until blood sugar drops to 250 mg%; then SC insulin may begin.
Test for Growth Hormone Secretion: Rapid IV injection.

Contraindications: Hypersensitivity to the type of insulin used (insulin animal protein).

Side Effects:
Primary: Hypoglycemia usually manifested as headache, tachycardia, hunger or nausea, cold sweat, pallor, fatigue, nervousness, palpitations, delirium, inability to concentrate, irritability, apprehension, and visual disturbances.
Secondary: Seizure or anaphylaxis.

Nursing Implications: Only regular insulin should be given IV.

Insulin produced by the same manufacturing process should be used consistently on a patient (recombinant DNA versus animal-source insulin). If a change is made, there may need to be a change in dosage.

Insulin is measured in units and should be drawn up only with an insulin syringe.

Insulin comes primarily in concentrations of 100 u/ml but is also available in 500, 80, and 40 u/ml. It is important that the corresponding u500, u100, u80, or u40 syringe be used or there will be an error in dosage.

When insulin is given as a continuous infusion, an infusion pump should be used.

When preparing a continuous insulin infusion, the insulin should be added slowly, and the first 50 ml of solution should be discarded, because insulin adheres to plastic and glass. This method allows for saturation of the tubing with insulin and thus prevents fluctuations in solution concentration.

Monitor blood glucose hourly or at least every 2 hours.

When insulin is changed from a continuous IV infusion to SC, the SC insulin should be given 15 minutes before the infusion is stopped to insure continuous insulin coverage and prevent excess rebound hyperglycemia.

If the blood glucose level is dropped too rapidly, the patient may experience signs of cerebral edema. Ideally the glucose should fall at a rate of 75–100 mg/dl/hour.

When IV insulin is used to assess growth hormone production:

1. The patient should be eating nothing by mouth.
2. A qualified person must be available to administer 25% or 50% glucose IV if the patient experiences severe hypoglycemia.
3. The blood sugar should be 40 mg% or lower to get maximum growth hormone production.
4. The patient should be constantly attended by a qualified nurse, because symptoms of severe hypoglycemia may be exhibited very rapidly and immediate intervention is necessary.
5. Assure that blood for growth hormone, cortisol, and glucose are drawn as ordered.
6. The peak effect of the insulin, when given as a bolus, is usually seen 20–30 minutes after injection.
7. Because such a small amount of insulin is given, it is recommended that the insulin be diluted with insulin diluent, l/u/l/ml.

Generic Name: IRON DEXTRAN

Trade Name: IMFERON

Classification: Hematinic

Actions: Treatment of iron-deficiency anemia. The iron in iron dextran is bound to transferrin after being absorbed into the bloodstream. It is then used to synthesize hemoglobin in the bone marrow.

Indications: Iron-deficiency anemia. Injectable iron should only be used when oral route is impossible.

Dosage:
Neonatal: (under 4.5 kg): No more than 25 mg/day.
Pediatric: (4.5–9 kg): No more than 50 mg/day.
Adult:
Less Than 50 kg: No more than 100 mg/day.
More Than 50 kg: No more than 250 mg/day.

Preparation: Injectable form available as 50 mg of iron per ml; 2-ml ampules for IM or IV use, 10-ml ampule for IM use *only*.

Compatibilities: Compatible with normal saline.

Administration: A test dose of 0.5 ml should be given IM or IV before the therapeutic dose. Anaphylactic reaction can occur immediately after administration or up to 1 hour later. If it has not occurred after this time, the remainder of the therapeutic dose can be given.

Neonatal: IM dose should be given Z-track. IV dose should be given slowly at a rate of 1 ml or less per minute.
Pediatric: See neonatal administration.
Adult: IM dose should be given Z-track. IV dose should be given slowly at a rate of 1 ml or less per minute.

Contraindications: Hypersensitivity, any diagnosed anemia other than iron-deficiency anemia.

Side Effects:
Primary: Hypotension, flushing with rapid IV administration, tachycardia, urticaria, anaphylaxis.
Secondary: Soreness, inflammation or skin discoloration at IM injection site, local phlebitis when given IV, headache, metallic taste, nausea.

Nursing Implications: Monitor vital signs for any type of reaction. Reactions can vary from pain of inflammation to anaphylactic shock.

Iron dextran for IM administration should be injected deeply into muscle of the buttock (upper outer quadrant) using Z-track method.

Emergency equipment should be readily available in case of drug reaction.

Monitor patient closely during test dose.

IV or IM sites should be rotated.

Laboratory tests should be monitored before, during, and after therapy. This includes complete blood count, hemoglobin, hematocrit, and reticulocyte count.

Generic Name: ISOPHOSPHAMIDE

Trade Name: HOLOXAN, IFOSFAMIDE

Classification: Antineoplastic alkylating agent

Actions: Binds to proteins and DNA and causes breaks in DNA. It is cell-cycle nonspecific.

Indications: Lung cancer, Hodgkin's and non-Hodgkin's lymphoma, ovarian and breast cancer, acute and chronic leukemias.

Dosage:
Neonatal: Not applicable.
Pediatric: 700–1200 mg/m^2 IV daily for 5 days every 3 weeks or 4 gm/m^2 by IV drip every 3 weeks or 900 mg/m^2 by IV push every week or 1200 mg/m^2 by continuous IV drip daily for 5 days. Doses should be reduced when administered with other chemotherapeutic agents and in patients undergoing radiation therapy.
Adults: See pediatric dosage.

Preparation: Available in 1-g vials that should be diluted with 20 ml of sterile water or saline and in 3-g vials that should be diluted with 30 ml of sterile water or saline.

Home Stability: Unopened vials are stable when stored in the refrigerator or at a room temperature of less than 35°C for 5 years. Prepared solutions are stable for 7 days at room temperature but should be used within 8 hours since the diluents do not contain a preservative.

Compatibilities: The activity of isophosphamide may be increased by phenobarbital, phenytoin, and chloral hydrate. Isophosphamide may also interact with drugs that are incompatible with cyclophosphamide.

Administration:
Neonatal: Not applicable.
Pediatric: Infuse in D$_5$W or normal saline over at least 30 minutes or by continuous IV drip over 5 days.
Adult: See pediatric administration.

Contraindications: Patients who cannot tolerate large hydration volumes.

Side Effects:
Primary:
Nephrotoxicity: Hematuria, dysuria, frequency, and hemorrhagic cystitis may occur without 2–3 liters of hydration and proper doses of ascorbic acid (see Cyclophosphamide for further information). Kidney damage may also occur. Bladder irrigation with neomycin sulfate may be required 48 hours after administration of single doses.
Gastrointestinal: Nausea and vomiting may occur especially with IV push administration, beginning in a few hours and lasting up to 3 days.
Cutaneous: Hair loss that is reversible usually occurs, especially with large IV push doses. Phlebitis and even slight necrosis may occur with extravasation.
Secondary: With high doses, bone marrow depression, lethargy, and confusion; increased liver enzymes. Risk of teratogenesis, infertility, and secondary malignancy is unknown.

Nursing Implications: Make sure the patient is well hydrated the day before therapy, during therapy, and for 3 days after therapy.

Monitor blood urea nitrogen levels.

Medicate with antiemetics as needed.

Administer 250 mg of ascorbic acid three times daily and 500 mg at bedtime.

Test all urine for blood and observe for gross blood.

Instruct patient to void at first sign of bladder fullness.

Inform patient of possible hair loss.

Monitor IV site for patency at least every hour during continuous infusions and instruct patient to report any feelings of burning or discomfort at the venipuncture site.

Continue safe-handling precautions for 4 days after isophosphamide is given.

Generic Name: ISOPROTERENOL HYDROCHLORIDE

Trade Name: ISUPREL

Classification: Adrenergic

Actions: Produces a potent inotropic and chronotropic effect on the myocardium, relaxes bronchial and gastrointestinal smooth muscle while showing little pressor effect.

Indications: Shock, cardiac standstill, cardiac arrhythmias.

Dosage:
Neonatal: Not applicable.
Pediatric: Give one-tenth to one-half of initial adult dose.
Adult: Initially 0.02–0.06 mg with subsequent doses of 0.01–0.2 mg or continuous infusion of 0.5–5.0 μg/minute.

Preparation: 1- or 5-ml ampules containing 0.2 mg/ml.

Home Stability: Not applicable.

Compatibilities: Infuse with 5% dextrose in water.

Administration:
Neonatal: Not applicable.
Pediatric: For direct IV administration, dilute in 10 ml of normal saline and give 0.02 mg/minute. For continuous infusion, dilute 2 mg in 500 ml of diluent (or less if desired) and titrate to patient's response.
Adult: See pediatric administration.

Contraindications: Tachycardia caused by digitalis intoxication, pre-existing tachycardia, concurrent epinephrine therapy. Use with caution in patients with coronary artery disease, myocardial infarction, diabetes, hyperthyroidism, and sensitivity to sympathomimetic amines. Propranolol and other beta blockers may block bronchodilating effects.

Side Effects:
Primary: Tachycardia, palpitations, angina, hypertension followed by hypotension, headache.
Secondary: Mild tremor, weakness, dizziness, nervousness, insomnia, nausea, vomiting, hyperglycemia, sweating, flushing of face, bronchial edema, inflammation.

Nursing Implications: Continuous cardiac monitoring is essential. Document rhythm changes. If heart rate exceeds 110 beats/minute it may be advisable to decrease or temporarily discontinue infusion. Doses sufficient to increase heart rate above 130 beats/minute may induce ventricular arrhythmias.

Continuous blood pressure monitoring is preferred; if not possible, check every 1–3 minutes until stable, then every 5–10 minutes during infusion.

Monitor hemodynamic profile if available.

Monitor urinary output hourly; notify physician if inadequate.

Monitor arterial blood gases for acidosis; ventilation/perfusion abnormalities may be aggravated during therapy.

Infuse via automatic infusion pump. Assess IV site frequently for signs of infiltration.

Be prepared to initiate emergency measures (cardiopulmonary resuscitation, countershock) if heart rhythm deteriorates further.

Assess patient carefully for side effects; notify physician.

Generic Name: KANAMYCIN SULFATE

Trade Name: KANTREX, KLEBCIL

Classification: Antibiotic (aminoglycoside)

Actions: Semisynthetic aminoglycoside derivative from *Streptomyces Kanamyceticus* with neuromuscular blocking action. Inhibits protein synthesis in bacterial cell and is bactericidal. Effective against a wide variety of gram-negative bacilli: *Escherichia coli,* Enterobacter, *Klebsiella pneumoniae,* and most strains of Proteus, *Serratia marcescens,* and Acinetobacter. Also effective against *Staphylococcus aureus* but is not the drug of choice.

Indications: Bacteremia and septicemia, including neonatal sepsis; serious infections such as infections of the urinary or respiratory tract, bones, joints, and central nervous system, including meningitis; burns and postoperative infections.

Dosage:
Neonatal:
Premature or Full-Term Neonates 1 Week of Age or Less: 15 mg/kg/day divided into 2 equal doses every 12 hours.
Over 1 Week of Age: 15 mg/kg/day divided into 3 equal doses every 8 hours.
Pediatric: 15 mg/kg/day divided into 3 equal doses every 8 hours.
Adult: Usual dose: 15 mg/kg/day divided into 3 equal doses every 8 hours. Dosage is based on ideal body weight.
General: Dosage is highly individualized and should be based on therapeutic drug monitoring.
 Therapeutic serum level: 8–16 μg/ml.
 Toxic serum level (peak): more than 35 μg/ml.
 Duration of therapy: 7–10 days.

Preparation: Supplied as a colorless solution, which does not require refrigeration, in 37.5- and 250-mg/ml vials.

Home Stability: Stable at room temperature as prepared by the manufacturer for at least 2 years.

Compatibilities: Compatible with solutions containing dextrose, saline, KCl, Ringer's, or lactated Ringer's. Compatible with aminophylline, dopamine, sodium bicarbonate, and total parenteral nutrition.

Administration:
Neonatal: Infuse over 1–2 hours. Administer at appropriate IV site based on infusion rate. Dilution should be based on fluid volume needs.
Pediatric: Infuse over 30–60 minutes. Administer at appropriate IV site based on infusion rate. Dilution should be based on fluid volume needs.
Adult: Dilute in 50–200 ml (1 mg/ml) IV solution and administer over 30–120 minutes.

Contraindications: Known sensitivity. Use with caution in clients with impaired renal function, eighth cranial nerve impairment, dehydration, fever, myasthenia gravis, parkinsonism, or hypocalcemia. Should not be administered concurrently with penicillins. If concurrent administration is prescribed, administer the drugs 2 hours apart. The neuromuscular blockade effects are enhanced with combined administration of the following drugs: decamethonium, ether, succinylcholine, tubocurarine, or related anesthetics. Cephalosporins may potentiate the nephrotoxic effects of kanamycin. Concurrent administration of other aminoglycosides, ethacrynic acid, or furosemide may enhance the ototoxic effects.

Side Effects:
Primary:
Nephrotoxicity: Proteinurea, presence of red and white blood cells in the urine; granular casts; azotemia; oliguria; urinary frequency; frank hematuria; increase in BUN and serum creatinine; decrease in creatinine clearance and specific gravity; renal damage and failure.
Ototoxicity: Auditory: high frequency hearing loss; complete hearing loss (occasionally permanent); tinnitus; fullness, ringing, or buzzing in ears. Vestibular: dizziness, vertigo; ataxia; nausea, vomiting; nystagmus.
Neurotoxicity: Drowsiness, headache, unsteady gait, weakness, clumsiness, paresthesias, tremors, muscle twitching and weakness, convulsions, neuromuscular blockade with respiratory depression.

Secondary: Nausea, vomiting, stomatitis, skin rash, urticaria, pruritus, generalized burning sensation, drug fever, arthralgia, eosinophilia, anemia, leukopenia, granulocytopenia, thrombocytopenia, unusual thirst, difficult breathing, superinfections, peripheral neuritis.

Nursing Implications: Monitor serum blood levels initially and throughout therapy.

Document the *exact* time of medication administration for determination of blood levels.

Assess renal function prior to initial administration via baseline BUN, creatinine and creatinine clearance, specific gravity, and urine analysis.

Monitor renal function throughout therapy via assessment of BUN, creatinine and creatinine clearance, specific gravity, urine analysis, and strict intake and output.

Encourage hydration of client to reduce chemical irritation to renal tubules.

Assess eighth cranial (vestibulocochlear) nerve function prior to initial administration and throughout therapy and upon discharge via audiometric tests and assessment of vestibular disturbance.

Monitor for overgrowth infection as evidenced by diarrhea, anogenital itching, vaginal discharge, stomatitis, or glossitis.

Antidote: Peritoneal dialysis or hemodialysis will assist in removal of the drug from the bloodstream.

Generic Name: LABETALOL HYDROCHLORIDE

Trade Name: NORMODYNE

Classification: Antihypertensive

Actions: Selectively competes for alpha-adrenergic sites and nonselectively competes for beta-adrenergic receptor sites, thereby blocking beta and selective alpha stimulation. This results in reduction of cardiac output, decreased release of renin from the kidney, and blocking of the vasoconstrictive actions of norepinephrine.

Indications: Severe hypertension.

Dosage:
Neonatal: Not applicable.
Pediatric: Not applicable.
Adult: 20 mg, with repeated doses of 40–80 mg or a continuous infusion of 2 mg/minute.

Preparation: Available in 20-ml ampules containing 5 mg/ml (total 100 mg).

Home Stability: Not applicable.

Compatibilities: May use with Ringer's, lactated Ringer's, or solutions containing dextrose, saline, or both. Not compatible with 5% sodium bicarbonate injection.

Administration:
Neonatal: Not applicable.
Pediatric: Not applicable.
Adult: Give bolus doses over a 2-minute period at 10-minute intervals until a desired blood pressure is achieved or 300 mg have been injected. For continuous infusion, dilute in 160–250 ml of an appropriate solution.

Contraindications: Bronchial asthma, overt cardiac failure, greater than first-degree heartblock, cardiogenic shock, severe bradycardia. Use with caution in patients with cardiac disease, diabetes mellitus, hypoglycemia, and pheochromocytoma.

Side Effects:
Primary: Orthostatic hypotension, hypotension, dizziness, nausea.
Secondary: Vivid dreams, fatigue, hallucination, peripheral vascular disease, nasal stuffiness, vomiting, diarrhea, sexual dysfunction, urinary retention, rash, increased airway resistance.

Nursing Implications: Continuous blood pressure monitoring is preferred. If not possible, obtain baseline blood pressure and check every 3–5 minutes during administration of bolus and until pressure is stabilized. Hourly checks should then be continued.

Continuous cardiac monitoring is needed. Observe for ischemic changes and arrhythmias.

Assess heart tones, jugular venous distension, peripheral edema, lung sounds, dyspnea, and capillary refill every 4 hours and as needed to ascertain effectiveness of treatment.

Fluid status should be monitored via hourly urine outputs, intake, and daily weights.

Keep patient supine for 3 hours after administration; then observe for and teach patient about orthostatic hypotension.

Generic Name: LATRODECTUS MACTANS ANTIVENIN

Trade Name: BLACK WIDOW SPIDER ANTIVENIN

Classification: Antivenin

Actions: Acts to neutralize venom of black widow spider and to provide symptomatic relief. The venom will cause motor paralysis and destroy nerve endings by acting on myoneural junctions or individual nerve endings. The first symptoms of envenomization occur within 15 minutes to several hours after the bite. They include local muscle cramps in shoulder, back, and thigh. After a period of time pain increases and abdominal rigidity develops, with thoracic respiration. The patient is restless and anxious and may develop a feeble pulse and cold, clammy skin. Small children are likely to develop convulsions. The acute stage of poisoning lasts from several hours to a day and then symptoms gradually subside, although there are exceptional fatal cases. Treatment with antivenin may not be necessary.

Indications: Treatment of black widow spider bite. Most effective when administered as soon as possible after the bite. For healthy patients between the ages of 16 and 60, treatment with antivenin may be deferred and treatment with muscle relaxants considered.

Dosage: A test for sensitivity to horse serum should be done prior to administration.
Children under 12, Severe Cases, or Shock: Contents of vial given slowly by IV.
Children over 12 and Adults: Contents of vial given IM.

Preparation: Combination package contains antivenin, 2.5-ml vial of sterile diluent, and 1-ml vial of normal horse serum (1:10 dilution) for sensitivity testing.

Compatibilities: Compatible with saline solution.

Administration: After sensitivity testing to horse serum with negative results:
Children under 12, Severe Cases, or Shock: Dilute in 10–50 ml of saline and administer IV over 15 minutes. It may be necessary to administer a second dose in some cases.
Children over 12 and Adults: 1 vial given IM in the anterolateral thigh.

Side Effects:
Primary: Hypersensitivity reaction to the horse serum along with anaphylaxis can occur immediately.
Secondary: Serum-sickness-like condition can develop 8–12 days after administration of antivenin.

Nursing Implications: Obtain description of the spider, bite location, symptoms, and time since bite.
Obtain medical history of the patient, especially allergy history. This is very important in preventing hypersensitivity reactions.
Monitor and document patient's vital signs and assessment of neurologic, respiratory, and cardiovascular system.
Emergency equipment and medications should be readily available for use. This is especially important during administration of the antivenin.
Supportive therapy may include the use of warm baths, muscle relaxants, or a narcotic analgesic for the relief of pain from muscle cramps. IV doses of 10% calcium gluconate may also relieve the muscle cramps.

Generic Name: LEUCOVORIN CALCIUM

Trade Name: LEUCOVORIN CALCIUM FOR INJECTION, WELLCOVORIN

Classification: The calcium salt of folinic acid, an active metabolite of folic acid

Actions: A form of folic acid that competes with methotrexate for transport into cells and so can "rescue" normal cells from the toxicities of high-dose methotrexate.

Indications: Administered as a rescue after high-dose methotrexate and antidote for toxic effects of folic acid antagonists and used experimentally in high doses to increase the effectiveness of fluorouracil. Used in treatment of folate deficiency megaloblastic anemias when oral folic acid not possible.

Dosage:
Neonatal: Not applicable.
Pediatric: 15–25 mg/m² by IV, IM, or by mouth every 6 hours × 8 up to 100 mg/m² every 3 hours × 12–24. May be given 2–24 hours after high-dose methotrexate has infused.
Adult: See pediatric dosage.

Preparation: Supplied in 50-mg/10-ml vials that should be mixed with 5 ml of sterile water (2.5

ml is the minimum diluent). Also comes in 5- 10-, 15-, and 25-mg tablets.

Home Stability: Unopened vials are stable for 2 years at room temperature. Diluted solutions are stable for 7 days at room temperature. Tablets should be stored in a dry place at room temperatures less than 86°F and should be protected from light.

Compatibilities: No known incompatibilities.

Administration: Infuse by IV push or drip at a reasonable rate. May also give by IV, IM, or mouth.

Side Effects:
Primary: Mild nausea and vomiting (primarily with oral doses).
Secondary: Possible hypersensitivity or allergic reactions.

Nursing Implications: Make sure this drug is given on time, every time, to avoid lethal toxicity from high-dose methotrexate. If patient is taking oral doses at home, this important point must be emphasized. If oral doses cannot be kept down, the physician should be notified immediately.

Generic Name: LEVALLORPHAN TARTRATE

Trade Name: LORFAN

Classification: Narcotic antagonist

Actions: Narcotic antagonist that also has some agonist activity. It can increase respiratory depression induced by non-narcotic medications. Narcotic antagonists are antidotes for overdoses of narcotics. They will prevent or reverse the effects of narcotics by competing for the same receptor sites. Their duration of action may be shorter than that of the narcotic, so repeated doses may be necessary. Because they have some agonist actions that can increase respiratory depression, naloxone is the drug of choice to treat respiratory depression induced by narcotics.

Indications: Asphyxia neonatorum; may be used to treat the side effects of narcotic overdose, but if the respiratory depression is not due to narcotics, this drug may cause further difficulty.

Dosage:
Neonatal: 0.05–0.1 mg into vein of umbilical cord, IM or SC. This may be repeated in 5–10 minutes.
Pediatric: 0.02 mg/kg IV. If further action is needed, 0.01–0.02 mg/kg may be given in 10–15 minutes.
Adult: 1 mg IV, then 0.5 mg in 10–15-minute intervals as needed. Maximum dose is 3 mg.

Preparation: Injectable form available as 1 mg/ml.

Compatibilities: This drug is given by direct IV push in emergencies and not mixed with other solutions.

Administration:
Neonatal: Given into umbilical vein directly after birth. May also be administered IM or SC.
Pediatric: The most rapid action will be seen with IV administration.
Adult: IV administration only.

Contraindications: Hypersensitivity; mild respiratory depression. Should not be used in narcotic addicts, because it may precipitate withdrawal symptoms.

Side Effects:
Primary: Increased respiratory depression when not due to narcotic overdose, lethargy, dizziness, restlessness. The sudden inversion of narcotic depression may cause nausea, vomiting, tachycardia, and increased blood pressure.
Secondary: Hallucinations, disorientation, infant irritability with tendency for increased crying.

Nursing Implications: Determine, when possible, nature of drug and time taken in cases of suspected narcotic overdose.

Assess vital signs and blood pressure at least every 5 minutes and maintain patent airway. Have resuscitation equipment available for immediate use.

Continue to monitor and assess patient until a response is observed. Do not leave unattended.

Patient must be monitored for further depression for the duration of the *narcotic* activity. Several doses of antagonist may be necessary, because its effects are shorter in duration than those of narcotics.

Vital signs may be monitored every 10–15 minutes after response from the antagonist is noted.

Generic Name: LEVORPHANOL TARTRATE

Trade Name: LEVO-DROMORAN

Classification: Narcotic analgesic, Schedule II controlled substance

Actions: Drugs in this class act to relieve moderate to severe pain and provide preoperative sedation. A patient's perception of pain is altered by preventing or changing the transmission of painful stimuli along the sensory pathways in the central nervous system. These pathways are specific to the patient's perception and emotional response to pain. In addition, these drugs suppress the respiratory and cough centers of the brain and have an antiperistaltic effect on the smooth muscle of the intestine. Because of their actions, narcotics can produce physical and psychological dependence. When used to treat severe pain, as in terminal illness, these medications should be given around the clock to maximize the relief of pain and the anxiety produced by the pain.

Indications: Management of moderate to severe pain due to a diversity of causes. It should not be used in cases of mild pain or pain that can be relieved by non-narcotic analgesics.

Dosage:
Neonatal: Not recommended.
Pediatric: Not recommended.
Adult: 2 mg by mouth or SC, with a maximum of 3 mg per dose every 6–8 hours.

Preparation: Injectable form available as 2 mg/ml.

Compatibilities: Not compatible when mixed directly with the following: diazepam, phenytoin, sodium bicarbonate, heparin, methicillin, iodides, barbiturates, and aminophylline. Use with caution in patients taking monoamine oxidase inhibitors, because drug interaction can precipitate unpredictable and possibly fatal reactions. This is possible up to 14 days after taking a monoamine oxidase inhibitor.

Administration:
Neonatal: Not recommended.
Pediatric: Not recommended.
Adult: By mouth or SC every 6–8 hours as needed. It is possible to give by slow IV push, but a narcotic antagonist should be readily available in case of respiratory arrest.

Contraindications: Known hypersensitivity, bronchial asthma, acute alcoholism. Use with caution in patients with head injuries, increased intracranial pressure, shock, central nervous system and respiratory depression, chronic obstructive pulmonary disease, in patients receiving other narcotic analgesics, during delivery of a premature infant, in patients taking MAO inhibitors or who have taken them within 14 days.

Side Effects:
Primary: Respiratory depression and apnea during IV administration, sensitivity reactions, hypotension, bradycardia, nausea, vomiting, dizziness, sedation, sweating.
Secondary: Constipation can occur because of the effect on the smooth muscle of the bowel; urinary retention, pain at the injection site, and phlebitis are possible after IV administration; physical dependence.

Nursing Implications: Because of the chance for respiratory depression, a narcotic antagonist should be available for rapid administration, especially if the route of choice is IV. Naloxone is the antagonist most often used.

Monitor vital signs frequently: IV dose, every 5–10 minutes; SC every 15–30 minutes.

Supportive equipment should be readily available in case of cardiac or respiratory arrest. A patent airway should be maintained.

Monitor infants when the drug is used during labor and delivery.

Monitor intake and output when the drug is given repeatedly, because it may cause urinary retention.

To augment the use of narcotic analgesics, give before severe pain occurs. Nursing actions also include the use of emotional support and patient comfort measures. Because of the depression of the respiratory centers, postoperative use in the management of pain should include the patient's turning, coughing, and deep breathing to prevent pulmonary complications.

Patients should be warned to avoid activities that require alertness.

Assist patient with ambulation. This medication may also cause orthostatic hypotension.

Generic Name: LEVOTHYROXINE SODIUM

Trade Name: LEVOTHROID, SYNTHROID

Classification: Thyroid agent

Actions: Exogenous thyroid hormone whose effect is to increase the metabolic rate of body tissues. The precise mechanism of action is not known. In children, thyroid hormone is necessary for the proper growth and differentiation of tissues, especially to assure ossification of the epiphyses and proper growth and development of the brain.

Indications: Diminished or absent thyroid function resulting from primary atrophy, functional deficiency, partial or complete absence of the gland, or from the effects of surgery, antithyroid agents, or radiation; in simple nonendemic goiter or chronic lymphocytic thyroiditis, to suppress the production of thyrotropin; as a diagnostic agent in suppression tests to diagnose suspected mild hyperthyroidism or thyroid gland autonomy. Given with antithyroid drugs to treat thyrotoxicosis, it may prevent goiter and hypothyroidism. This usage is particularly important during pregnancy. It is the drug of choice to treat congenital hypothyroidism (cretinism).

Dosage:
Neonatal:
Less than 2000 g Except for Those at Risk for Cardiac Failure: 20 μg/24 hours each day.
Over 2000 g: 20–40 μg/24 hours each day.
Pediatric:
4 Weeks–1 Year: 40 μg/24 hours each day.
Over 1 Year: Oral dose is 3–5 μg/kg/24 hours; as IV, give 75 percent of the oral dose.
Adult: Starting dose is 200–500 μg (in patients without severe cardiac disease) followed 24 hours later by 100–300 μg. A rapid increase in metabolism may be risky in the patient with severe cardiac disease, so a smaller initial dose should be used.

Preparation: Supplied as a lyophilized powder in vials containing 200 or 500 μg with 15 mg of mannitol.

Home Stability: Use immediately after reconstituted.

Compatibilities: Compatible with normal saline. Not compatible with *bacteriostatic* sodium chloride or other IV solutions.

Administration:
Neonatal: See pediatric administration.
Pediatric: Reconstitute to concentration of 100 μg/ml in 0.9% sodium chloride and given as a single bolus IV infusion.
Adult: Initial dose is given, followed 24 hours later by a second smaller dose.

Contraindications: Acute myocardial infarction, untreated thyrotoxicosis, history of adverse reactions to any of the ingredients. It may cause acute adrenal crisis if given to patients with uncorrected adrenal insufficiency. Use with caution in patients with cardiovascular disease, diabetes mellitus, diabetes insipidus, hypertension, or adrenal cortical insufficiency, as it can increase symptoms and affect overall management of these conditions. Use with caution in patients with corrected adrenal insufficiency or ischemic states.

Use with caution in patients with arteriosclerosis, as they may experience angina, coronary occlusion, or stroke.

Side Effects:
Primary: Rare.
Secondary: Usually occur as a result of therapeutic overdose. Weight loss, palpitations, nervousness and anxiety, abdominal cramps and diarrhea, sweating, tachycardia, angina, tremors, arrhythmias, insomnia, headaches, intolerance of heat, change in appetite, nausea, leg cramps, fever, menstrual irregularities.

Nursing Implications: Observe the patient for evidence of thyroid hormone toxicity: chest pain, palpitations, excessive sweating, tachycardia, heat intolerance, and nervousness.

In patients with diabetes mellitus, antidiabetic

medication may need to be increased with administration of levothyroxine and decreased if the dose of levothyroxine is decreased.

Levothyroxine may affect the dosage of anticoagulants given.

Children may experience hair loss in the initial months of therapy.

In pediatric cases of cretinism, therapy should begin as soon as possible to prevent developmental delay.

Generic Name: LIDOCAINE HYDROCHLORIDE

Trade Name: **XYLOCAINE**

Classification: Antiarrhythmic

Actions: Local anesthetics prevent the initiation and transmission of impulses to the central nervous system by stabilizing neuronal membranes. Because most topical anesthetics cause vasodilation, a vasoconstrictor (epinephrine) is added to the compound. This delays absorption, prolongs the action, and controls bleeding from the site.

Indications: Among many others, peripheral nerve block, central nerve block, caudal and saddle block.

Dosage: Varies with age and weight of patient, procedure to be performed, and amount of block needed. A 0.5% or 1.0% solution is suggested.

Preparation: Available in a variety of solutions and concentrations, with and without epinephrine.

Administration: Varies with procedure and site of block.

Contraindications: Hypersensitivity to epinephrine or lidocaine, also paraben preservatives and amide-type local anesthetics. Use with caution for anesthesia of oropharyngeal mucosa, because suppression of gag reflex could result in aspiration.

Side Effects:
Primary: Hypersensitivity and rash may result from excessive dosage or rapid absorption. Hypersensitivity reactions include nervousness, dizziness, tremors, drowsiness, convulsion, and possible cardiac/respiratory arrest.
Secondary: Nausea, vomiting, chills, cardiovascular reactions and arrest, urinary retention (spinal block), headache.

Nursing Implications: Check label carefully for proper solution and concentration.

If an extremity is involved, protect from injury because of loss of sensation.

Monitor vital signs as appropriate and observe for adverse reactions.

Generic Name: LINCOMYCIN HYDROCHLORIDE

Trade Name: LINCOCIN

Classification: Antibiotic

Actions: Interferes with protein synthesis of bacterial organisms and is bactericidal against *Staphylococcus aureus* and *epidermidis* (formerly *albus*), beta-hemolytic streptococci, *Streptococcus viridans* and *pneumoniae*, *Clostridium tetani* and *perfringens*, *Corynebacterium diphtheriae* and *acnes*.

Indications: Treatment of serious infections due to susceptible strains of streptococci, pneumococci, and staphylococci when penicillin is not the drug of choice because of allergy or penicillin-resistant gram-positive infections.

Dosage:
Neonatal: Not recommended for infants under 1 month of age.
Pediatric (Over 1 Month): 10–20 mg/kg in equally divided doses every 8–12 hours based on severity of infection.
Adult: 600–1000 mg/day in equally divided doses every 8–12 hours. Total doses of 4–8 g/day have been given for life-threatening infections.

Preparation: Supplied as a liquid in 300 mg/ml ampules.

Compatibilities: Compatible with sodium chloride, glucose, Ringer's, sodium lactate, dextran in 6% saline, B-complex, and B-complex with ascorbic acid. Compatible with the following antibiotics: penicillin G, cephalothin, tetracycline hydrochloride, colistimethate, ampicillin, methicillin, chloramphenicol, polymyxin B sulfate. Do not mix with any other drug.

Administration:
Neonatal: Not applicable.
Pediatric (Over 1 Month): Do not administer by IV injection; cardiac arrest has been reported. Dilute dose in a minimum of 100 ml of solution and infuse via infusion pump over at least 1 hour. If 4 g or more are administered, dilute in 500 ml.
Adult: See pediatric administration.

Contraindications: Hypersensitivity to lincomycin, clindamycin, or erythromycin; monilial infections unless concurrently being treated; minor bacterial or viral infections; pre-existing liver disease; in newborns, pregnancy, and lactation.

Side Effects:
Primary: Pseudomembranous colitis, cardiac arrest, glossitis, stomatitis, diarrhea, allergic reactions, nausea, vomiting.
Secondary: Jaundice and abnormalities in hepatic function tests, neutropenia, leukopenia, agranulocytosis, thrombocytopenia purpura. Aplastic anemia and pancytopenia have been reported.

Nursing Implications: Prior to and during therapy, culture and sensitivity tests should be completed.

Monitor for hypersensitivity reactions: hypotension, facial edema, dyspnea, and restlessness may indicate pending anaphylactic reaction. Contact physician if these symptoms should occur.

Monitor for symptoms of pseudomembranous colitis. Record frequency of bowel movements; note if blood, pus, or mucus is present. Withhold drug if abdominal cramping or diarrhea occurs, and contact physician.

Monitor baseline and periodic renal, hematologic, and hepatic functions.

Monitor for superinfection: fever, redness, soreness, pain, swelling, drainage, monilial rash in perineal area, change in cough, diarrhea.

Monitor respiratory functions in clients receiving concurrent neuromuscular blocking agents. Lincomycin may potentiate their effects.

Generic Name: LORAZEPAM

Trade Name: ATIVAN

Classification: Benzodiazepine, Schedule IV controlled substance

Actions: The benzodiazepines act to reduce anxiety by depressing the central nervous system at the subcortical level. The effects are sedation, anticonvulsing action, and skeletal muscle relaxation with antianxiety and sedative effects. Lorazepam specifically is used to relieve preoperative anxiety. It also eliminates recall of happenings on the day of surgery. The patient is able to respond to simple commands but remains sedated. The optimum time for surgery is 2 hours after IM administration and 15–20 minutes after IV administration. Lorazepam will not increase the respiratory depressant effects of meperidine provided the patient remains alert enough to respond. A dose greater than that recommended can produce heavy sedation.

Indications: Preanesthetic medication that produces sedation and relief of anxiety. Also used to relieve anxiety, agitation, and tension due to neuroses or organic disorders.

Dosage:
Neonatal: Not recommended for those under the age of 18.
Pediatric: See neonatal dosage.
Adult: 2–4 mg IM or IV.

Preparation: Injectable form available as 2 and 4 mg/ml.

Home Stability: Any solution that has been diluted should be refrigerated.

Compatibilities: Compatible with sterile water, sodium chloride, and 5% dextrose; narcotic analgesics; atropine; muscle relaxants; and frequently used anesthetics. Not compatible with cimetidine.

Administration:
Neonatal: Not recommended.
Pediatric: Not recommended.
Adult: IM dose may be given undiluted but should be given deep into the muscle. IV dose must be diluted with a compatible IV solution 1:1. It can then be given directly to the patient, but the rate of infusion should not exceed 2 mg/minute.

Contraindications: Sensitivity to benzodiazepines or diluents (polyethylene glycol, propylene glycol, and benzyl alcohol); acute narrow-angle glaucoma; myasthenia gravis; psychosis. Use with caution in patients with renal or hepatic impairment or organic brain syndrome.

Side Effects:
Primary: Sedation, depression, slurred speech, nervousness, difficulty in concentration, bradycardia, cardiovascular collapse.
Secondary: Nausea, constipation, weakness, changes in libido, urinary retention.

Nursing Implications: Assess patient for adverse side effects (oversedation) during peak action periods.

Monitor vital signs and maintain patent airway. Emergency equipment should be readily available.

Lorazepam should not be mixed with alcohol or other depressants.

Assess patient for central nervous system response to drug and assist with ambulation as required.

After long-term therapy, dosage should be decreased gradually to prevent withdrawal symptoms.

Generic Name: MAGNESIUM SULFATE

Trade Name: EPSOM SALT

Classification: Anticonvulsant

Actions: Anticonvulsant, mechanism of action unknown. Believed to produce depression of the central nervous system by decreasing the amount of acetylcholine available from motor nerve terminal, in effect producing a peripheral neuromuscular blockade. It also depresses smooth, skeletal, and cardiac muscle. The rate of sinoatrial node impulse formation is slowed, and conduction time is prolonged. Large doses produce vasodilation by direct action on blood vessels.

Indications: Treatment of acute magnesium deficiency, control and prevention of seizures, control of hypertension.

Dosage: Titrate according to need. These are guidelines only.
Pediatric:
Seizures or Tetany (Hypomagnesemia): 0.2 ml/kg (50% solution) IM, every 12 hours (in severe cases, every 4–8 hours may be necessary).
Acute Hypomagnesemia: 0.1–0.2 ml/kg IM or well diluted IV every 12 hours.
Hypertension/Seizures in Acute Nephritis: 0.2 ml/kg IM every 4–6 hours as needed.
Adult: 1–4 g of 10–20% solution IV or 1–5 g of 20–50% solution 6 times a day as needed.

Preparation: Injectable (IV, IM) 10%, 25%, or 50% solutions.

Compatibilities: Compatible with D_5W or normal saline. Avoid solutions with calcium or phosphate.

Administration:
Pediatric: IV rate not to exceed 150 mg/minute.
Adult: With 10–20% solution, do not exceed 1.5 ml/minute.

Contraindications: Myocardial damage, heart block, IV administration 2 hours before delivery. Use with caution in patients with impaired renal function, digitalized patients, and patients receiving other central nervous system depressants.

Side Effects:
Primary: Hypermagnesemia, flushing, sweating, thirst, hypotension, depressed reflexes, muscle weakness, complete heart block, depressed cardiac function, circulatory and respiratory collapse. Symptoms become more life-threatening as the drug level in the blood rises.
Secondary: Drowsiness, hypothermia, hypocalcemia.

Nursing Implications: Any patient receiving parenteral magnesium sulfate should be monitored carefully. Document effect of drug on patient's condition.

Monitor plasma levels. Normal value is 1.8–3.0 mEq/L.

Assess patient's vital signs, reflexes, and output prior to each IV dose.

Document intake and output.

Emergency resuscitation equipment should be readily available. *Antidote:* calcium gluconate or calcium gluceptate.

Monitor newborns of treated mothers for signs of overdose.

Maintain a safe environment for patient experiencing central nervous system depression.

Generic Name: MANNITOL

Trade Name: OSMITROL

Classification: Diuretic

Actions: Osmotic diuretic, distributed in the body's extracellular compartments. Especially effective in reducing cerebrospinal and intraocular fluids.

Indications: Reduction of intracranial and intraocular pressure; edema; ascites. May be used to treat oliguria.

Dosage:
Neonatal: Not applicable.
Pediatric: 1–2 g/kg/day or 30–60 g/m^2/day as a 15–20% solution.
Adult: 1–2 g/kg/day, not to exceed 6 g/kg/day (1 g equal to 5.5 mOsm).

Preparation: Available in solutions of 25% (12.5 g/50 ml or 1375 mOsm/L), 20% (50 g/250 ml or 1100 mOsm/L), 15% (22.5 g/150 ml or 825 mOsm/L), 10% (50 g/500 ml or 550 mOsm/L), and 5% (50 g/L or 275 mOsm/L).

Compatibilities: May infuse with dextrose, saline, or a combination of the two.

Administration:
Neonatal: Not applicable.
Pediatric: 1–2 g/kg over 30–90 minutes. Test or loading doses of 200 mg/kg can be given over 3–5 minutes.
Adult: 1–2 g/kg over 30–90 minutes. Test or loading doses of 200 mg/kg can be given over 3–5 minutes.

Contraindications: Anuria, fluid and electrolyte depletion, pregnancy, severe congestive heart failure, severe dehydration, severe renal impairment.

Side Effects:
Primary: Dehydration, dizziness, nausea, thirst, thrombophlebitis, hyponatremia, hypochloremia.
Secondary: Backache, blurred vision, chest pain, chills, convulsions, dryness of mouth, edema, fever, headache, hypertension, hypotension, pulmonary edema, rhinitis, tachycardia, urinary retention.

Nursing Implications: Potential for volume and electrolyte depletion, leading to profound water loss, dehydration, reduction in blood volume, and circulatory collapse. Therefore monitor intake and output, serum electrolytes, blood pressure, and pulse rate frequently.

Assess for signs of hypokalemia (muscle weakness and cramping). Teach patients about potassium-rich foods (citrus fruits, tomatoes, bananas, dates, apricots). Be especially careful in patients receiving digitalis because of the increased risk of digitalis toxicity.

Assess for signs of congestive heart failure during treatment.

Caution patient to change position slowly due to orthostatic hypotension.

Monitor BUN and creatinine for signs of deteriorating renal function.

Administer in the morning to prevent nocturia.

Elderly patients are especially susceptible to excessive diuresis.

Generic Name: MECHLORETHAMINE HYDROCHLORIDE (NITROGEN MUSTARD)

Trade Name: MUSTARGEN

Classification: Antineoplastic alkylating agent

Actions: Destroys tumors by causing miscoding in the DNA, cross-linking DNA pairs, causing breaks in the DNA chain, clinging to a DNA base component, and inhibiting RNA-directed protein synthesis and other cell membrane and metabolic processes. Because of its multiple mechanisms of cell destruction, mechlorethamine is cell-cycle nonspecific.

Indications: Hodgkin's and non-Hodgkin's lymphoma, lung cancer, malignant pleural effusions, mycosis fungoides, psoriasis.

Dosage:
Neonatal: Not applicable.
Pediatric: 0.4 mg/kg IV every 4–6 weeks or 6 mg/m² IV on days 1 and 8 every 2 weeks; 10–30 mg diluted to 50–100 ml for pleural effusion instillation and intraperitoneally; 10–20 mg given intrapericardially; 10 mg dissolved in 50–60 ml of tap water or 10% ointment for topical use. Special preparations have been made for intralesional injections into mycosis fungoides.
Adult: See pediatric dosage.

Preparation: Available in 10-mg vials that should be diluted with 10 ml of sterile water without preservative.

Home Stability: Undiluted vials may be stored at room temperature. However, once the drug is mixed it should be used within a half-hour.

Compatibilities: As with most antineoplastic agents, it is advisable not to administer drug with other admixture solutions.

Administration:
Neonatal: Not applicable.
Pediatric: Administer by slow IV push into the side arm of a free-flowing IV, checking patency every 2–3 minutes to avoid extravasation of this severe vesicant.
Adult: See pediatric administration.

Contraindications: Pregnancy, presence of infection, especially herpes zoster. Use with caution in patients with bone marrow metastasis and chronic lymphocytic leukemia.

Side Effects:
Primary:
Hematopoietic: Decreased lymphocytes within 24 hours; decreased granulocytes and platelets within 6–8 days, lasting for 10–20 days.
Cutaneous: Thrombosis or thrombophlebitis that may be diminished by Solu Cortef; extravasation produces pain, swelling, redness, hardness, and tissue damage. Hypersensitivity reactions, hyperpigmentation, rashes, dry skin, and itching may occur with topical use, especially with the aqueous solution.
Gastrointestinal: Nausea and vomiting within 1–3 hours, lasting up to 8 hours; anorexia, metallic taste immediately after drug injection, and diarrhea.
Reproductive: Teratogenesis and infertility are definite. Menstrual irregularity may occur.
Electrolyte: Hyperuricemia secondary to rapid cell death if allopurinol is not given, especially in patients with leukemia and lymphoma.
Secondary: Skin rashes, weakness, drowsiness, headache, fever, chills, tinnitus, deafness, possible contribution to amyloidosis, reversible aphasia, hair loss. Cardiac arrhythmias may occur with intrapericardial use. Allergic and anaphylactic reactions are rare. Avoid direct eye contact. The possibility of a secondary malignancy increases when used with other chemotherapy drugs or radiation therapy.

Nursing Implications: Monitor complete blood count.

Instruct patient and family on infection and bleeding precautions during the second and third weeks after the treatment is given.

Establish and maintain good venous access, checking for patency every 2–3 minutes during IV push administration and instructing the patient to report any sensations of burning or pain. Have mechlorethamine's antidote, sodium thiosulfate 10%, available for extravasations or accidental spills.

Premedicate with antiemetics and continue them for about 12 hours.

Obtain an order for an antidiarrheal if necessary.

Discuss with patient the likelihood of menstrual irregularities, temporary or permanent sterility, and birth defects if pregnancy occurs while taking drug.

Monitor uric acid levels and instruct patient on importance of taking allopurinol and maintaining adequate hydration.

Instruct and/or assist the patient in changing positions (side to side, Trendelenburg to reverse Trendelenburg) every 5–10 minutes for 1 hour after intrapleural or intraperitoneal administration.

Inform patient of the likelihood of hypersensitivity reactions with topical application of drug.

Continue safe-handling precautions for 1 day after drug is given.

Generic Name: MENADIOL SODIUM DIPHOSPHATE (VITAMIN K₃)

Trade Name: SYNKAYVITE, KAPPADIONE

Classification: Vitamin

Actions: Essential for hepatic synthesis of clotting factors II, VII, IX, and X. Used to treat coagulation disorders caused by faulty formation of these factors. Vitamin K does not negate the pharmacologic effects of heparin. This form of vitamin K is a synthetic water-soluble form of menadione and is not recommended for neonatal administration.

Indications: Treatment of hypoprothrombinemia that is secondary to the limited absorption or synthesis of vitamin K. Some examples of this are biliary fistula, obstructive jaundice, ulcerative colitis, intestinal obstruction, and antibacterial therapy.

Dosage:
Neonatal: Not recommended.
Pediatric: 5–10 mg once or twice daily.
Adult: 5–15 mg once or twice daily.

Preparation: Injectable form contains 5, 10, or 37.5 mg/ml.

Home Stability: Store at room temperature. Does not need to be refrigerated.

Administration:
Neonatal: Not recommended.
Pediatric: SC, IM, IV.

Adult: SC, IM, IV. The rate of IV administration should not exceed 1 mg/minute. The action of vitamin K will be more rapid with IV administration, but the duration of action will be longer when given SC or IM. A single dose will usually correct hypoprothrombinemia, but if laboratory work does not show improvement the dosage may be repeated.

Contraindications: Hypersensitivity; treatment of oral anticoagulant overdose, hepatocellular disease, heparin-induced bleeding. Should not be given to mothers in the last few weeks of pregnancy, since it may cause severe side effects in the baby.

Side Effects:
Primary: Headache, nausea, vomiting, pruritus, hyperbilirubinemia in newborns, which can lead to kernicterus.
Secondary: Erythrocyte hemolysis in patients with G-6-PD deficiency; may depress liver function in patients with liver disease.

Nursing Implications: Observe patient for signs of bleeding. Monitor laboratory work such as prothrombin time, bleeding time, hemoglobin, and complete blood count.

During and after administration, watch for signs of allergic reaction.

Instruct patient that pain, swelling, or tenderness at injection site is possible.

Generic Name: MEPERIDINE HYDROCHLORIDE

Trade Name: DEMEROL

Classification: Narcotic analgesic, Schedule II controlled substance

Actions: Drugs in this class act to relieve moderate to severe pain and provide preoperative sedation. A patient's perception of pain is altered by preventing or changing the transmission of painful stimuli along the sensory pathways in the central nervous system. These pathways are specific to the perception and emotional response of the patient to pain. In addition, these drugs suppress the respiratory and cough centers of the brain and have an antiperistaltic effect on the smooth muscle of the intestine. Because of their actions, narcotics can produce physical and psychological dependence. When used to treat severe pain, as in terminal illness, these medications should be given around the clock to maximize the relief of pain and the anxiety produced by the pain.

Indications: Management of moderate to severe pain due to a diversity of causes. It should not be used in cases of mild pain or pain that can be relieved by non-narcotic analgesics.

Dosage:
Neonatal: See pediatric dosage.
Pediatric: 1 mg/kg, IM or SC every 4–6 hours or 6 mg/kg/day, IM or SC every 4 hours. Maximum is 100 mg/dose. IV administration causes respiratory depression; use caution if administering by this route.
Adult: 50–150 mg, IM or SC, every 4 hours. Any IV dose, pediatric or adult should be diluted before slow IV administration.
General: Dosage must be decreased if given by IV method.

Preparation: Available in injectable multidose vials of 50 or 100 mg/ml and in single-dose vials, syringes, and ampules with 25, 50, 75, and 100 mg/dose.

Compatibilities: Not compatible when directly mixed with the following: diazepam, phenytoin, sodium bicarbonate, heparin, methicillin, iodides, barbiturates, aminophylline. Use with caution in patients taking MAO inhibitors; it can precipitate unpredictable and possibly fatal reactions. This is possible up to 14 days after taking a MAO inhibitor.

Administration:
Neonatal: See pediatric administration.
Pediatric: Avoid IV route if possible, because it will cause significant respiratory depression. Dilute and give slowly when given parenterally.
Adult: Give IM or SC. IV dose can cause severe respiratory depression. If given IV, dilute before administration and give slowly.

Contraindications: Hypersensitivity; during delivery of a premature infant; in patients taking monoamine oxidase inhibitors or who have taken them within 14 days. Use with caution in patients with head injuries, increased intracranial pressure, shock, central nervous system and respiratory depression, chronic obstructive pulmonary disease, and in patients receiving other narcotic analgesics.

Side Effects:
Primary: Respiratory depression and apnea during IV administration, sensitivity reactions, hypotension, bradycardia, nausea, vomiting, dizziness, sedation, sweating.
Secondary: Constipation can occur because of the effect on the smooth muscle of the bowel. Urinary retention, pain at injection site, and phlebitis are possible after IV administration. Physical dependence.

Nursing Implications: Because of the chance for respiratory depression, a narcotic antagonist should be available for rapid administration, especially if the route of choice is IV. Naloxone is the antagonist most often used.

Monitor vital signs frequently. For IV dose, every 5–10 minutes; for IM and SC dose, every 15–30 minutes.

Supportive equipment should be readily available in case of cardiac or respiratory arrest. A patent airway should be maintained.

Monitor infants when the drug is used during labor and delivery.

Monitor intake and output when the drug is given repeatedly; it may cause urinary retention.

To augment the use of narcotic analgesics, give before severe pain occurs. Nursing actions also include the use of emotional support and patient comfort measures. Because of depression of respiratory centers, postoperative use in management of pain should include the patient's turning, coughing, and deep breathing to prevent pulmonary complications.

Patients should be warned to avoid activities that require alertness.

Assist patient with ambulation. This medication may also cause orthostatic hypotension.

Generic Name: MEPHENTERMINE SULFATE

Trade Name: WYAMINE

Classification: Vasopressor

Actions: Increases systolic and diastolic blood pressure by increasing cardiac output and vasoconstriction.

Indications: Treatment of shock and hypotension. Safe for hypotension following spinal anesthesia during obstetric procedures and otherwise.

Dosage:
Neonatal: Not applicable.
Pediatric: 0.4 mg/kg.
Adult: 0.5 mg/kg. Maintenance infusion may be titrated.
During Obstetric Procedures: 15 mg IV as needed.
Other Hypotensions: 30–45 mg in a single injection, then 30 mg repeated as needed.

Preparation: Available as 30 mg in 1-ml Tubex.

Home Stability: Not recommended for home use.

Compatibilities: May infuse with 5% dextrose in water, saline, or any combination thereof.

Administration:
Neonatal: Not applicable.
Pediatric: Can give undiluted at a rate of 30 mg/ minute. Mix maintenance infusion 16.6 ml mephentermine (30 mg/ml) in 500 ml 5% dextrose in water.
Adult: See pediatric administration.

Contraindications: Concealed hemorrhage or hypotension from hemorrhage (except in emergencies), concurrent use of phenothiazines, use of MAO inhibitors within 2 weeks. Use with caution in patients with arteriosclerosis, cardiovascular disease, hyperthyroidism, hypertension, or chronic illness. Hypercapnia, hypoxia, and acidosis may reduce effectiveness or increase adverse effects.

Side Effects:
Primary: Arrhythmias, hypertension, euphoria, nervousness, anxiety, tremor, incoherence, drowsiness, convulsions.
Secondary: Anorexia.

Nursing Implications: Obtain baseline blood pressure and heart rate and rhythm.
Check blood pressure every 2 minutes during infusion until stabilized, then every 5 minutes.
Observe for side effects; report to physician.
IV drug is not irritating to tissue and extravasation is not dangerous.
May increase uterine contractions during third trimester of pregnancy.

Generic Name: MERSALYL AND THEOPHYLLINE

Trade Name: FOYURETIC, MERCUTHEOLIN, MARSA, MERSALYN, THEO-SYL-R

Classification: Diuretic

Actions: Releases mercury ions, which irritate renal tubular cells, preventing reabsorption of sodium, chlorides, and water.

Indications: Treatment of edema and ascites in cardiac and cardiorenal diseases, nephrosis, cirrhosis of the liver, and thrombophlebitic and thyrocardiac edema.

Dosage:
Neonatal: Not applicable.
Pediatric: Half of the recommended adult dose.
Adult: 0.5 ml. May repeat every 24 hours with 0.5–1.0 ml if no side effects occur. Desired dose is 1–2 ml twice weekly.

Compatibilities: Compatible with dextrose or saline solutions.

Administration:
Neonatal: Not applicable.
Pediatric: Dilute with 5–10 ml of sterile water and infuse at a rate of 0.5 ml of actual medication over 2 minutes.
Adult: See pediatric administration.

Contraindications: Acute nephritis, chronic kidney disease, hypersensitivity to mercury, pregnancy and lactation, severe liver disease, ulcerative colitis. Use with extreme caution in patients with myocardial infarction, urologic disease, or renal or hepatic insufficiency.

Side Effects:
Primary: Alkalosis, blood volume reduction, circulatory collapse, cyanosis, dyspnea, excessive diuresis, hypokalemia, nephrotoxicity, hypotension, thrombophlebitis, vascular thrombosis, ventricular arrhythmias, death.
Secondary: Cutaneous eruption, dehydration, diarrhea, fever, flushing, gingivitis, hematuria, increased salivation, muscle cramps, nausea, stomatitis, vertigo, vomiting.

Nursing Implications: Do not give unless patient's EKG is monitored. Observe closely for sudden onset of arrhythmias.

Assess vital signs before treatment begins, then hourly until stable.

Monitor serum electrolyte levels closely. Hypokalemia can potentiate cardiac irritability, especially in conjunction with digitalis therapy.

Assess IV site frequently; infiltration can cause necrosis.

Monitor daily weight, intake and output, and skin turgor during therapy—urine output may reach 8 or 9 L in 24 hours.

Generic Name: METARAMINOL BITARTRATE

Trade Name: ARAMINE

Classification: Vasopressor

Actions: Potent sympathomimetic amine that increases both systolic and diastolic blood pressure, exerts a positive inotropic effect on the heart, and vasoconstricts peripheral vessels.

Indications: Severe shock, hypotension.

Dosage:
Neonatal: Not applicable.
Pediatric: 0.01 mg/kg as a single injection; for continuous infusion, 1 mg/25 ml and titrate.
Adult: 0.5–5.0 mg by direct IV injection for severe shock; for continuous infusion, 15–100 mg/500 ml and titrate.

Preparation: Available in 1- or 10-ml vials containing 10 mg of metaraminol per milliliter.

Home Stability: Not applicable.

Compatibilities: May infuse with 5% dextrose, normal saline, Ringer's, lactated Ringer's, dextran 6% in saline, Normosol-R, and Normosol-M in D_5W.

Administration:
Neonatal: Not applicable.
Pediatric: May give up to 5 mg undiluted over 1 minute as a single injection. Follow injection, if given, with continuous infusion, allowing at least 10-minute intervals between titration of dosage.
Adult: See pediatric administration.

Contraindications: Uncorrected hypotension resulting from blood volume deficits, pregnancy, peripheral or mesenteric thrombosis, pulmonary edema, hypercarbia, acidosis, and concurrent use with cyclopropane and halogenated hydrocarbon anesthetics. Use with caution in patients with hypertension, thyroid disease, diabetes, cirrhosis, or malaria, and when used concurrently with digitalis. May cause hypertensive crisis when used with MAO inhibitors.

Side Effects:
Primary: Metabolic acidosis in hypovolemia, increased body temperature, respiratory distress.
Secondary: Hypertension, hypotension, precordial pain, arrhythmias (including sinus or ventricular tachycardia), bradycardia, premature supraventricular beats, atrioventricular dissociation, apprehension, restlessness, dizziness, headache, tremors, weakness, nausea, vomiting, decreased urinary output, hyperglycemia, flushing, pallor, sweating.

Nursing Implications: Record baseline heart rate and rhythm, blood pressure, quality of pulses, and color, temperature, and capillary refill of extremities before beginning infusion.

Monitor blood pressure every 5 minutes during titration until stabilized, then every 15 minutes.

Monitor heart rhythm and rate continuously. Document and report any changes to physician.

Assess pulse quality. Assess color, temperature, and capillary refill of extremities.

Monitor urinary output. It may decrease initially but should increase with resumption of normal blood pressure. Report persistent low output.

Infuse via automatic infusion pump. Titrate according to physician's guidelines, avoiding an excessive blood pressure response, which can cause acute pulmonary edema, arrhythmias, and cardiac arrest.

Discontinue drug slowly, monitoring vital signs every 5 minutes until drug is stopped and blood pressure is stabilized.

Monitor blood sugar levels in diabetics for possible adjustment of insulin requirements.

Atropine reverses bradycardia caused by metaraminol; phentolamine decreases vasopressor effects.

Infuse via the largest vein possible and assess IV site frequently for signs of infiltration or blanching along the course of the infused vein.

Generic Name: METHICILLIN SODIUM

Trade Name: STAPHCILLIN, CELBENIN

Classification: Antibiotic (penicillin)

Actions: Semisynthetic penicillin bactericidal against penicillinase-producing strains of staphylococci, beta-hemolytic streptococci, and *Streptococcus pneumoniae*.

Indications: Infections caused by penicillinase-producing staphylococci, *Streptococcus pneumoniae*, group A beta-hemolytic streptococci, and penicillin G–resistant and penicillin G–sensitive staphylococci.

Dosage:
Neonatal:

0–14 Days of Age and 2000 g or Less: 50 mg/kg/day divided into equal doses every 12 hours.

0–14 Days of Age and over 2000 g: 75 mg/kg/day divided into equal doses every 8 hours.

15–30 Days of Age and 2000 g or Less: 75 mg/kg/day divided into equal doses every 8 hours.

15–30 Days of Age and over 2000 g: 100 mg/kg/day divided into equal doses every 6 hours.

Pediatric: 100–400 mg/kg/day in divided doses every 4–6 hours.

Adult: 1 g every 6 hours. In severe infections, higher doses may be appropriate.

Preparation: Supplied as a powder. Reconstitute with sterile water or sodium chloride for injection as follows:

VIAL SIZE	DILUENT	CONCENTRATION
1 g	1.5 ml	500 mg/ml
4 g	5.7 ml	500 mg/ml
6 g	8.6 ml	500 mg/ml

Home Stability: Use solution within 24 hours of reconstitution if kept at room temperature or within 4 days if kept refrigerated.

Compatibilities: Compatible with solutions containing dextrose, saline, KCl, Ringer's, or lactated Ringer's. Compatible with aminophylline, heparin, and total parenteral nutrition. Do not mix with any other antibiotic; may inactivate or become inactivated by antibiotics.

Administration:
Neonatal: Dilute to 20 mg/ml and give by slow IV push over 5 minutes if dosage is less than 500 mg. Do not exceed rate of 200 mg/minute.
Pediatric: Dilute to 50 mg/ml and give by slow IV push at the Y-site over 5 minutes. If dosage exceeds 500 mg, administer as for adult, below.
Adult: Dilute to 20 mg/ml in IV solution and infuse by IV piggyback over 30–60 minutes.

Contraindications: Hypersensitivity to penicillins. A cross-allergic reaction may occur with cephalosporins. Anaphylaxis may occur. Safety in pregnancy has not been established.

Side Effects:
Primary: Hypersensitivity reactions such as skin rash, pruritus, anaphylaxis, urticaria, serum sickness, interstitial nephritis, febrile reactions; superinfections; pain and thrombosis of the IV site; oral lesions (glossitis, stomatitis).
Secondary: Neuropathy and bone marrow depression; anemia, neutropenia, granulocytopenia, agranulocytopenia.

Nursing Implications: Prior to and during therapy, culture and sensitivity tests should be completed.

Monitor for allergic reactions.

Monitor for signs and symptoms of interstitial nephritis for 2–4 weeks following therapy: spiking fever, anorexia, skin rash, oliguria, hematuria, cloudy urine, eosinophilia.

Monitor baseline and periodic renal, hepatic, and hematologic functions, especially in long-term therapy.

Monitor for superinfection. Assess for oral lesions (stomatitis, glossitis); rectal or vaginal itching; vaginal discharge; loose, foul-smelling stools; unusual odor to urine.

Monitor infusion site hourly for signs of thrombophlebitis.

Monitor methicillin blood levels closely in infants; urinary excretion is slower because of undeveloped renal function.

Generic Name: METHOCARBAMOL

Trade Name: DELAXIN, ROBAXIN

Classification: Skeletal muscle relaxant

Actions: Acts centrally to produce sedation and muscle relaxation by blocking spinal polysynaptic reflexes. Doses are absorbed rapidly, whether orally or parenterally administered.

Indications: Oral doses are used to relieve acute, painful muscle spasms, either localized or due to inflammation or trauma. Parenteral administration is indicated in tetanus or other acute spasms. It is not used for long-term therapy.

Dosage: IV or IM.
Pediatric: 15 mg/kg IV every 6 hours. Maximum dose: 1.8 g/m^2/day for 3 consecutive days.
Adult: Range: 1–3 g daily. Do not exceed 300 mg/minute. Infusion: Mix 1 g in not more than 250 ml NaCl or D$_5$W. Maximum dose: 3 g/day for 3 consecutive days.

Preparation: Available in 10-ml single-dose vials of 100 mg/ml.

Compatibilities: Compatible with sodium chloride and D$_5$W.

Administration:
Pediatric: Do not exceed 6 mg/kg/minute.
Adult: Do not exceed 300 mg/minute.

Contraindications: Renal impairment, hypersensitivity, central nervous system depression, or acidosis, in comatose patients. Safe use in pregnant and lactating women, children, and women of childbearing potential has not been established.

Side Effects:
Primary: Drowsiness and dizziness, vertigo, hypotension, anaphylactic reaction, blurred vision, bradycardia.
Secondary: Metallic taste in mouth, thrombophlebitis, pain at injection site, flushing.

Nursing Implications: Monitor patient carefully after administration for side effects. Obtain a baseline set of vital signs.
Carefully monitor infusion rate.
Inform patient of possible drowsiness or dizziness. Maintain a safe environment for patient. Assist with ambulation.
Monitor IV site carefully for signs of extravasation. This drug may cause severe tissue damage.
Do not administer subcutaneously. Rotate IM injection sites.

Generic Name: METHOTREXATE SODIUM

Trade Name: FOLEX

Classification: Antineoplastic antimetabolite

Actions: Folic acid antagonist that binds to a cellular enzyme resulting in blockage of DNA, RNA, and protein synthesis. Cell-cycle specific in the S phase.

Indications: Acute leukemias; trophoblastic tumors; Burkitt's lymphoma; lymphosarcoma; mycosis fungoides; osteogenic sarcoma; epidermoid carcinoma of the head and neck; multiple myeloma; lung, breast, and ovarian cancers; psoriasis.

Dosage:
Neonatal: Not applicable.
Pediatric: 15–30 mg IM or by mouth daily for 5 days every 1–2 weeks for 3–5 courses or 30 mg/m² IM or by mouth 2 times a week or 2.5 mg/kg IV every 2 weeks or 10–25 mg by mouth 4–8 times every 7–10 days or 2.5–10 mg by mouth daily for several weeks or 50 mg IM once a week for several weeks or 25 mg IM 2 times a week for several weeks. High-dose therapy consists of 100 mg–2–3 g/m² IV every 1–3 weeks. Intrathecal doses range from 10–15 mg/m². The recommended dose into an Ommaya Reservoir is 1 mg every 12 hours for 6 times.
Adult: See pediatric dosage.

Preparation: Available in 20-mg, 50-mg, 500-mg, and 1-g vials that can be diluted with sterile water, D_5W, normal saline, or Elliott's B solution in the amounts of 20 ml or less, 5, 9.6, and 20 ml respectively. Oral methotrexate comes in 2.5- and 50-mg tablets.

Home Stability: Unopened vials and tablets are stable at room temperature for 2 years. Once in solution, methotrexate is stable for a week at room temperature, but it should be used within 24 hours since it contains no preservative.

Compatibilities: Effectiveness may be decreased if given with prednisolone, indomethacin, vitamins with folic acid, asparaginase, and Ara-C. Toxicity may be increased by salicylates, probenecid, sulfonamides, phenytoin ethyl alcohol, triamterene, chloral hydrate, alcohol, phenylbutazone, penicillins, thiazide diuretics, pyrimethamine, and para-aminobenzoic acid. Toxicity is decreased by asparaginase and thymidine. May potentiate oral anticoagulants like warfarin. Amphotericin B may potentiate methotrexate's cytotoxicity. High-dose methotrexate may be synergistic with fluorouracil if given 12–24 hours before the latter. Direct admixture with Ara-C and fluorouracil must be avoided. As with most antineoplastic agents, it is advisable not to administer methotrexate with other admixture solutions.

Administration:
Neonatal: Not applicable.
Pediatric: Infuse regular dose by IV push, preferably through side arm of free-flowing IV, or drip at a convenient rate. Infuse high dose over 6–42 hours.
Adult: See pediatric administration.

Contraindications: Signs of gastrointestinal bleeding. Dosage reduction required if creatinine clearance is less than 60 mg/minute. Use with caution in the very young or old and in patients with aplasia, infection, bleeding, anemia, peptic ulcer, ulcerative colitis, debility, or hepatic dysfunction.

Side Effects:
Primary:
Hematopoietic: Decreased red and white blood cells and platelets in 2–13 days with recovery in 9–19 days.
Gastrointestinal: Stomatitis, pharyngitis, diarrhea (presence requires discontinuing the drug); moderate nausea and vomiting; anorexia.
Hepatotoxicity: Increased SGOT, BUN, prothrombin, and bilirubinemia with a decrease in plasma factor VII and possible liver atrophy, necrosis, fibrosis, and cirrhosis.
Cutaneous: Rashes, itching, changes in pigmentation, photosensitivity, vasculitis, acne, reversible alopecia.
Neurotoxicity: Dizziness, blurred vision, headache, sleepiness, seizures, encephalopathy.
Nephrotoxicity: Renal failure, especially without hydration, and urine alkalization with high doses.

Reproductive: Teratogenesis, menstrual dysfunction.

Secondary: Chills, fever, malaise, osteoporosis, pneumonitis, pulmonary fibrosis. Intrathecal use may result in severe headache, nuchal rigidity, fever, vomiting, motor dysfunction of the limbs (spasticity), cranial nerve palsies, convulsions, dementia, coma, Guillain-Barré-type syndrome, and chronic brain injury. Hypersensitivity reactions with wheezing, itching, rashes, decreased blood pressure, and anaphylaxis are infrequent. Infertility is unlikely but possible. The risk of secondary malignancy is unknown.

Nursing Implications: Monitor complete blood count.

Instruct patient and family on infection and bleeding precautions during the first to third weeks after treatment. Teach the patient ways to conserve energy by pacing activities.

Instruct patient on good oral hygiene with a soft-bristled toothbrush after meals and at bedtime. Report early signs of mouth sores.

Premedicate with antiemetics with high doses.

Guaiac all emesis and stools and report diarrhea to the physician.

Monitor SGOT, prothrombin, bilirubin, and plasma factor VII. Report any signs of jaundice.

Instruct patient on the possibility of skin changes and reversible hair loss.

Instruct patient to report any headache, blurred vision, or dizziness.

With high-dose therapy, maintain prehydration of 1.5 L/m^2 with 100 mEq bicarbinate and 10–20 mEq potassium for 12 hours before therapy and continue as posthydration at 3 L/m^2 for 24 hours. Check urine pH with each void and obtain an order for more Diamox or sodium bicarbonate if the pH is not above 7.0. Leucovorin calcium *must* be given on schedule every time. Monitor methotrexate levels and obtain orders for more leucovorin if the levels are not less than:

$5 \times 10 - 6$ at 24 hours
$5 \times 10 - 7$ at 48 hours
$5 \times 10 - 8$ at 72 hours

Instruct patient to take no medications without first checking with physician.

Inform patient of possibility of menstrual dysfunction and of birth defects if pregnancy occurs while taking methotrexate.

Continue safe-handling precautions for 2 days after last dose of methotrexate.

Generic Name: METHOXAMINE HYDROCHLORIDE

Trade Name: VASOXYL

Classification: Vasopressor

Actions: Potent prolonged vasoconstriction without increase in heart rate.

Indications: For support, restoration, or maintenance of blood pressure during anesthesia.

Dosage:
Neonatal: Not applicable.
Pediatric: Not applicable.
Adult: 3–5 mg. May repeat after at least 10 minutes, then follow with continuous or intermittent IV drip or IM administration.

Preparation: Available as 20 mg in 1-ml ampules.

Home Stability: Not recommended for home use.

Compatibilities: Compatible with 5% dextrose in water.

Administration:
Neonatal: Not applicable.
Pediatric: Not applicable.
Adult: IV: Give undiluted slowly or mix 40 mg in 250 ml of 5% dextrose in water.

Contraindications: Hypersensitivity. Not to be used to prolong the effects of local anesthetics. Use with caution in patients with hyperthyroidism, hypertension, congestive heart failure, and cardiac disease, and with concurrent use of ergot alkaloids. Safe for use with cyclopropane anesthesia.

Side Effects:
Primary: Bradycardia, hypertension, severe headache, pilomotor response, projectile vomiting, desire to void.

Nursing Implications: May supplement IV route with IM administration for a prolonged effect.
  Monitor blood pressure and heart rate every 2 minutes until stabilized, then every 5 minutes.
  Bradycardia may be reversed with atropine.
  Assess heart tones, jugular venous distension, peripheral edema, lung sounds, dyspnea, and capillary refill every 4 hours and as needed.
  Assess IV site frequently; infiltration can cause tissue necrosis. If extravasation has occurred, infiltrate area with phentolamine.

Generic Name: METHYLDOPATE HYDROCHLORIDE

Trade Name: ALDOMET

Classification: Antihypertensive

Actions: Stimulation of central inhibitory alpha-adrenergic receptors, decreasing sympathetic outflow, resulting in lowered peripheral and renal vascular resistance.

Indications: Mild to severe hypertension.

Dosage:
Neonatal: Not applicable.
Pediatric: 20–40 mg/kg every 6 hours. Maximum dose: 65 mg/kg or 3.0 g daily (whichever is less).
Adult: 250–500 mg every 6 hours. Maximum dose: 1.0 g every 6 hours.

Preparation: Available as 5-ml vials containing 250 mg.

Home Stability: Not recommended for home use.

Compatibilities: Compatible with solutions containing dextrose, saline, or both.

Administration:
Neonatal: Not applicable.
Pediatric: Dilute in 100 ml of 5% dextrose and give over 30–60 minutes.
Adult: See pediatric administration.

Contraindications: Hypersensitivity, active hepatic disease, history of liver disorders with previous methyldopa therapy. Use with caution in patients with impaired hepatic function and in concurrent therapy with MAO inhibitors or other hypertensives. Norepinephrine, phenothiazine, tricyclic antidepressants, and amphetamines may cause hypertensive effects when used with methyldopa.

Side Effects:
Primary: Hemolytic anemia, hepatic necrosis, sedation, decreased mental acuity, orthostatic hypotension, edema, weight gain, dry mouth, nasal stuffiness.
Secondary: Reversible granulocytopenia, thrombocytopenia, headache, asthenia, weakness, dizziness, psychic disturbances, depression, nightmares, bradycardia, aggravated angina, myocarditis, diarrhea, pancreatitis, involuntary choreoathetoid movements, gynecomastia, lactation, skin rash, impotence, drug-induced fever.

Nursing Implications: Monitor blood pressure and heart rate every 30 minutes until stabilized, then hourly.
Monitor complete blood count before and during therapy.
Fluid status should be monitored via hourly urine outputs, intake, and daily weights.
Teach patient to rise or change positions slowly to minimize orthostatic hypotension.
Offer ice chips, sour hard candy, or sugarless chewing gum to relieve dry mouth.
If blood transfusions are required during treatment, obtain both a direct and indirect Coombs' test to avoid cross-matching difficulties.
Assess for side effects; notify physician if they occur.
After dialysis, monitor for hypertension, since methyldopa is removed during dialysis.

Generic Name: METHYLERGONOVINE MALEATE

Trade Name: METHERGINE

Classification: Synthetic oxytocic

Actions: Synthetic oxytocic that increases the strength, duration, and frequency of uterine contractions and decreases uterine bleeding following placental delivery. This is achieved by directly stimulating the smooth muscle of the uterus and vasoconstricting the uterine vessels.

Indications: For routine management after delivery of the placenta; postpartum atony; hemorrhage; subinvolution. Under obstetric supervision, may be given in the second stage of labor following delivery of the anterior shoulder.

Dosage:
Adult: 0.2 mg after delivery of the placenta, after delivery of the anterior shoulder, or during the puerperium every 2–4 hours.

Compatibilities: Specific information is not available. Do not mix with any other medication.

Administration:
Adult: Administer at IV site via stopcock or T-connector undiluted. IV route is reserved for lifesaving measures. Administer over at least 60 seconds.

Contraindications: Hypersensitivity, hypertension, toxemia, prior to the third stage of labor in pregnancy. Use with caution in clients with sepsis, obliterative vascular disease, or hepatic or renal involvement.

Side Effects:
Primary: Hypertensive or cardiovascular accidents.
Secondary: Nausea, vomiting, dizziness, headache, tinnitus, diaphoresis, palpitation, temporary chest pain, dyspnea.

Nursing Implications: Assess blood pressure prior to administration and every 3–5 minutes after administration.

Assess uterine response every 15 minutes after administration.

Assess client's calcium level; uterine response may be poor in calcium-deficient clients. Administer a calcium supplement if ordered.

Generic Name: METHYLPREDNISOLONE

Trade Name: MEDROL

Classification: Corticosteroid

Actions: The members of this family have many and varied effects because they influence almost every cell in the body. Some of these actions are accelerated protein metabolism, which results in muscle weakness and wasting, suppression of immune response and impaired wound healing, redistribution of fat and increase in adipose tissue formation. The levels of blood glucose increase because it is utilized less. This causes an increase in the release of insulin. Steroids suppress the body's immune response by affecting histamine release and inhibit the chain of events that leads to the inflammatory response. Finally, they have an effect on the reabsorption and distribution of some electrolytes and other elements necessary for normal body function. Any patient who has been on long-term therapy should have steroids withdrawn slowly to prevent development of acute adrenal insufficiency.

Indications: Steroids are indicated in the treatment of many disorders, including (but not limited to) inflammatory, endocrine, collagen, dermatologic, rheumatic, allergic, respiratory, hematologic, gastrointestinal, and nervous system disorders.

Dosage: Varies from 4–48 mg/day. As with other steroids, the dose is highly dependent on the condition under treatment.

Preparation: Available as 20, 40, and 80 mg/ml.

Administration:
All Ages: IM or by mouth.

Contraindications: Hypersensitivity, systemic fungal infections. The smallest dose for the shortest period of time should be used because of the chance of side effects. May stunt growth in children. Do not give immunizations during therapy. Use with caution in patients with active infections, congestive heart failure, hypertension, osteoporosis. May aggravate diabetes mellitus, Cushing's syndrome, and optic nerve damage.

Side Effects: Many effects are dependent on dose or length of therapy. The following side effects are related to the effects of the drug itself.

Primary: Fluid and electrolyte disturbances, osteoporosis, long bone fractures, effects on central nervous system, increased incidence of infections, impaired wound healing, ocular effects, endocrine effects.

Secondary: Abrupt withdrawal may lead to withdrawal syndrome or adrenal insufficiency.

Nursing Implications: Obtain baseline information—height, weight, vital signs, physical assessment, and laboratory results.

Check label carefully—some solutions should not be administered IV, only IM.

Any patient who has been on long-term therapy *must* have dose tapered. Observe for clinical symptoms of withdrawal.

Continuing assessment includes weight, vital signs, and laboratory follow-up. Assess for side effects.

Patient at home should be instructed to avoid contact with any person with an active infection because of decreased resistance.

Dietary adjustments may be necessary for the diabetic patient. Any patient on long-term therapy may need to increase protein intake.

Monitor patient for improvement in condition under therapy. Document observations.

Additional patient teaching may be needed regarding the occurrence of diarrhea or tarry stools, the avoidance of exposure to infection and reporting of any possible infections and unhealed cuts, and the need for periodic eye examinations and routine laboratory tests.

Generic Name: METOCLOPRAMIDE HYDROCHLORIDE

Trade Name: REGLAN

Classification: Gastrointestinal

Actions: Stimulates motility of the upper gastrointestinal tract but does not increase gastric, biliary, or pancreatic secretions. Exact mode of action not known but may sensitize tissue to acetylcholine. Other effects include improvement of gastric contractions and increased peristalsis of duodenum and jejunum.

Similar in action to phenothiazines, it may produce some extrapyramidal effects and sedation.

Indications: Relief of delayed gastric emptying time associated with diabetic gastroparesis.

Dosage: The following are all single doses.
Neonatal: IV: 0.1 mg/ kg.
Pediatric:
Under 6 Years: IV: 0.1 mg/kg.
6–14 Years: IV: 2.5–5mg.
Adult: IV, IM: 10 mg.

Preparation: Available as injectable 10 mg/2 ml.

Compatibilities: Compatible with D_5W, sodium chloride, D5.45 sodium chloride, Ringer's, or lactated Ringer's.

Administration: Give IV or IM for severe symptoms. IV administration: Direct IV bolus over 1–2 minutes or infusion over 15–20 minutes. Protect from light. IV infusion method is usually used to combat the nausea and vomiting of cisplatin administration. The dose is repeated every 2 hours times 2, then every 3 hours times 3. For relief of symptoms of gastroparesis, administer 30 minutes before meals and at bedtime.

Contraindications: Hypersensitivity, conditions in which stimulation of gastric motility is dangerous, as in obstruction, pheochromocytoma, epilepsy, or in patients receiving other medications that may cause extrapyramidal reactions.

Side Effects:
Primary: Restlessness, drowsiness, fatigue.
Secondary: Dizziness, headache, extrapyramidal reactions.

Nursing Implications: Complete assessment with description of symptoms.

Observe for any adverse reactions such as involuntary movement of extremities or facial movements.

Assist patient with ambulation as necessary because of dizziness or drowsiness. Caution patient about doing tasks that require alertness.

Record and evaluate drug response, relief of nausea, vomiting, intake and output.

Generic Name: METOPROLOL TARTRATE

Trade Name: LOPRESSOR

Classification: Beta-adrenergic blocker

Actions: Selective beta-1 adrenoreceptor blocking agent acting primarily on cardiac muscle with some effect on beta-2 adrenoreceptors (bronchial and vascular musculature) at higher doses.

Indications: Myocardial infarction to reduce cardiovascular mortality.

Dosage:
Neonatal: Not applicable.
Pediatric: Not applicable.
Adult: 5-mg bolus injections: maintenance with 50-mg oral preparations.

Preparation: Available in 5-ml ampules containing 5 mg of drug.

Home Stability: Not applicable.

Compatibilities: Compatible with dextrose or saline.

Administration:
Neonatal: Not applicable.
Pediatric: Not applicable.
Adult: Give 5-mg injections by IV push at 2-minute intervals for a total of 3 doses; 15 minutes after third injection, give 50 mg by mouth and repeat every 6 hours for 48 hours.

Contraindications: Heart rate less than 45 beats/minute, heart block greater than first degree, systolic blood pressure less than 100 mmHg, moderate to severe cardiac failure, bronchospastic disease. Use with caution in patients with hepatic dysfunction. Catecholamine-depleting drugs (e.g., resperine) may have an additive effect when used concurrently with metoprolol tartrate. Excessive bradycardia and increased depressant effect may be observed when used with cardiac glycosides. Barbiturates and rifampin increase metabolism of metoprolol. Chlorpromazine and cimetidine decrease metabolism of metoprolol.

Side Effects:
Primary: Bradycardia, hypotension, congestive heart failure.
Secondary: Fatigue, lethargy, nausea, vomiting, diarrhea, rash, fever.

Nursing Implications: Continuous cardiac monitoring is essential during therapy. Notify physician of any changes in rate or rhythm. Document strips.

Assess heart tones, jugular venous distension, peripheral edema, lung sounds, dyspnea, and capillary refill before therapy begins and hourly until stable.

Continue to monitor patient for chest pain or discomfort.

Generic Name: METRONIDAZOLE HYDROCHLORIDE

Trade Name: FLAGYL IV, FLAGYL IV RTU. (READY TO USE)

Classification: Synthetic antibiotic

Actions: Synthetic antibiotic with bactericidal activity against Bacteroides, Clostridium, Eubacterium, Peptococcus, Peptostreptococcus, and Fusobacterium.

Indications: Treatment of the following serious infections caused by susceptible gram-positive and gram-negative anaerobic bacteria: intraabdominal infections, infections of the skin and soft tissues, gynecological infections, septicemia, endocarditis, and infections of the bones, joints, central nervous system, and lower respiratory tract.

Dosage:
Neonatal: Not recommended.
Pediatric: Not recommended.
Adult: Loading dose: 15 mg/kg administered over 1 hour. Maintenance dose: 7.5 mg/kg administered 6 hours after the loading dose and then every 6 hours. Maximum dosage in a 24-hour period is 4.0 g. *Reduced dosage is indicated in clients with severe hepatic disease.*

Preparation: Supplied in single-dose vials containing 500 mg of drug or in 100-ml ready-to-use vials containing 500 mg of reconstituted solution. Reconstitute the 500-mg vials with 4.4 ml of sterile water for injection, normal saline, or bacteriostatic normal saline. Solution after mixing will be clear, pale yellow, or yellow-green in color.

Home Stability: Stable at room temperature for 96 hours after initial reconstitution. Final concentration is stable for 24 hours. Do not refrigerate final concentration.

Compatibilities: Compatible with normal saline, 5% dextrose, and lactated Ringer's. Not compatible with any other medication. *Do not administer with aluminum needles or hubs.*

Administration:
Neonatal: Not recommended.
Pediatric: Not recommended.
Adult: To reconstitute, dilute, and neutralize: Dilute dose with a compatible solution for a final concentration of no more than 8 mg/ml. Add 5 mEq of sodium bicarbonate injection for each 500 mg of drug. Reconstituted solution may be added to glass or plastic IV container. Administer over 1 hour via infusion pump. Ready-to-use form does not require further dilution or neutralization. Administer over 1 hour via infusion pump. Do not use plastic containers in series connections such as a primary and secondary IV line. Disconnect the primary solution during metronidazole infusion.

Contraindications: Hypersensitivity to metronidazole or other nitroimidazole derivatives. Use in pregnancy only when the benefits outweigh the risks. Not indicated during lactation or in children.

Side Effects:
Primary: Seizures, peripheral neuropathy (numbness or paresthesia of an extremity), nausea with headache, anorexia, vomiting, diarrhea, epigastric distress, abdominal cramping, constipation, proctitis, sharp and unpleasant metallic taste, modification of taste of alcoholic beverages, furry tongue, glossitis, stomatitis, vaginitis (associated with sudden overgrowth of Candida), flattening of the T-wave, hypersensitivity reaction.
Secondary: Dizziness, vertigo, incoordination, ataxia, confusion, irritability depression, weakness, insomnia, headache, syncope, reversible neutropenia, dysuria, cystitis, polyuria, incontinence, sense of pelvic pressure, dyspareunia, decreased libido, fleeting joint pains resembling serum sickness.

Nursing Implications: Prior to and during therapy, culture and sensitivity tests should be completed.

Monitor for hypersensitivity reactions as evidenced by urticaria, erythematous rash, flushing, nasal congestion, dryness of mouth (or vagina or vulva), fever.

Monitor baseline and periodic renal, hepatic,

and hematologic functions, especially in long-term therapy.

Monitor for superinfection. Assess for the onset of black, hairy tongue; oral lesions (stomatitis, glossitis); rectal or vaginal itching; vaginal discharge; loose, foul-smelling stools; unusual odor to urine.

Monitor infusion site hourly for signs of thrombophlebitis.

Sodium concentration must be taken into consideration in clients on a sodium-restricted diet or those predisposed to edema or congestive heart failure.

Assess client for signs of seizure activity or peripheral neuropathy. Report findings to the physician immediately and take seizure precautions.

Assess clients for bleeding episodes and prolongation of prothrombin time.

Generic Name: MEZLOCILLIN SODIUM

Trade Name: MEZLIN

Classification: Antibiotic (penicillin)

Actions: Extended-spectrum penicillin bactericidal against gram-positive and gram-negative, aerobic and anaerobic strains, especially Klebsiella and Pseudomonas. Also has broad-spectrum bactericidal action against Bacteroides, Enterobacter, Escherichia, Hemophilus, Proteus, Serratia, and *Streptococcus faecalis.*

Indications: Severe infections such as urinary, respiratory, intra-abdominal, gynecologic, skin, and soft tissue infections and septicemia caused by susceptible organisms.

Dosage: Usual duration of therapy is 7–10 days.
Neonatal (Under 1 Month): Limited information available.
Pediatric (Over 1 Month): 300 mg/kg/day every 4 hours.
Adult: 200–300 mg/kg/day every 4–6 hours, not to exceed 24 g/24 hours.

Preparation: Supplied as a powder. Reconstitute with sterile water. Dilute each gram with 10 ml of diluent. If precipitation occurs, warm to 37°C (98.6°F) in a water bath for 20 minutes and shake vigorously.

Home Stability: Stable in IV solution at room temperature for 72 hours.

Compatibilities: Compatible with dextrose, saline, KCl, Ringer's, or lactated Ringer's. Do not mix with any other antibiotic.

Administration:
Neonatal (Under 1 Month): Not applicable.

Pediatric (Over 1 Month): Infuse over 3–5 minutes by IV push or IV Y-site. More rapid infusion can result in seizures.
Adult: Infuse over 30 minutes by IV piggyback.

Contraindications: Hypersensitivity to penicillin derivatives or cephalosporins. Individuals with a history of allergic problems are more susceptible to untoward reactions. Safety in pregnancy has not been established.

Side Effects:
Primary: Hypersensitivity reactions such as skin rash, pruritus, anaphylaxis, urticaria, and febrile reactions; superinfections; pain and thrombosis of the IV site.
Secondary: Neutropenia; leukopenia; eosinophilia; thrombocytopenia; hypokalemia; increase in SGOT, SGPT, alkaline phosphatase, serum bilirubin, creatinine, BUN; decrease in hematocrit and hemoglobin; seizures; neuromuscular hyperirritability; nausea; vomiting; diarrhea; abnormal taste sensations.

Nursing Implications: Prior to and during therapy, culture and sensitivity tests should be completed.
Monitor for allergic reactions.
Monitor baseline and periodic renal, hepatic, and hematologic functions, especially in long-term therapy.
Monitor for superinfection. Assess for the onset of black, hairy tongue; oral lesions (stomatitis, glossitis); rectal or vaginal itching; vaginal discharge; loose, foul-smelling stools; unusual odor to urine.
Monitor infusion site hourly for signs of thrombophlebitis.
Sodium concentration must be taken into consideration in clients on a sodium-restricted diet.

Generic Name: MICONAZOLE

Trade Name: MONISTAT IV

Classification: Antifungal agent

Actions: Fungicidal against *Coccidioides immitis*, *Candida albicans*, *Cryptococcus neoformans*, *Petriellidium boydii*, and *Paracoccidioides brasiliensis*.

Indications: Treatment of severe systemic fungal infections.

Dosage:
Neonatal: Safety in children under 1 year of age has not been established.
Pediatric (Over 1 Year): 20–40 mg/kg/day divided into 3 equal infusions administered every 8 hours, not to exceed 15 mg/kg per infusion.
Adult: Dosage varies with diagnosis and fungal infection, as shown below.

INFECTION	TOTAL DAILY RANGE (mg)	DURATION OF THERAPY (WEEKS)
Coccidioidomy-cosis	1800–3600	3–20 +
Cryptococcosis	1200–2400	3–12 +
Petriellidiosis	600–3000	5–20 +
Candidiasis	600–1800	1–20 +
Paracoccidiodo-mycosis	200–1200	2–16 +

Each daily dose is divided into 3 equal infusions administered every 8 hours. *Administer with caution to clients with hepatic or renal impairment who may not be able to metabolize adequately.*

Preparation: Supplied in 20-ml ampules as 10 mg/ml.

Home Stability: Use immediately after dilution.

Compatibilities: Compatible with 0.9% sodium chloride or 5% dextrose in water. Do not administer with any other medications or IV solutions.

Administration:
Neonatal: Not indicated.
Pediatric (Over 1 Year): Dilute dose in amount ordered by the physician and infuse via infusion pump over 30–60 minutes.
Adult: Dilute in at least 200 ml of 0.9% normal saline or 5% dextrose in water and infuse over 30–60 minutes.

Contraindications: Hypersensitivity; clients under 1 year of age. Safety in pregnancy has not been established.

Side Effects:
Primary: Thrombophlebitis, pruritus, rash, nausea, vomiting, febrile reactions, drowsiness.
Secondary: Transient increases in hematocrit following infusion, thrombocytopenia, aggregation of erythrocytes and rouleau formation on blood smears, hyperlipemia, electrophoretic abnormalities of the lipoprotein.

Nursing Implications: Prior to and during therapy, culture and sensitivity tests should be completed.
Monitor for hypersensitivity reactions. A physician should be present for the initial administration.
Monitor baseline and periodic renal, hepatic, and hematologic functions, specifically hemoglobin, hematocrit, electrolytes, triglycerides, and cholesterol.
Monitor intake-output ratio. Report oliguria, hematuria, and changes in intake-output ratio.
Monitor for superinfection. Assess for the onset of black, hairy tongue; oral lesions (stomatitis, glossitis); rectal or vaginal itching; vaginal discharge; loose, foul-smelling stools; unusual odor to urine.
Monitor infusion site hourly for signs of thrombophlebitis.
Assess clients for bleeding episodes and prolongation of prothrombin time.
Notify the physician if a rash occurs. Symptomatic relief includes cool room temperatures, soapless baths, and medications as ordered.

Generic Name: MICRURUS FULVIUS ANTIVENIN

Trade Name: NORTH AMERICAN CORAL SNAKE ANTIVENIN

Classification: Antivenin

Actions: Treatment of envenomization by eastern and Texas coral snakes. Venom of the Arizona and Sonoran coral snakes is not neutralized by this agent. The bite of a coral snake does not produce edema or necrosis at the site. There may be one or several tooth marks, but they can be difficult to find. Pain may be present, and it can radiate across extremities to the chest area. Numbness or weakness may develop within 2 hours, but no symptoms may develop for 8 hours or more. Symptoms include drowsiness, apprehension, weakness, tremor of tongue, excessive salivation, and difficulty swallowing. Because the poison is neurotoxic in action, the patient may also develop dyspnea and paralysis. Treatment should be started as soon as possible after the bite occurs.

Indications: Treatment of the venomous bite of the eastern and Texas coral snakes. Not effective for the bite of the Arizona or Sonoran coral snakes.

Dosage: A test for sensitivity to horse serum should be done prior to administration. The dosage is not based on size or weight.
Adults and Children: Administer contents of 3–5 vials of antivenin. For severe poisoning, 7–10 vials may be needed.

Preparation: Combination package includes one vial of lyophilized antivenin and one 10-ml vial of bacteriostatic water for injection.

Compatibilities: Compatible with normal saline.

Administration: Give the patient the first 1–2 ml over 3–5 minutes and observe for hypersensitivity reaction. Further rate of administration (if no reaction occurs) depends on the patient's fluid status. The remaining antivenin may be given by slow IV push directly into the line or mixed into the bottle or bag of normal saline used for infusion.

Side Effects:
Primary and Secondary: Hypersensitivity reactions, both immediate and delayed. Usual symptoms are shock and anaphylaxis. A delayed serum-sicknesslike reaction can occur 5–24 days after administration. Some symptoms are malaise, fever, urticaria, and joint pain.

Nursing Implications: Immobilization of patient may help to prevent spread of venom.

Assessment of patient includes allergy history, location of the bite, time passed since the bite, presenting symptoms, and description of the snake.

Monitor vital signs and blood pressure frequently. Document observations of increasing or decreasing severity of symptoms.

Avoid use of sedatives and narcotics, which may further depress respiration.

Emergency equipment and medications should be available for immediate use. This is especially important during administration of the antivenin.

Generic Name: MINOCYCLINE HYDROCHLORIDE

Trade Name: MINOCIN, VECTRIN

Classification: Antibiotic (tetracycline)

Actions: Long-acting tetracycline bactericidal against Rickettsia; *Mycoplasma pneumoniae;* agents of psittacosis and ornithosis; agents of lymphogranuloma venereum and granuloma inguinale; the spirochetal agent of relapsing fever (*Borrelia recurrentis*); infections caused by the following gram-negative organisms: *Hemophilus ducreyi, Pasteurella pestis* and *tularensis,* Bartonella *bacilliformis,* Bacteroides, and Brucella; and infections caused by the following gram-positive organisms: selective streptococci and *Staphylococcus aureus* for skin and soft tissues. When penicillin is contraindicated, minocycline hydrochloride is an alternate therapy for infections caused by *Neisseria gonorrhoeae, Treponema pallidum,* and *pertenue, Listeria monocytogenes,* Clostridium, *Bacillus anthracis, Fusobacterium fusiforme,* and Actinomyces.

Indications: Treatment of infections caused by the above-stated organisms when sensitivity testing shows susceptibility.

Dosage:
Neonatal: Not recommended.
Pediatric (8 Years and Over): 2–4 mg/kg/day in divided doses every 12 hours. Use of this drug during the years of tooth development can cause permanent discoloration of the teeth and enamel hypoplasia. Do not use tetracyclines with this age group or in pregnancy unless other drugs are ineffective or contraindicated.
Adult: 200 mg as a loading dose, then 100 mg every 12 hours. Maximum dosage: 400 mg in 24 hours.
General: Normal renal function is indicated for these dosages.

Preparation: Supplied as a powder in vials of 100 mg. Reconstitute with sterile water for injection. Add 5 ml of diluent to a 100-mg vial.

Home Stability: Infuse within 24 hours of preparation. Darkening solution indicates deterioration and should be discarded.

Compatibilities: Compatible with solutions containing dextrose, saline, Ringer's, or lactated Ringer's. Do not administer with total parenteral nutrition or any other medication.

Administration: Administration should be continued for at least 24–48 hours after symptoms and fever have subsided.
Neonatal: Not recommended.
Pediatric (8 Years and Over): Further dilute the drug to a concentration of 10 mg/100 ml and infuse over 1 hour.
Adult: Further dilute the drug to a concentration of 10 mg/ml and infuse over 1 hour. May give as a continuous infusion by diluting the prescribed dose in 500–1000 ml of a compatible IV solution and infusing over 12 hours.

Contraindications: Hypersensitivity. Not recommended in clients with renal insufficiency or in pregnancy or lactation.

Side Effects:
Primary: Hypersensitivity reactions including anaphylaxis, liver damage, photosensitivity, systemic moniliasis, thrombophlebitis, renal toxicity including a rise in BUN.
Secondary: Anorexia, nausea, vomiting, diarrhea, glossitis, dysphagia, enterocolitis, *Candida albicans* overgrowth in the perineal area (Monilia) and mouth (thrush), hemolytic anemia, thrombocytopenia. In infants, bulging fontanels, papilledema, which usually disappears with discontinuation of the drug.

Nursing Implications: Prior to and during therapy, culture and sensitivity tests should be completed.
Monitor for allergic reactions.
Monitor baseline and periodic renal, hepatic, and hematologic functions.
Monitor for superinfection. Assess for the onset of black, hairy tongue; oral lesions (stomatitis, glossitis); rectal or vaginal itching; vaginal discharge; loose, foul-smelling stools; unusual odor to urine.

Monitor infusion site for signs of thrombophlebitis.

Clients on anticoagulants may require lower doses of those drugs while on minocycline.

Monitor intake-output ratios. Notify physician of gastrointestinal disturbance or change in renal status.

Notify physician of signs of increasing intracranial pressure.

Generic Name: MITOMYCIN

Trade Name: MUTAMYCIN

Classification: Antineoplastic antibiotic

Actions: Inhibits DNA synthesis by binding to DNA and cross-linking it at high doses; RNA synthesis is also affected. Although cell-cycle nonspecific, mitomycin is more effective in the late G_1 and early S phases.

Indications: Adenocarcinomas of the stomach, breast, colon, and pancreas; head and neck cancers; bladder cancer; melanoma; biliary, ovarian, lung, and cervical squamous cell cancers; osteogenic and soft tissue sarcomas; chronic myelogenous leukemia.

Dosage:
Neonatal: Not applicable.
Pediatric: IV: 10–20 mg/m^2 in a single dose every 6–8 weeks or 2 mg/m^2 daily for 5 days with 2 days off and repeat or 0.05 mg/kg daily for 6 days, then every other day until 50 mg or 15 mg/m^2 on day 1, 10 mg/m^2 on day 8, then 5 mg/m^2 every 4 weeks. Into the bladder: 20–60-mg/20-ml dose 3 times a week for 20 weeks. A wide variety of doses are given intra-arterially.
Adult: See pediatric dosage.

Preparation: Available in 5- and 20-mg vials that should be diluted with 10 ml of D$_5$W, normal saline, or sterile water per 5 mg of drug. Gentle shaking and standing at room temperature may be required to dissolve the drug, which is a blue-gray color.

Home Stability: Unopened vials can be stored at room temperature. The solution is stable for 7 days at room temperature and 14 days in the refrigerator if protected from light. If exposed to light, the drug must be used within 24 hours.

Compatibilities: Compatible with heparin. Dextran sulfate and urokinase may increase the cytotoxicity of mitomycin. As with most antineoplastic agents, it is advisable not to administer mitomycin with other admixture solutions.

Administration:
Neonatal: Not applicable.

Pediatric: IV: Administer by slow IV push into the side arm of a free-flowing IV, checking patency every 2–3 minutes to avoid extravasation of this severe vesicant. Into the bladder: Instill and retain for as long as possible, at least 3 hours.
Adult: See pediatric administration.

Contraindications: Previous allergy to mitomycin; pregnancy; low blood counts or coagulation disorders. Do not administer if serum creatinine is greater than 1.7 mg/dl.

Side Effects:
Primary:
Hematopoietic: A delayed and possibly cumulative decrease in red and white blood cells and platelets occurs 3–8 weeks after administration and may last as long as 8 weeks.
Gastrointestinal: Moderate nausea, vomiting, and anorexia within 1–2 hours and lasting for 2–3 hours, stomatitis, diarrhea.
Cutaneous: Purple colored bands in the nailbeds that correspond to each dose of the drug, chemical phlebitis, cellulitis at venipuncture site, severe tissue damage if extravasated. Extravasation may occur at sites other than the current venipuncture site, even a previous venipuncture site in the other arm.
Nephrotoxicity: Delayed renal failure.
Reproductive: Teratogenesis.
Secondary: Increased BUN and serum creatinine; reversible alopecia; fatigue; weight loss; weakness; drowsiness; lethargy; confusion; skin changes (a palmar rash may develop with bladder instillation; treat with antihistamines or topical steroids); fever; interstitial pneumonia and pulmonary fibrosis, which require discontinuing the drug; possible cardiotoxicity, especially in patients with previous doxorubicin therapy. A syndrome of hemolytic anemia, decreased platelets, renal failure, and increased blood pressure has occurred, especially with fluorouracil. Risk of hypersensitivity reactions is very low. Risk of infertility or secondary malignancy is unknown.

Nursing Implications: Monitor complete blood count and serum creatinine.
Instruct patient and family on infection and bleeding precautions during third to eighth weeks after treatment is given.

Premedicate with antiemetics and continue them for 8 hours afterward.

Warn patient of possible nailbed changes.

Establish and maintain good venous access, checking for patency every 2–3 minutes during IV push administration and instructing the patient to report any sensations of burning or pain.

Inform patient of the possibility of birth defects if pregnancy occurs while taking mitomycin.

Continue safe-handling precautions for 1 day after the last dose of mitomycin.

Generic Name: MORPHINE SULFATE

Trade Name: MORPHINE

Classification: Narcotic analgesic, Schedule II controlled substance

Actions: Drugs in this class act to relieve moderate to severe pain and provide preoperative sedation. A patient's perception of pain is altered by preventing or changing the transmission of painful stimuli along the sensory pathways in the central nervous system. These pathways are specific to the perception and emotional response of the patient to pain. In addition, these drugs suppress the respiratory and cough centers of the brain and have an antiperistaltic effect on the smooth muscle of the intestine. Because of their actions, narcotics can produce physical and psychological dependence. When used to treat severe pain, as in terminal illness, these medications should be given around the clock to maximize the relief of pain and anxiety.

Indications: Treatment of severe pain such as that of myocardial infarction. Also used to treat dyspnea associated with pulmonary edema and acute left ventricular failure. Should not be used in cases of mild pain or pain that can be relieved by non-narcotic analgesics.

Dosage:
Neonatal: See pediatric dosage.
Pediatric: IM, SC: 0.1–0.2 mg/kg/dose every 4 hours as needed. Maximum of 15 mg/dose. IV: one-half the IM dose.
Adult: IM, SC: 10 mg/70 kg with a range of 5–20 mg. IV: 4–10 mg given slowly.

Preparation: Injectable form available in 1- or 2-ml syringes or ampules, for IV, IM, or SC use in concentrations of 2, 4, 8, 10, and 15 mg/ml.

Home Stability: Stable at room temperature.

Compatibilities: Compatible with sterile water or normal saline. Not compatible when mixed directly with diazepam, phenytoin, sodium bicarbonate, heparin, methicillin, iodides, barbiturates, and aminophylline.

Administration:
Neonatal: See pediatric administration.
Pediatric: IV: Dilute with sterile water or normal saline and give slowly over 2–5 minutes.
Adult: Give IV doses slowly over 2–5 minutes. Rapid administration increases the incidence of side effects. Morphine may be given by continuous IV drip to treat acute or chronic pain. The dosage range is 0.5–275 mg/hour. Patient should be monitored carefully during continuous infusion, especially with large doses.

Contraindications: Hypersensitivity; during delivery of a premature infant; in patients taking MAO inhibitors or who have taken them within 14 days. Use with caution in patients with head injuries, increased intracranial pressure, shock, central nervous system and respiratory depression, chronic obstructive pulmonary disease, and in patients receiving other narcotic analgesics.

Side Effects:
Primary: Respiratory depression and apnea during IV administration. Also known sensitivity to narcotic analgesics, hypotension, bradycardia, nausea, vomiting, dizziness, sedation, sweating.
Secondary: Constipation can occur because of the effect on smooth muscle of the bowel. Urinary retention, pain at injection sites, and phlebitis are possible after IV administration. Physical dependence.

Nursing Implications: Because of the chance for respiratory depression, a narcotic antagonist should be available for rapid administration, especially if the route of choice is IV. Naloxone is the antagonist most often used.

Monitor vital signs frequently. For IV dose, every 5–10 minutes; for SC dose, every 15–30 minutes.

Supportive equipment should be readily available in case of cardiac or respiratory arrest. A patent airway should be maintained.

Monitor infants when the drug is used during labor and delivery.

Monitor intake and output when the drug is given repeatedly, because it may cause urinary retention.

To augment the use of narcotic analgesics,

give before severe pain occurs. Nursing actions also include the use of emotional support and patient comfort measures. Because of depression of the respiratory centers, postoperative use in the management of pain should include the patient's turning, coughing, and deep breathing to prevent pulmonary complications.

Patients should be warned to avoid activities that require alertness.

Assist patient with ambulation. This medication may also cause orthostatic hypotension.

Generic Name: MOXALACTAM DISODIUM

Trade Name: MOXAM

Classification: Antibiotic (cephalosporin)

Actions: Third-generation cephalosporin antibiotic with antibacterial action against a wide range of gram-positive and gram-negative organisms and anaerobes. Effective against *Streptococcus pneumoniae, Hemophilus influenzae,* Klebsiella, *Staphylococcus aureus,* beta-hemolytic streptococci, *Proteus morganil* and *vulgaris,* Providencia rettgeri, Enterobacter, Citrobacter, Serratia, Clostridium, Peptococcus, Peptostreptococcus, *Bacteroides fragilis,* Fusobacterium, and Eubacterium.

Indications: Treatment of serious infections of the central nervous system and genitourinary and lower respiratory tracts; infections of the bones, joints, and intra-abdominal area; septicemia; skin and skin-structure infections.

Dosage:

Neonatal:

0–1 Week: 50 mg/kg every 12 hours.
1–4 Weeks: 50 mg/kg every 8 hours.
Infants Over 4 Weeks: 50 mg/kg every 6 hours.
Pediatric: 50 mg/kg every 6–8 hours; up to 200 mg/kg/24 hours. In gram-negative meningitis, an initial loading dose of 100 mg/kg is administered.
Adult: 2–4 g/24 hours in equally divided doses every 8 hours for 5–10 days up to 14 days.
Mild to Moderate Infection: 500–2000 mg every 12 hours.
Mild Skin and Skin Structure Infections and Uncomplicated Pneumonia: 500 mg every 8 hours.
Mild, Uncomplicated Urinary Tract Infections: 250 mg every 12 hours.
Persistent Urinary Tract Infections: 500 mg every 12 hours.
Serious Urinary Tract Infections: Up to 500 mg every 8 hours.
Life-Threatening Infections: Up to 4 g every 8 hours.
General: Lower doses are needed by renal-impaired clients.

Preparation: Supplied as a powder. Reconstitute each gram with 3 ml of sterile water for injection, bacteriostatic water for injection, 0.9% sodium chloride, or bacteriostatic sodium chloride.

Home Stability: After concentration, solution is stable for 24 hours at room temperature and 96 hours refrigerated.

Compatibilities: Compatible with solutions containing dextrose, saline, KCl, and lactated Ringer's. Do not mix with any other antibiotic.

Administration:

Neonatal: Dilute to 100 mg/ml and administer by IV push over 3–5 minutes.
Pediatric: Dilute to 100 mg/ml and administer by IV push or IV Y-site over 3–5 minutes.
Adult: Dilute to 100 mg/ml and administer by IV piggyback over 15–30 minutes.

Contraindications: Hypersensitivity to cephalosporins or penicillin derivatives. Individuals with a history of allergic problems are more susceptible to untoward reactions. Use in pregnancy only if absolutely necessary. Safety has not been established in pregnancy, and moxalactam is excreted through breast milk.

Side Effects:

Primary: Hypersensitivity reactions such as skin rash, pruritus, anaphylaxis, urticaria, and febrile reactions; superinfections; pain and thrombosis of the IV site, bleeding (moxalactam can interfere with hemostasis through hypoprothrombinemia).
Secondary: Nausea; vomiting; abdominal cramps; diarrhea; pseudomembranous colitis; neutropenia; thrombocytopenia; hypoprothrombinemia; positive Coombs' test; increase in SGOT, SGPT, alkaline phosphatase, BUN; decreased creatinine clearance.

Nursing Implications: Prior to and during therapy, culture and sensitivity tests should be completed.

Monitor for allergic reactions.

Monitor baseline and periodic renal function and prothrombin time. Assess for bleeding.

Monitor for superinfection. Assess for the onset of black, hairy tongue; oral lesions (stomati-

tis, glossitis); rectal or vaginal itching; vaginal discharge; loose, foul-smelling stools; unusual odor to urine.

Monitor infusion site hourly for signs of thrombophlebitis.

Observe clients closely for the first half-hour after initial dose for a wheal or redness at IV site and other signs of allergic reaction.

Report onset of diarrhea to the physician.

Monitor intake-output ratio. Report oliguria, hematuria, and changes in intake-output ratio. Use glucose oxidase reagents to check urine glucose. False positive reactions can occur wth Clinitest.

Instruct client to avoid all alcoholic beverages. A severe reaction including nausea, vomiting, and headache may occur.

Generic Name: MULTIVITAMINS

Trade Name: BEROCCA (IV)

Classification: Vitamin

Actions: Organic substances essential for normal metabolism, growth, and development. They are not protein, carbohydrates, or fats and do not serve as sources of energy. Commercial preparations contain different compounds and strengths of vitamins, some of which are:

Vitamin A-A: Fat-soluble vitamin essential for epithelial tissue integrity and normal tooth and bone development.

B Complex: Water soluble. Signs of deficiency include beriberi, pellagra, gastrointestinal manifestations, and anemia.

Ascorbic Acid (Vitamin C): Water-soluble vitamin essential for integrity of intracellular connective tissue. A deficiency will lead to scurvy.

Vitamin D: Fat-soluble vitamin essential for absorption of calcium and therefore normal bone integrity.

Vitamin E: Fat-soluble vitamin essential for human health but whose action is not yet completely understood.

Indications: To prevent deficiencies in clients with diets that do not meet daily requirements and those on parenteral nutrition.

Dosage: Varies for all age groups depending on strength of compound and condition under treatment.

Preparation: Infusion available in single or multidose vials of Berocca Parenteral Nutrition solution I and II.

Home Stability: Store unreconstituted product in refrigerator and protect from light. Mixed product (solutions I and II) is stable for 14 days in refrigerator. After it is added to IV fluids, it is stable for 24 hours under refrigeration.

Compatibilities: Compatible with 0.9% normal saline, 5% or 10% glucose or dextrose, and lactated Ringer's.

Administration:

All Ages: IV: Should not be given bolus but mixed with IV solution, 1 ml of solution I or II to at least 250 ml of IV fluid.

Contraindications: Hypersensitivity to any component of the solution.

Side Effects: Multivitamin preparations that provide normal doses are rarely toxic.

Primary: Large doses can cause significant accumulation of the fat-soluble vitamins. This may cause toxic side effects. Folic acid can mask pernicious anemia.

Secondary: Any other side effects will depend on specific combinations in given compounds and on the amount administered.

Nursing Implications: Assess patient for nutritional status and any signs and symptoms of vitamin deficiency.

During IV administration, monitor for signs of anaphylaxis.

Do not administer by IV bolus. Must be diluted and infused with IV solutions.

Monitor patient daily for improvement in any documented physical symptoms.

Provide nutritional counseling as indicated to patient and family.

Generic Name: NAFCILLIN SODIUM

Trade Name: NAFCIL, UNIPEN

Classification: Antibiotic (penicillin)

Actions: Semisynthetic penicillin bactericidal against the following gram-positive organisms: penicillin G–sensitive organisms, resistant strains of *Staphylococcus aureus,* pneumococci, and group A beta-hemolytic streptococci.

Indications: Treatment of infections caused by penicillinase-producing staphylococci, pneumococci, and group A beta-hemolytic streptococci.

Dosage:
Neonatal: 60 mg/kg/24 hours divided into 6 doses.
Pediatric: See neonatal dosage.
Adult: 500–1000 mg every 4 hours.

Preparation: Supplied as a powder. Do not use bacteriostatic diluent if drug is being administered to a neonate. Reconstitute with sterile water as follows:

VIAL SIZE	VOLUME DILUENT	CONCENTRATION
500 mg	1.7 ml	250 mg/ml
1 g	3.4 ml	250 mg/ml
2 g	6.7 ml	250 mg/ml

Home Stability: Reconstituted solutions are stable for 3 days at room temperature and 7 days when refrigerated. May be frozen for up to 3 months.

Compatibilities: Compatible with solutions containing dextrose, saline, KCl, Ringer's, or lactated Ringer's. Do not mix with any other antibiotic or with total parenteral nutrition.

Administration:
Neonatal: Dilute to 25 mg/ml and administer by IV push or IV Y-site over 5–10 minutes. Maximum infusion rate is 200 mg/minute.

Pediatric: See neonatal administration.
Adult: Dilute to 25 mg/ml in IV piggyback and infuse over 30–60 minutes. Dilute further if phlebitis occurs.

Contraindications: Hypersensitivity to penicillin derivatives or cephalosporins. Individuals with a history of allergic problems are more susceptible to untoward reactions. Safety in pregnancy has not been established.

Side Effects:
Primary: Hypersensitivity reactions such as skin rash, pruritus, anaphylaxis, urticaria, and febrile reactions. Superinfections, pain and thrombosis of the IV site.
Secondary: Neutropenia; leukopenia; eosinophilia; thrombocytopenia; hypokalemia; increase in SGOT, SGPT, alkaline phosphatase, serum bilirubin, creatinine, BUN; decrease in hematocrit and hemoglobin; seizures; neuromuscular hyperirritability; nausea; vomiting; diarrhea; abnormal taste sensations; nephritis.

Nursing Implications: Prior to and during therapy, culture and sensitivity tests should be completed.
Monitor for allergic reactions.
Monitor baseline and periodic renal, hepatic, and hematologic functions, especially in long-term therapy.
Monitor for superinfection. Assess for the onset of black, hairy tongue; oral lesions (stomatitis, glossitis); rectal or vaginal itching; vaginal discharge; loose, foul-smelling stools; unusual odor to urine.
Monitor infusion site hourly for signs of thrombophlebitis.
Sodium concentration must be taken into consideration in clients on a sodium-restricted diet.
Use glucose oxidase reagents to check urine glucose. False positive reactions can occur with Clinitest.

Generic Name: NALBUPHINE HYDROCHLORIDE

Trade Name: NUBAIN

Classification: Potent analgesic with narcotic agonist and antagonist effects.

Actions: Relieves moderate to severe pain, provides preoperative sedation. A patient's perception of pain is altered by preventing or changing the transmission of painful stimuli along the sensory pathways in the central nervous system. These pathways are specific to the perception and emotional response of the patient to pain. In addition, this drug suppresses the respiratory and cough centers of the brain. Less likely to cause physical dependence than narcotic analgesics but more potent than morphine, meperidine, and pentazocine.

Indications: Management of moderate to severe pain due to a diversity of causes. Should not be used in cases of mild pain or pain that can be relieved by other less potent non-narcotic analgesics.

Dosage:
Neonatal: Not recommended.
Pediatric: Not recommended.
Adult: IV, IM, SC: 10 mg/70 kg given every 3–6 hours as needed. Maximum daily dose: 160 mg.

Preparation: Injectable form available as 10 mg/ml.

Administration:
Neonatal: Not recommended.
Pediatric: Not recommended.
Adult: IV, IM, SC. Must be given by slow IV push. Naloxone should be readily available for administration in case of severe respiratory depression. Onset of action will occur 2–3 minutes after IV administration and less than 15 minutes after SC or IM.

Contraindications: Hypersensitivity, during delivery of a premature infant. Use with caution in clients with narcotic addiction or long-term narcotic usage, since its narcotic antagonist actions can precipitate withdrawal symptoms. Also use with caution in patients with head injuries, increased intracranial pressure, shock, central nervous system and respiratory depression, chronic obstructive pulmonary disease, ventricular dysfunction, acute myocardial infarction, coronary insufficiency, renal or hepatic dysfunction, and in patients receiving narcotic analgesics.

Side Effects:
Primary: Sedation, headache, nausea, clamminess, palpitations, blood pressure instability, respiratory depression.
Secondary: Dizziness, lethargy, lightheadedness, nervousness, unusual dreams, blurred vision, dry mouth.

Nursing Implications: Because of the chance for respiratory depression, a narcotic antagonist should be available for rapid administration, especially if the route of choice is IV. Naloxone is the antagonist most often used.

Monitor vital signs frequently. For IV dose, every 5–10 minutes; for SC dose, every 15–30 minutes.

Supportive equipment should be readily available in case of cardiac or respiratory arrest. A patent airway should be maintained.

Monitor infants when the drug is used during labor and delivery.

To augment the use of potent analgesics, give before severe pain occurs. Nursing actions also include emotional support and patient comfort measures. Because of depression of the respiratory centers, postoperative use should include the patient's turning, coughing, and deep breathing to prevent pulmonary complications.

Patients should be warned to avoid activities that require alertness and should be assisted with ambulation.

Generic Name: NALOXONE HYDROCHLORIDE

Trade Name: NARCAN

Classification: Narcotic antagonist

Actions: Pure narcotic antagonist with no agonist or other pharmacologic actions, which will not create physical dependence or tolerance. In cases of narcotic overdose, antagonists serve as antidotes by competing with the narcotics for the same receptor sites. This reverses effects including respiratory depression, sedation, and hypotension. These same effects may be caused by other classes of drugs such as barbiturates and by other sedative-hypnotics, but naloxone is effective only against narcotics.

Indications: To reverse the symptoms of narcotic depression, partially or completely; in diagnosis of suspected narcotic overdoses; to counteract respiratory depression in the neonate following delivery.

Dosage:
Neonatal: 0.01 mg/kg. May be repeated every 2–3 minutes.
Pediatric: 0.01 mg/kg. May be repeated every 2–3 minutes.
Adult: 0.4–2.0 mg. May be repeated every 2–3 minutes for 3 doses.

Preparation: Injectable form available as 0.4 mg/ml. Neonatal injectable form available as 0.02 mg/ml.

Home Stability: Not routinely used for home administration.

Compatibilities: Compatible with sterile water, normal saline, and 5% dextrose solutions. It should not be mixed with solutions containing bisulfite, metasulfite, or having an alkaline pH.

Administration:
Neonatal: IV, IM, SC. Should be given by IV push in an emergency situation for maximum immediate effect. May also be given by infusion in compatible solutions: 2 mg naloxone added to 500 ml equals 0.004 mg/ml. These solutions are stable for 24 hours.
Pediatric: IV as above.
Adult: IV as above.

Contraindications: Hypersensitivity; use in known narcotic addicts, since it may precipitate withdrawal symptoms. Use with caution in patients with known cardiovascular disease.

Side Effects: No real side effects, but sudden reversal of narcotic side effects can cause nausea, vomiting, hypertension, and tachycardia.

Nursing Implications: In cases of suspected narcotic overdose, determine, when possible, nature and time of drug administered.

Assess vital signs and blood pressure at least every 5 minutes and maintain patent airway. Have resuscitation equipment available for immediate use.

Continue to monitor and assess patient until response to drug is observed. Do not leave unattended.

Patient must be monitored for further depression for duration of *narcotic* activity. Several doses of antagonist may be necessary, because its effects are shorter in duration than those of narcotics.

Vital signs may be monitored every 10–15 minutes after response from the antagonist is noted.

Generic Name: NEOSTIGMINE

Trade Name: PROSTIGMIN

Classification: Cholinergic

Actions: Drugs in this classification act to facilitate transmission of impulses across the myoneural junction and inhibit the destruction of acetylcholine. They have a variety of onsets and durations of action.

Indications: Diagnosis and treatment of myasthenia gravis and as an antidote for curare. The duration of action is longer with neostigmine than with edrophonium.

Dosage:

Neonatal and Pediatric: Not available.

Adults:

Antidote for Curare Preparations: 0.5–2 mg slowly by IV. It is also recommended that atropine be given just prior to neostigmine (0.6–1.2 mg). The total dose of neostigmine is 5 mg.

Myasthenia Gravis: 0.5 mg SC or IM. Oral treatment with 15-mg tablets is preferred. The range is 15–375 mg/day, dependent on relief of symptoms.

Preparation: Available in concentrations of 1:1000, 1:2000, and 1:4000.

Administration: IM, SC, or slow IV. May also be administered orally.

Contraindications: Hypersensitivity, obstructions (mechanical intestinal and urinary), bradycardia, hypotension. Use with caution in patients with bronchial asthma or cardiac dysrhythmias. Atropine and epinephrine should be available in case of hypersensitivity reaction. Do not use neostigmine bromide in patients with a history of hypersensitivity to bromides or urinary tract infections.

Side Effects: The following side effects may occur but have not been observed with each agent.

Primary: Ocular changes; convulsions; dysphonia; dysphagia; respiratory changes including increased secretions, paralysis, and laryngospasm; arrhythmias; gastrointestinal disturbances; muscle weakness.

Secondary: Urinary frequency and incontinence, thrombophlebitis with IV use.

Nursing Implications: Complete assessment should be done of patient and symptoms observed.

Emergency equipment should be readily available in case of hypersensitivity reaction.

Observe myasthenic patient for any exacerbation of symptoms.

If drug is being administered as curare antagonist, observe patient for return of muscle movement.

If patient has myasthenia gravis, determine if in a crisis or in a cholinergic crisis. Because symptoms are so similar, it may be necessary to do an edrophonium test.

Monitor vital signs closely.

Patient teaching should include spacing activities to avoid fatigue, signs of drug overdosage or underdosage, and need for follow-up care and close medical supervision.

Generic Name: NETILMICIN SULFATE

Trade Name: NETROMYCIN

Classification: Antibiotic (aminoglycocide)

Actions: Semisynthetic aminoglycoside derivative from *Micromonospora purpurea,* with neuromuscular blocking action. It inhibits protein synthesis in bacterial cells and is bactericidal. It is effective against a wide variety of gram-negative bacilli: *Escherichia coli,* Enterobacter, Klebsiella pneumoniae, and most strains of *Pseudomonas aeruginosa, Proteus mirabilis,* Citrobacter, Salmonella, and Shigella. Also effective against Staphylococcus, *Streptococcus faecalis,* and gentamicin-resistant strains.

Indications: Treatment of serious infections such as septicemia, peritonitis, intra-abdominal abscesses, and infections of the urinary or respiratory tract, bones, joints, and skin.

Dosage:
Neonatal: 2–3.4 mg/kg every 12 hours.
Pediatric: 1.8–2.7 mg/kg every 8 hours or 2.7–4 mg/kg every 12 hours.
Adult: 1.3–2.2 mg/kg every 8 hours or 2–3.25 mg/kg every 12 hours.
General: Dosage is highly individualized and should be based on therapeutic drug monitoring.
Desired peak and trough:
Therapeutic serum peak: 6–10 μg/ml.
Trough serum level: 0.5–2 mcg/ml.
Duration of therapy: 7–14 days.

Preparation: Available as 100 mg/ml preserved with benzyl alcohol. Should not be used for neonates, infants, or children because of the preservative. Netromycin Pediatric Injection 25 mg/ml and Netromycin Neonatal Injection 10 mg/kg do not contain benzyl alcohol.

Home Stability: Stable for 72 hours when stored in a glass container at room temperature or refrigerated. Avoid freezing.

Compatibilities: Compatible with solutions containing dextrose, saline, KCl, Ringer's, or lactated Ringer's.

Administration:
Neonatal: Infuse over 30 minutes to 2 hours. Administer at appropriate IV site based on infusion rate. Dilution should be based on fluid volume needs.
Pediatric: See neonatal administration.
Adult: Dilute in 50–200 ml (1 mg/ml) of IV solution and administer over 30–120 minutes by IV piggyback.

Contraindications: Sensitivity to aminoglycosides, bisulfites, or benzyl alcohol; pregnancy; nursing infants. Use with caution in clients with impaired renal function; premature infants, neonates, and the elderly; clients with ascites, edema, dehydration, severe burns, fever, anemia, myasthenia gravis, parkinsonism, cystic fibrosis, a history of hearing problems; and in cases of infant botulism. Do not administer concurrently with penicillins. If concurrent administration is prescribed, administer the drugs 2 hours apart. The neuromuscular blockade effects are enhanced with combined administration of decamethonium, ether, succinylcholine, tubocurarine, and related anesthetics. Cephalosporins may potentiate the nephrotoxic effects of netilmicin. Concurrent administration of other aminoglycosides, ethacrynic acid, or furosemide may enhance the ototoxic effects.

Side Effects:
Primary:
Nephrotoxicity: Proteinurea, presence of red and white blood cells in the urine, granular casts, azotemia, oliguria, urinary frequency, frank hematuria, increase in BUN and serum creatinine, decrease in creatinine clearance and specific gravity, renal damage and failure.
Ototoxicity: Auditory: high-frequency hearing loss; complete hearing loss (occasionally permanent); tinnitus; fullness, ringing, or buzzing in ears. Vestibular: dizziness, vertigo; ataxia; nausea, vomiting; nystagmus.
Neurotoxicity: Drowsiness, headache, unsteady gait, weakness, clumsiness, paresthesias, tremors, muscle twitching and weakness, convulsions, neuromuscular blockade with respiratory depression.
Secondary: Nausea, vomiting, stomatitis, skin rash, urticaria, pruritus, generalized burning

sensation, drug fever, arthralgia, eosinophilia, anemia, leukopenia, granulocytopenia, thrombocytopenia, unusual thirst, difficult breathing, superinfections, peripheral neuritis.

Nursing Implications: Monitor serum blood levels initially and throughout therapy.

Document the *exact* time of medication administration and blood collection for determination of blood levels.

Assess renal function prior to initial administration via baseline BUN, creatinine and creatinine clearance, specific gravity, and urine analysis.

Monitor renal function throughout therapy via assessment of BUN, creatinine and creatinine clearance, specific gravity, urine analysis, and strict intake and output.

Encourage hydration of client to reduce chemical irritation to renal tubules.

Assess eighth cranial nerve function prior to initial administration, throughout therapy, and upon discharge via audiometric tests and assessment of vestibular disturbance.

Monitor for overgrowth infection as evidenced by diarrhea, anogenital itching, vaginal discharge or itching, stomatitis, or glossitis.

Antidote: Peritoneal dialysis or hemodialysis will assist in removal of the drug from the bloodstream.

Generic Name: NICOTINIC ACID

Trade Name: NIACIN

Classification: Vitamin

Actions: Part of coenzyme system that transports hydrogen and helps to metabolize carbohydrates. Occasionally used as oral vasodilator for some peripheral vascular diseases. If the patient is also receiving sympathetic-blocking agents for treatment of hypertension, it is possible to increase vasodilation and cause postural hypotension. Also used to reduce serum lipids in conjunction with dietary control of cholesterol.

Indications: Treatment of deficiency such as pellagra and in cases where diet and weight loss do not control serum cholesterol levels.

Dosage:
Neonatal: Not available.
Pediatric: Up to 300 mg by mouth or 100 mg IV daily, depending on severity of symptoms.
Adult: 10–20 mg by mouth, SC, IM, or IV daily, depending on severity of symptoms. Maximum dose of 500 mg should be divided into 10 doses.

Preparation: Injectable form available as 50 and 100 mg/ml.

Administration:
Neonatal: Not available.

Pediatric: By mouth or by slow IV.
Adult: IV, IM, or SC. Give slowly when administering by IV. IV method is the preferred parenteral route.

Contraindications: Hypersensitivity, active peptic ulcer, hepatic dysfunction, severe hypotension, hemorrhage or arterial bleeding. Use with caution in patients with gout, diabetes mellitus, and gallbladder disease.

Side Effects:
Primary: Peripheral vasodilation, diarrhea, nausea and vomiting, flushing, hypotension.
Secondary: Dizziness, hepatic dysfunction, pruritus, hyperglycemia.

Nursing Implications: Assess patient for nutritional status and signs of deficiency, including fatigue; weight loss; anorexia; redness and soreness of mouth, tongue, and lips; and confusion.

Provide nutritional counseling where appropriate.

Patient should be monitored for side effects for 2 hours after administration. Notify physician if effects become more severe.

Assess and document patient's response to therapy.

Generic Name: NIKETHAMIDE

Trade Name: CORAMINE

Classification: Respiratory stimulant

Actions: Central nervous system stimulant that has direct medullary effects and also stimulates peripheral chemoreceptors, which increases respirations. As an analeptic, it is less effective than doxapram. Its exact mode of action is not understood.

Indications: Treatment of central nervous system depression, respiratory depression, and circulatory failure.

Dosage: Variable, depending on condition under treatment and needs of patient. Most effective route is IV, but drug is also absorbed IM, SC, or by mouth. This drug has a very narrow therapeutic range, and patient must be observed closely for signs of overdose, which include coughing, sneezing, muscle tremors, and increase in heart rate and blood pressure. Muscle spasms and seizures may occur with a large overdose.

Preparation: Available as a 25% solution.

Compatibilities: Compatible with sterile water.

Administration: See Dosage.

Contraindications: Hypersensitivity.

Side Effects: Because the difference between an effective dose and a toxic dose is small, the following side effects could be the result of an overdose.
Primary: Burning or itching, especially in the back of the nose; flushing; sneezing; coughing; nausea; vomiting; restlessness; change in respirations.
Secondary: Sweating, feeling of warmth, increased heart rate and blood pressure.

Nursing Implications: Obtain a history of cause of resiratory depression.
Monitor vital signs closely. Obtain necessary laboratory results.
Maintain patent airway. Have emergency equipment available.
If seizures occur from an overdose, have short-acting barbiturate available for control (as ordered).
Assess level of consciousness and nature of respirations. Document effectiveness of therapy.

Generic Name: NITROFURANTOIN SODIUM

Trade Name: IVADANTIN

Classification: Antibacterial

Actions: Synthetic antibacterial agent for urinary tract infections, bactericidal against *Escherichia coli*, enterococci, *Staphylococcus aureus*, and some strains of Enterobacter, Klebsiella, and Proteus.

Indications: Treatment of urinary tract infections due to susceptible strains of gram-negative and gram-positive bacteria.

Dosage:
Neonatal: Not recommended for children under 1 month of age.
Pediatric: Safety in children under 12 years of age has not been established.
Under 120 Pounds: 3 mg/pound/day administered in 2 equally divided doses.
Over 120 Pounds: 180 mg administered in 2 equally divided doses twice a day.
Adult:
Under 120 Pounds: 3 mg/pound/day administered in 2 equally divided doses.
Over 120 Pounds: 180 mg administered in 2 equally divided doses twice a day.
General: Administer for at least 7 days and continue for 3 days after sterile urine is obtained.

Preparation: Supplied as a powder. Reconstitute 180-mg vial with 20 ml of 5% dextrose in water or sterile water for injection only. Reconstitute immediately prior to administration. Do not wipe vials with alcohol. Use a sterile needle with each step of dilution. Solutions containing methyl and propyl parabens, phenol, or cresol preservatives may cause the powder to precipitate out of solution.

Home Stability: Final dilution must be used within 24 hours. Protect from ultraviolet light by wrapping in foil.

Compatibilities: Compatible only with 5% dextrose in water, normal saline, and sterile water. Do not mix with other drugs or total parenteral nutrition.

Administration:
Neonatal: Not recommended.
Pediatric: Further dilute solution to a concentration of 1 ml of drug per 25 ml of parenteral solution. Dilute 180 mg in a minimum of 500 ml of parenteral solution. Infuse at a rate of 2–3 ml/minute at the Y-site or by continuous drip. Administer via infusion pump.
Adult: See pediatric administration.

Contraindications: Hypersensitivity, renal impairment, anuria, oliguria, a creatinine clearance under 40 ml/minute, in pregnancy and lactation.

Side Effects:
Primary: Acute pneumonitis, subacute and chronic fibrosis manifested by fever, chills, cough, chest pain, dyspnea, pulmonary infiltration with consolidation of pleural effusion on X-ray, and eosinophilia. (Discontinue therapy if the previous reactions occur; deaths have been reported. Hemolytic anemia appears to be linked to glucose-6-phosphate dehydrogenase deficiency, superinfections secondary to Pseudomonas, hepatitis, and peripheral neuropathy in clients with renal impairment, anemia, diabetes, electrolyte imbalance, vitamin B deficiency, and other debilitating conditions. Other sensitivity reactions include anaphylaxis, asthmatic attack, cholestatic jaundice, drug fever, and arthralgia. Most frequent adverse reactions are infusion-related and include anorexia, nausea, and emesis.
Secondary: Maculopapular, erythematous, or eczematous eruption, pruritus, urticaria, angioedema, hemolytic anemia, granulocytopenia, leukopenia, eosinophilia, megaloblastic anemia, transient alopecia, superinfections by resistant organisms.

Nursing Implications: Prior to and during therapy, culture and sensitivity tests should be completed.
Monitor for allergic reactions.
Monitor for the onset of an acute pulmonary hypersensitivity reaction. Notify physician of the onset of any symptoms.
Monitor for the onset of hemolytic anemia. Notify the physician of the onset of any symptoms.

Monitor for signs and symptoms of peripheral neuropathy. Notify the physician of the onset of any symptoms.

Warn the client that urine will turn brown and that alopecia is a transient possibility.

Monitor baseline and periodic renal, hepatic, and hematologic functions.

Monitor for superinfection.

Monitor infusion site hourly for signs of thrombophlebitis or infiltration.

Generic Name: NITROGLYCERIN

Trade Name: NITRO-BID IV, NITROSTAT IV, TRIDIL

Classification: Vasodilator

Actions: Vasodilation of venous vasculature predominates, but some arterial relaxation occurs, resulting in a reduction mainly in preload but also in afterload.

Indications: Control of blood pressure in preoperative hypertension and congestive heart failure associated with acute myocardial infarction, treatment of angina pectoris, production of controlled hypotension during surgical procedures.

Dosage:
Neonatal: Not applicable.
Pediatric: Initial dose is 5 μg/minute; no maximum dose.
Adult: Initial dose is 5 μg/minute; no maximum dose.

Preparation: Available in ampules containing 50 mg/10 ml.

Home Stability: Not applicable.

Compatibilities: Compatible with dextrose or saline in glass bottles only.

Administration:
Neonatal: Not applicable.
Pediatric: Dilute solution as ordered. Titrate initial infusion in 5-μg/minute increments every 3–5 minutes until 20 μg/minute is reached; then in 10–20-μg/minute increments every 3–5 minutes.

Once a blood pressure response is observed, titration should proceed more slowly. Infusion should be through nonpolyvinyl-chloride tubing only.
Adult: See pediatric administration.

Contraindications: Hypersensitivity, hypotension, uncorrected hypovolemia, increased intracranial pressure, cerebral hemorrhage, severe anemia, constrictive pericarditis, pericardial tamponade. Use with caution in patients with severe liver or renal disease.

Side Effects:
Primary: Headache, hypotension, tachycardia, orthostatic hypotension, dizziness.
Secondary: Weakness, fainting, nausea, vomiting, cutaneous vasodilation.

Nursing Implications: Continuous monitoring of blood pressure is preferred. If not possible, take blood pressure before each titration and every 5 minutes after each titration until stabilized.

Assess patient's chest pain frequently.

Monitor EKG for changes, especially in the ST segment; document strips.

Assess heart tones, jugular venous distension, peripheral edema, lung sounds, dyspnea, and capillary refill every 4 hours and as needed to ascertain effectiveness of treatment.

Headaches can be annoying to severe; medicate as ordered and assess pain relief.

If hemodynamic monitoring is available, monitor pulmonary wedge pressure frequently. A decrease in this parameter will precede the onset of arterial hypotension.

Generic Name: NITROPRUSSIDE SODIUM

Trade Name: NIPRIDE

Classification: Antihypertensive

Actions: Potent vasodilator affecting both arterial and venous smooth muscle.

Indications: Hypertensive crisis requiring immediate reduction in blood pressure; during anesthesia to produce hypotension to reduce bleeding; to reduce preload and afterload in cardiac pump failure or cardiogenic shock.

Dosage:
Neonatal: Not applicable.
Pediatric: 1.4 μg/kg/minute adjusted slowly to patient response.
Adult: Range: 0.5–10 μg/kg/minute. Average: 3 μg/kg/minute.

Preparation: Reddish-brown powder supplied in a 5-ml amber-colored vial containing 50 mg of drug.

Home Stability: Not applicable.

Compatibilities: Compatible only with 5% dextrose in water.

Administration:
Neonatal: Not applicable.
Pediatric: Dissolve contents of 50-mg vial in 2–3 ml of dextrose in water, then dilute in 250–1000 ml of 5% dextrose in water. Promptly wrap bag in aluminum foil or other opaque materials to protect from light. Titrate to patient response.
Adult: See pediatric administration.

Contraindications: Do not use for treatment of compensatory hypertension or during surgery on patients with known inadequate cerebral circulation. Use with caution in patients with hepatic insufficiency or renal disease.

Side Effects:
Primary: Headache, dizziness, restlessness, muscle twitching, diaphoresis, vomiting, nausea, abdominal pain.
Overdosage: Metabolic acidosis, tolerance to the drug, headache, vomiting, dizziness, ataxia, loss of consciousness, coma, absent reflexes, dilated pupils, distant heart sounds, weak pulse, dyspnea, palpitations, pink color, shallow breathing.

Nursing Implications: Fresh solution has a brownish tint; replace if infusion is any other color (blue, green, or dark red). Discard after 24 hours.

Obtain baseline vital signs before beginning the infusion; check every 5 minutes during titration of the drug, then every 15 minutes. Continuous blood pressure monitoring via arterial line is recommended.

If hypotension occurs, slowing or stopping the drug will result in a return to baseline values within 1–10 minutes.

Assess skin color and temperature, pulses, jugular venous distension, heart sounds, lung sounds, level of consciousness, and capillary refill every 4 hours and as needed.

Obtain hemodynamic profiles before beginning the infusion and as ordered during titration of the drug if available.

Check serum thiocyanate levels every 72 hours. Assess for symptoms of overdosage every 4 hours and as needed.

Infuse via automatic infusion pump. Assess IV site frequently for signs of infiltration.

Generic Name: NOREPINEPHRINE (FORMERLY LEVARTERENOL BITARTRATE)

Trade Name: LEVOPHED

Classification: Adrenergic

Actions: Potent sympathomimetic amine that increases both systolic and diastolic blood pressure, exerts a positive inotropic effect on the heart, and vasoconstricts peripheral vessels.

Indications: Restoration of blood pressure in acute hypotensive states and as an adjunct in the treatment of cardiac arrest and profound hypotension.

Dosage:
Neonatal: Not applicable.
Pediatric: Not applicable.
Adult: Initially 8–12 μg/minute by continuous infusion, then titrate. Average maintenance dose is 2–4 μg/minute.

Preparation: Available as 4-ml ampules containing 4 mg of drug.

Home Stability: Not applicable.

Compatibilities: Compatible with 5% dextrose or dextrose and saline combinations. Not compatible with plain saline solution.

Administration:
Neonatal: Not applicable.
Pediatric: Not applicable.
Adult: Titrate according to patient response within physician guidelines.

Contraindications: Uncorrected hypotension resulting from blood volume deficits, pregnancy, peripheral or mesenteric thrombosis, pulmonary edema, hypercarbia, acidosis, and concurrent use with cyclopropane and halogenated hydrocarbon anesthetics. Use with caution in patients with hypertension, thyroid disease, diabetes, cirrhosis, malaria, and in concurrent use with digitalis. May cause hypertensive crisis when used with MAO inhibitors.

Side Effects:
Primary: Ventricular tachycardia and fibrillation, headache, decreased urinary output, metabolic acidosis.
Secondary: Anxiety, weakness, dizziness, tremor, restlessness, insomnia, bradycardia, severe hypertension, marked increase in peripheral vascular resistance, decreased cardiac output, arrhythmias, atrioventricular dissociation, precordial pain, hyperglycemia, increased glycogenolysis, fever, respiratory difficulty.

Nursing Implications: Record baseline heart rate and rhythm, blood pressure, quality of pulses, and color, temperature, and capillary refill of extremities before beginning infusion.

Monitor blood pressure every 2 minutes during titration until stabilized, then every 5 minutes.

Monitor heart rhythm and rate continuously. Document and report any changes to physician.

Assess pulse quality, color, temperature, and capillary refill of extremities.

Monitor urinary output hourly, reporting decreased output to physician immediately.

Infuse via automatic infusion pump. Titrate according to physician's guidelines, avoiding an excessive blood pressure response.

Discontinue drug slowly, monitoring vital signs every 5 minutes until drug is stopped and blood pressure is stabilized.

Monitor blood sugar levels in diabetics for possible adjustment of insulin requirements.

Atropine reverses bradycardia caused by norepinephrine; phentolamine decreases vasopressor effects; propranolol should be given for arrhythmias.

Infuse via largest vein possible and assess IV site frequently for signs of infiltration or blanching along course of infused vein. If extravasation occurs, infiltrate site with 5–10 mg of phentolamine within 12 hours.

Generic Name: ORPHENADRINE CITRATE

Trade Name: DISIPAL

Classification: Skeletal muscle relaxant

Actions: Analgesic and anticholinergic. Exact mechanism of action unknown.

Indications: Adjunct to physical therapy and other measures used to relieve discomfort of muscle spasm.

Dosage: Not recommended in pediatric patients. Safety has not been established.
Adult: 60 mg IM or IV. Can be repeated every 12 hours.

Preparation: Available in 2-ml ampules of 60 mg/ampule.

Compatibilities: Compatible with normal saline.

Administration: IM or IV.

Contraindications: Glaucoma, duodenal or pyloric obstruction, any obstruction of the bladder neck, stenosing peptic ulcers, myasthenia gravis, hypersensitivity. Use with caution in patients with cardiac disease and in pregnancy.

Side Effects:
Primary: Tachycardia, palpitations, urinary retention, blurred vision, drowsiness.
Secondary: Dry mouth, disorientation, restlessness, headache, hypersensitivity reactions.

Nursing Implications: Complete an initial assessment prior to administering the drug to establish a baseline of information. Assess client after administration to determine effectiveness.

Monitor for side effects. Notify physician as appropriate.

Maintain a safe environment because of possible disorientation. Caution patient to avoid hazardous activities until the drug reaction is known.

Generic Name: OXACILLIN SODIUM

Trade Name: PROSTAPHLIN, BACTOCILL

Classification: Antibiotic (penicillin)

Actions: Semisynthetic penicillin bactericidal against gram-positive organisms, penicillin G-sensitive organisms, resistant strains of *Staphylococcus aureus,* pneumococci, and group A beta-hemolytic streptococci.

Indications: Treatment of infections caused by penicillinase-producing staphylococci, pneumococci, and group A beta-hemolytic streptococci.

Dosage:
Neonatal: 50 mg/kg/day in divided doses every 6 hours.
Pediatric:
Under 40 kg: 50–100 mg/kg/day in divided doses every 6 hours.
Over 40 kg: 50–200 mg/kg/day in divided doses every 4–6 hours.
Adult: (over 40 kg): 50–200 mg/kg/day in divided doses every 4–6 hours.

Preparation: Supplied as a powder. Reconstitute with sterile water or sodium chloride for injection. Do not use bacteriostatic diluent if drug is being administered to a neonate. Reconstitute as follows:

VIAL SIZE	VOLUME DILUENT	CONCENTRATION
250 mg	1.4 ml	167 mg/ml
500 mg	2.7 ml	167 mg/ml
1 g	5.7 ml	167 mg/ml
2 g	11.5 ml	167 mg/ml
4 g	23.0 ml	167 mg/ml

Home Stability: Reconstituted solutions are stable for 7 days when refrigerated.

Compatibilities: Compatible with solutions containing dextrose, saline, KCl, Ringer's, or lactated Ringer's. Do not mix with any other antibiotic or with total parenteral nutrition.

Administration:
Neonatal: Dilute to 50 mg/ml and administer by IV push or IV Y-site over 10 minutes. Maximum infusion rate is 100 mg/minute.
Pediatric: See neonatal administration.
Adult: Dilute to 50 mg/ml in IV piggyback and infuse over 30–60 minutes. Dilute further if phlebitis occurs.

Contraindications: Hypersensitivity to penicillin derivatives or cephalosporins. Individuals with a history of allergic problems are more susceptible to untoward reactions. Safety in pregnancy has not been established.

Side Effects:
Primary: Hypersensitivity reactions such as skin rash, pruritus, anaphylaxis, urticaria, and febrile reactions; superinfections; pain and thrombosis of the IV site.
Secondary: Neutropenia, leukopenia, eosinophilia, thrombocytopenia; increase in SGOT, SGPT, hepatitis, intestinal nephritis, transient hematuria, albuminuria, azotemia, nausea, vomiting, diarrhea.

Nursing Implications: Prior to and during therapy, culture and sensitivity tests should be completed.
Monitor for allergic reactions.
Monitor baseline and periodic renal, hepatic, and hematologic functions, especially in long-term therapy.
Monitor for superinfection. Assess for the onset of black, hairy tongue; oral lesions (stomatitis, glossitis); rectal or vaginal itching; vaginal discharge; loose, foul-smelling stools; unusual odor to urine.
Monitor infusion site hourly for signs of thrombophlebitis.
Sodium concentration must be taken into consideration in clients on a sodium-restricted diet.
Use glucose oxidase reagents to check urine glucose. False positive reactions can occur with Clinitest.

Generic Name: OXYMORPHONE HYDROCHLORIDE

Trade Name: NUMORPHAN

Classification: Narcotic analgesic

Actions: Drugs in this class act to relieve moderate to severe pain and provide preoperative sedation. A patient's perception of pain is altered by preventing or changing the transmission of painful stimuli along the sensory pathways in the central nervous system. These pathways are specific to the perception and emotional response of the patient to pain. In addition, these drugs suppress the respiratory and cough centers of the brain and have an antiperistaltic effect on the smooth muscle of the intestine. Because of their actions, narcotics can produce physical and psychological dependence. When used to treat severe pain, as in terminal illness, these medications should be given around the clock to maximize the relief of pain and anxiety.

Indications: Management of moderate to severe pain from a diversity of causes. Should not be used in cases of mild pain or pain that can be relieved by non-narcotic analgesics.

Dosage:
Neonatal: Safe use for children under 12 has not been established.
Pediatric: See neonatal dosage.
Adult: IV: 0.5 mg every 4–6 hours as needed. IM or SC: 1–1.5 mg every 4–6 hours as needed.

Preparation: Injectable form available as 1 and 1.5 mg/ml.

Administration:
Neonatal: Not recommended.
Pediatric: Not recommended.
Adult: Usually given IM or SC. When given by IV route, administer by IV push over several minutes to avoid an increase in side effects, especially respiratory depression.

Contraindications: Sensitivity to narcotic analgesics; during delivery of a premature infant; in patients taking MAO inhibitors or who have taken them within 14 days. Use with caution in patients with head injuries, increased intracranial pressure, shock, central nervous system and respiratory depression, chronic obstructive pulmonary disease, and in patients receiving other narcotic analgesics.

Side Effects:
Primary: Respiratory depression and apnea during IV administration, hypotension, bradycardia, nausea, vomiting, dizziness, sedation, sweating.
Secondary: Constipation can occur because of the effect on the smooth muscle of the bowel. Urinary retention, pain at injection site, and phlebitis are possible after IV administration. Physical dependence.

Nursing Implications: Because of the chance for respiratory depression, a narcotic antagonist should be available for rapid administration, especially if the route of choice is IV. Naloxone is the antagonist most often used.

Monitor vital signs frequently. For IV dose, every 5–10 minutes; for SC dose, every 15–30 minutes.

Supportive equipment should be readily available in case of cardiac or respiratory arrest. A patent airway should be maintained.

Monitor infants when the drug is used during labor and delivery.

Monitor intake and output when the drug is given repeatedly, because it may cause urinary retention.

To augment the use of narcotic analgesics, give before severe pain occurs. Nursing actions also include emotional support and patient comfort measures. Because of depression of respiratory centers, postoperative use in management of pain should include patient's turning, coughing, and deep breathing to prevent pulmonary complications.

Patients should be warned to avoid activities that require alertness.

Assist patient with ambulation. This medication may cause orthostatic hypotension.

Generic Name: OXYTETRACYCLINE HYDROCHLORIDE

Trade Name: TERRAMYCIN IV

Classification: Antibiotic

Actions: Broad-spectrum antibiotic bactericidal against Rickettsia, *Mycoplasma pneumoniae,* agents of psittacosis and ornithosis, agents of lymphogranuloma venereum and granuloma inguinale, the spirochetal agent of relapsing fever (*Borrelia recurrentis*), and infections caused by the gram-negative organisms *Hemophilus ducreyi, Pasteurella pestis* and *tularensis, Bartonella bacilliformis,* Bacteroides, *Vibrio comma* and *fetus,* and Brucella.

Indications: Treatment of infections caused by the following organisms when sensitivity testing shows susceptibility. *Gram-negative: Escherichia coli, Enterobacter aerogenes,* Shigella, *Acinetobacter calcoaceticus,* Hemophilus influenzae (in respiratory infections), Klebsiella (in respiratory and urinary infections), Mima, and Herellae. *Gram-positive: Streptococcus pneumoniae* (not indicated for rheumatic fever prophylaxis), *Diplococcus pneumoniae.* When penicillin is contraindicated, oxytetracycline hydrochloride is indicated for the treatment of *Neisseria gonorrhoeae* and *menigitidis, Treponema pallidum* and *pertenue* (syphilis and yaws), *Listeria monocytogenes,* Clostridium, *Bacillus anthracis, Fusobacterium fusiforme* (Vincent's infection), Actinomyces, and amebicides.

Dosage:
Neonatal: Not recommended for neonates, but 10–15 mg/kg every 12 hours has been used.
Pediatric:
8 Years and Under: 10–15 mg/kg/day in divided doses every 12 hours.
8 Years and Over: 10–20 mg/kg/day in divided doses every 12 hours.
Use of this drug during the years of tooth development can cause permanent discoloration of the teeth and enamel hypoplasia. Do not use tetracyclines in this age group or in pregnancy unless other drugs are ineffective or contraindicated. Oxytetracycline is excreted in breast milk.
Adult: 250–500 mg every 6 hours. Maximum dosage: 500 mg every 6 hours.
General: In clients with renal impairment, dosage adjustment must be made.

Preparation: Supplied as a powder. Reconstitute with sterile water for injection. Add 10 ml of diluent to both the 250- and 500-mg vial.

Home Stability: Store in the refrigerator and discard after 48 hours. Administer within 12 hours at room temperature.

Compatibilities: Compatible with dextrose, saline, Ringer's, or lactated Ringer's. Not compatible with total parenteral nutrition or any other medication. Infusion must be completed within 6 hours when administered with lactated Ringer's.

Administration: Administration should be continued for at least 24–48 hours after symptoms and fever have subsided.
Neonatal: Infuse each 100 mg or fraction thereof over a minimum of 5 minutes by IV push, IV Y-site, or continuous infusion.
Pediatric: Further dilute the drug with 100 ml of compatible IV solution and infuse over 1 hour. May give as continuous infusion over 6–12 hours.
Adult: See pediatric administration.

Contraindications: Hypersensitivity. Not recommended in clients with renal insufficiency; in pregnancy or lactation; or in neonates.

Side Effects:
Primary: Hypersensitivity reactions including anaphylaxis; liver damage; photosensitivity; systemic moniliasis; thrombophlebitis; renal toxicity including a rise in BUN.
Secondary: Anorexia, nausea, vomiting, diarrhea, glossitis and dysphagia, enterocolitis, *Candida albicans* overgrowth in the perineal area (Monilia) and mouth (thrush), hemolytic anemia, thrombocytopenia. In infants: bulging fontanels and papilledema, which usually disappears with discontinuation of the drug.

Nursing Implications: Prior to and during therapy, culture and sensitivity tests should be completed.
Monitor for allergic reactions.
Monitor baseline and periodic renal, hepatic, and hematologic functions.
Monitor for superinfection. Assess for the on-

set of black, hairy tongue; oral lesions (stomatitis, glossitis); rectal or vaginal itching; vaginal discharge; loose, foul-smelling stools; unusual odor to urine.

Monitor infusion site for signs of thrombophlebitis.

Clients on anticoagulants may require lower doses of those drugs while on tetracyclines.

Monitor intake-output ratios. Notify physician of gastrointestinal disturbance or changes in renal status.

Notify physician of signs of increasing intracranial pressure.

Generic Name: OXYTOCIN INJECTION

Trade Name: PITOCIN, SYNTOCINON

Classification: Synthetic oxytocic hormone

Actions: Synthetic posterior pituitary derivative that increases or stimulates uterine contractions.

Indications: To initiate or increase uterine contractility for labor, to control postpartum bleeding, and for treatment of incomplete or inevitable abortion.

Dosage:
Adult:
Induction or Stimulation of Labor: Titrate dosage as follows. Initial dosage: 1–2 mU/minute; gradually increase dose in increments of no more than 1–2 mU/minute at 15–30-minute intervals until a satisfactory uterine contraction pattern has been seen. Maximum dosage: 20 mU/minute. Discontinue infusion immediately in the event of fetal distress or uterine hyperactivity.
Control of Uterine Bleeding: 10–40 U in 1000 ml of 5% dextrose in water. Titrate rate to uterine firmness. Initial dosage is 1–2 mU/minute increased by 1–2 mU/minute.
Incomplete or Inevitable Abortion: 10 units of oxytocin in 0.9% sodium chloride infused at a rate of 2–4 ml/minute (20–40 mU/minute).

Preparation: Supplied in ampules in concentrations of 5 U/0.5 ml, 10 U/1 ml, and 100 U/10 ml and in disposable syringes containing 10 U/1 ml.

Home Stability: Not indicated.

Compatibilities: Compatible with 5% dextrose in water and normal saline. Do not administer with any other medication.

Administration:
Adult:
Extreme Emergencies: Dilute dose in 5 ml of sodium chloride and inject slowly by IV push.

Titration for Uterine Contractility: Dilute 10 U in 1000 ml of 5% dextrose in water. Administer via infusion pump. A secondary IV line should be established for use when oxytocin is discontinued.

Contraindications: Significant cephalopelvic disproportion; unfavorable fetal positions; in emergencies where the benefit-to-risk ratio for fetus or mother favors surgical intervention; in fetal distress where delivery is not imminent; prolonged use in uterine inertia or severe toxemia; hypertonic uterine patterns; hypersensitivity; in cases where vaginal delivery is contraindicated. Probably should not be administered in cases of fetal distress, prematurity, placenta previa, abruptio placentae, borderline disproportion, or any situation where uterine rupture is possible, such as in patients who have previously undergone cesarean section.

Side Effects:
Primary: Tetanic uterine contraction, uterine rupture and pelvic hematomas, hypotension, arrhythmias, water intoxication, hypertensive episodes leading to cardiovascular accident or subarachnoid hemorrhage, hypersensitivity, fetal bradycardia, neonatal jaundice, postpartum hemorrhage, fatal afibrinogenemia.
Secondary: Chest pain, anxiety, dyspnea, hypersensitivity.

Nursing Implications: Assess maternal blood pressure and pulse and fetal heart rate and determine uterine activity (strength, duration, frequency of contractions) before initiating oxytocin and at least every 15 minutes thereafter.

Notify physician immediately of any change in fetal heart rate or any evidence of fetal distress; change in rate, rhythm, or frequency of uterine contractions; or change in maternal vital signs.

If hypertonic contractions occur or fetal distress is noted, discontinue IV oxytocin but continue maintenance IV.

Monitor fluid balance by measuring intake-output ratio.

Generic Name: **PANCURONIUM BROMIDE**

Trade Name: *PAVULON*

Classification: Neuromuscular blocker

Actions: Causes skeletal muscle paralysis by preventing acetylcholine from reaching its receptor sites at the myoneural junctions. Five times stronger than tubocurarine; does not alter consciousness or pain perception. Length of action is dose-related but is usually 30–45 minutes. First effects are seen 2–3 minutes after administration.

Indications: To facilitate anesthesia by relaxing skeletal muscles and in the management of patients on ventilators.

Dosage:
All Ages: 0.04–0.1 mg/kg. Dose may vary depending on patient and needs.
Neonatal: A test dose of 0.02 mg/kg may be given. Length of action in this group is short.
Pediatric: Not recommended for children under 10 years but has been used safely at the above dosage.

Preparation: Injectable 1 and 2 mg/ml.

Administration:
All Ages: IV.
Pediatric: IV, IM.

Contraindications: Hypersensitivity to drug or bromides. Use with caution in patients with thyroid disorders, myasthenia gravis, or renal or hepatic impairment.

Side Effects:
Primary: Skeletal muscle weakness, respiratory depression, apnea, tachycardia, paralysis.
Secondary: Excess salivation (pediatric), sweating.

Nursing Implications: Before administration, intubation and supportive equipment must be available.

Monitor patient for recovery from anesthesia. Observe for muscle movement, return of swallow and gag reflexes.

If used for patient on controlled ventilation, maintain skin integrity by turning, etc. Insure lubrication of eyes.

Drug has no analgesic/sedative actions. Other medication may be required.

Generic Name: PARALDEHYDE

Trade Name: PARACETALDEHYDE, PARAL

Classification: Sedative, hypnotic, anticonvulsant, Schedule IV controlled substance

Actions: Depresses various levels of the central nervous system with effects similar to those of barbiturates, chloral hydrate, and alcohol. Can be used to control convulsions or induce basal anesthesia in pediatric clients. Should not be used to control pain—has no analgesic effects unless given to produce an anesthetic state.

Indications: For fast-acting control of acute seizures. It is readily absorbed orally or rectally, and effects can be seen in 5–15 minutes.

Dosage: Varies depending on use.
Pediatric: IV administration not recommended. If used, dilute well and give no faster than 1 ml/minute.
Oral (for sedation or hypnosis): 0.15 ml/kg/dose. This can be doubled for hypnosis.
Rectal (for seizures): 0.15–3.0 ml/kg/dose by high rectal tube (retention enema). Be sure to clear tube with normal saline. Mix dose with equal parts of oil.
For sedation: 0.15 ml/kg/dose.
Adult: Oral and rectal: For sedation: 5–10 ml. For hypnosis: 10–30 ml.
IM or IV. IM dose: 5 ml. IV dose: 3–5 ml.

Preparation: Available in 2-, 5-, and 10-ml ampules. 30-ml bottles (non-sterile).

Administration: Oral: Dose may be diluted in milk or iced fruit juice.
Rectal: Dilute with at least equal parts of mineral, cottonseed, vegetable, or olive oil.
IV: Dilute in at least 100 ml of 0.9% sodium chloride. Give no faster than 1 ml/minute.

Contraindications: Hypersensitivity. Avoid oral doses in patients with peptic ulcer, gastrointestinal inflammation, respiratory disease, or severe hepatic impairment.

Side Effects:
Primary: Irritation of the mucous membranes, nausea, vomiting. High doses can cause hypotension or respiratory failure. IV administration can cause pulmonary edema or hemorrhage.
Secondary: Unpleasant taste and odor, hangover, ataxia, dizziness, skin rash. IM administration can cause sterile abscesses. IV administration can cause thrombophlebitis, necrosis, or severe tissue damage upon infiltration.

Nursing Implications: Protect from light, heat, or air—these will oxidize the drug. Solution should be clear and colorless. Drug has strong odor and burning, unpleasant taste.
Drug should not be used if open for more than 24 hours. Always use glass when administering or measuring drug.
IV dose has many side effects, including hypotension, respiratory depression, and pulmonary edema, and may also cause circulatory collapse. Patient should be monitored carefully. A physician should be readily available in case of emergency or to administer the drug itself.
Maintain a safe environment because of possible confusion or dizziness.
Patient's room should be well ventilated. Some of the drug is excreted by the lungs, and it gives off a strong odor.
Addiction may result from prolonged use. Drug should be withdrawn slowly.
Assess patient's condition before and after administration and any noted effects. Note type of seizure activity.

**Generic Name: PENICILLIN G POTASSIUM
PENICILLIN G SODIUM**

Trade Name: PENICILLIN G POTASSIUM, PFIZERPEN

Classification: Antibiotic (penicillin)

Actions: Natural derivative of *Penicillium notatum* and related molds, bactericidal against gram-positive cocci (nonpenicillinase-producing staphylococci, streptococci including *Streptococcus pneumoniae*), gram-negative cocci (*Neisseria gonorrhoeae* and *meningitidis*), gram-positive bacilli (*Bacillus anthracis,* Clostridium, Corynebacterium, Erysipelothrix, Listeria), gram-negative bacilli (Fusobacterium, Pasteurella, streptobacillus, Bacteroides, *Escherichia coli, Proteus mirabilis,* Salmonella, Shigella, *Enterobacter aerogenes, Alcaligenes faecalis*), spirochetes (*Treponema pallidum* and *pertenue*, Leptospira), and actinomycetes (*Actinomyces bovis* and *israelii*).

Indications: Actinomycosis, anthrax, diphtheria, empyema, erysipelas, gas gangrene, gonorrheal infections, leptospirosis, mastoiditis, meningitis, osteomyelitis, otitis media, pneumonia, staphylococcal and streptococcal infections (scarlet fever, syphilis, tetanus, urinary tract infections), and Vincent's gingivostomatitis.

Used prophylactically in clients with rheumatic or congenital heart disease.

Dosage:
Neonatal: Do not exceed 250,000 u/kg/day. Administer dosage every 6 hours for meningitis.
0–7 Days: 50,000–150,000 u/kg/day every 12 hours.
Over 7 Days: 75,000–250,000 u/kg/day every 8 hours.
Pediatric: 75,000–250,000 u/kg/day every 8 hours. *Do not exceed* 250,000 u/kg/day. Administer dosage every 6 hours for meningitis.
Adult: 200,000 to 4 million u every 6–8 hours.

Preparation: Supplied as a powder in vial sizes of 1, 5, 10, and 20 million u. Reconstitute with sterile water. Dilute as follows:

VIAL SIZE	DILUENT	CONCENTRATION
1,000,000	9.6	100,000
5,000,000	23.0	200,000
10,000,000	15.4	500,000
20,000,000	31.6	500,000

Home Stability: After reconstitution, store in refrigerator and use within 1 week.

Compatibilities: Compatible with solutions containing dextrose, saline, KCl, Ringer's, or lactated Ringer's, and with total parenteral nutrition. Do not mix with any other antibiotic.

Administration:
Neonatal: Doses under 75,000 u: Dilute to 25,000 u/ml and administer by IV push over 5–10 minutes.
Doses 75,000–250,000 u: Dilute to 25,000 u/ml and administer by IV Y-site over 5–10 minutes.
Pediatric: Doses under 75,000 units: Dilute to 25,000 u/ml and administer by IV push over 5–10 minutes.
Doses 75,000–250,000 units: Dilute to 25,000 u/ml and administer by IV Y-site over 5–10 minutes.
Over 250,000 u: Dilute in IV solution to 25,000 units per milliliter and administer by IV piggyback over 30 minutes.
Adult: Dilute in IV solution to 25,000 u/ml and administer by IV piggyback over 30 minutes.

Contraindications: Hypersensitivity to penicillin derivatives or cephalosporins, use of penicillin G sodium in sodium-restricted clients. Individuals with a history of allergic problems are more susceptible to untoward reactions. Infants may be sensitized through breast milk of mothers receiving penicillin G.

Side Effects:
Primary: Hypersensitivity reactions such as skin rash, itching palms or axilla, pruritus, anaphylaxis, urticaria, and febrile reactions; superinfections; pain and thrombosis of the IV site; electrolyte imbalance: hyperkalemia (penicillin G potassium), hypokalemia, alkalosis, hypernatremia, congestive heart failure (penicillin G sodium), diarrhea.
Secondary: Bone marrow depression, granulocytopenia, seizures, neuromuscular hyperirritability, Jarisch-Herxheimer reaction (syphilis).

Nursing Implications: Prior to and during therapy, culture and sensitivity tests should be completed.
Monitor for allergic reactions.
Monitor baseline and periodic renal, hepatic,

and hematologic functions, especially in long-term therapy.

Monitor for superinfection. Assess for the onset of black, hairy tongue; oral lesions (stomatitis, glossitis); rectal or vaginal itching; vaginal discharge; loose, foul-smelling stools; unusual odor to urine.

Monitor infusion site hourly for signs of thrombophlebitis.

Sodium concentration must be taken into consideration in clients on a sodium-restricted diet.

Observe clients closely for the first half-hour after initial dose for a wheal or redness at IV site and other allergic reactions.

Monitor intake-output ratio. Report oliguria, hematuria, and changes in intake-output ratio.

Use glucose oxidase reagents to check urine glucose. False positive reactions can occur with Clinitest.

Monitor for signs of neurotoxicity when high doses of penicillin therapy are being administered.

Monitor for signs of electrolyte imbalance and congestive heart failure.

Generic Name: PENTAZOCINE HYDROCHLORIDE

Trade Name: TALWIN

Classification: Narcotic analgesic

Actions: Drugs in this class act to relieve moderate to severe pain and provide preoperative sedation. A patient's perception of pain is altered by preventing or changing the transmission of painful stimuli along the sensory pathways in the central nervous system. These pathways are specific to the perception and emotional response of the patient to pain. In addition, these drugs suppress the respiratory and cough centers of the brain and have an antiperistaltic effect on the smooth muscle of the intestine. Because of their actions, narcotics can produce physical and psychological dependence. When used to treat severe pain, as in terminal illness, they should be given around the clock to maximize the relief of pain and anxiety.

Indications: Management of moderate to severe pain from a diversity of causes. Should not be used in cases of mild pain or pain that can be relieved by non-narcotic analgesics.

Dosage:
Neonatal: Safe administration in patients under 12 has not been established.
Pediatric: See neonatal dosage.
Adult: 30 mg IM, SC, or IV every 3–4 hours as needed. Doses over 30 mg IV or 60 mg IM are not recommended. Total maximum daily dose is 360 mg. Administration SC can cause severe tissue damage.

Preparation: Injectable form available as 30 mg/ml.

Compatibilities: Will precipitate when mixed with soluble barbiturates.

Administration:
Neonatal: Safety when given to patients under age 12 has not been established.
Pediatric: See neonatal administration.
Adult: SC, IV, IM. When given slowly by IV push, effects are seen within 2–3 minutes. Effects are seen in 20–30 minutes after SC or IM administration. Avoid repeated SC doses because they may cause severe tissue damage. Rotate injection sites when given IM.

Contraindications: Sensitivity to narcotic analgesics, during delivery of a premature infant, in patients taking MAO inhibitors or who have taken them within 14 days. Use with caution in patients with head injuries, increased intracranial pressure, shock, central nervous system and respiratory depression, chronic obstructive pulmonary disease, and in patients receiving other narcotic analgesics.

Side Effects:
Primary: Respiratory depression and apnea during IV administration. Also known sensitivity to narcotic analgesics; hypotension, bradycardia, nausea, vomiting, dizziness, sedation, sweating.
Secondary: Constipation can occur because of the effect on the smooth muscle of the bowel. Urinary retention, pain at injection site, and phlebitis are possible after IV administration. Physical dependence.

Nursing Implications: Because of the chance for respiratory depression, a narcotic antagonist should be available for rapid administration, especially if the route of choice is IV. Naloxone is the antagonist most often used.

Monitor vital signs frequently. For IV dose, every 5–10 minutes; for SC dose, every 15–30 minutes.

Supportive equipment should be readily available in case of cardiac or respiratory arrest. A patent airway should be maintained.

Monitor infants when the drug is used during labor and delivery.

Monitor intake and output when the drug is given repeatedly, because it may cause urinary retention.

To augment the use of narcotic analgesics, give before severe pain occurs. Nursing actions also include emotional support and patient comfort measures. Because of depression of respiratory centers, postoperative use in management of pain should include patient's turning, coughing, and deep breathing to prevent pulmonary complications.

Patients should be warned to avoid activities that require alertness.

Assist patient with ambulation. This medication may cause orthostatic hypotension.

Generic Name: PENTOBARBITAL SODIUM

Trade Name: NEMBUTAL

Classification: Sedative, hypnotic

Actions: Members of the barbiturate family can produce a variety of effects on the central nervous system, from excitation to sedation to deep coma. They act at the level of the thalamus to depress cortex functioning, which decreases motor activity and produces sedation. They also produce respiratory depression, but its severity is dose dependent. Barbiturates have limited usefulness as sedatives. They decrease the amount of time spent in the dreaming stage of sleep. Much of their sleep-producing effect disappears after about 2 weeks, so they are not indicated for long-term treatment of insomnia.

Indications: Short-term treatment of insomnia, preanesthetic medication, treatment of acute convulsive episodes.

Dosage: Varies with use, patient age, weight, and other factors. Following are guidelines only.
Neonatal:
Over 2 Years: 3 mg/kg/dose IM every 8 hours.
Pediatric: 3–5 mg/kg/dose IM.
Adult: 150–200 mg IM.

Preparation: Injectable available as 50 mg/ml.

Administration:
Neonatal: IM. IV only when impossible to give by another route. Continuous infusion possible for increased intracranial pressure at 2 mg/kg/hour.
Pediatric: See neonatal administration.
Adult: IM. When administering IM, give deep into muscle. IV only if other routes impossible.

Contraindications: Hypersensitivity, hepatic dysfunction, severe respiratory depression and distress.

Side Effects:
Primary: Somnolence, agitation, ataxia, central nervous system depression, anxiety, dizziness, respiratory depression, hypotension, bradycardia.
Secondary: Skin rashes, constipation, nausea, vomiting, tissue necrosis from extravasation, headache, fever.

Nursing Implications: Monitor vital signs.

Have supportive equipment available in case of severe respiratory depression.

Do not administer closely with a narcotic analgesic.

Maintain a safe environment for patient because of depressant effects on the central nervous system. Raise side rails of bed, assist with ambulation, etc.

Generic Name: PERPHENAZINE

Trade Name: TRILAFON

Classification: Antipsychotic

Actions: Mechanism of action not completely understood, but agents in this classification block postsynaptic dopamine receptors in the brain. By inhibiting or altering dopamine release and increasing the firing rate of neuronal cells in the midbrain, antipsychotic drugs suppress the clinical signs of schizophrenia. These medications may also depress control of basic body functions such as metabolism, body temperature, level of consciousness, and hormonal balance. These drugs are widely distributed and stored in the tissues and may be eliminated in the urine for up to 6 months after therapy is discontinued.

Drugs in this family differ in the severity of side effects. Major side effects are sedation, extrapyramidal effects, and orthostatic hypotension. These can be minimized by changing from one drug to another.

Indications: Treatment and management of psychotic disorders; may be used in treatment of severe nausea and vomiting.

Dosage:

Neonatal and Pediatric: Dosage has not been established.

Adult: Usual IM dose is 5 mg every 6 hours. Daily dose should not exceed 15 mg for ambulatory patients and 30 mg for hospitalized patients. Parenteral form more potent than tablet form.

Preparation: Injectable form available as 16 mg/5 ml or 5 mg/ml.

Administration: May be administered orally, IM, or IV, but oral administration is used for maintenance therapy. Parenteral administration provides more active drug than oral doses.

Neonatal and Pediatrics: For children over 12, see adult administration.

Adult: IM initially in acute situation or when oral administration is not possible. After initiation of therapy, oral administration is begun.

IV form should only be used when absolutely necessary to control severe vomiting.

Contraindications: In patients who are comatose or experiencing central nervous system depression; blood dyscrasias; presence of hepatic disease, coronary artery disease, or convulsive disorders.

Side Effects: All side effects listed have not been observed in the use of this drug, but because of the similarities of the phenothiazines, they are listed for all drugs in this group.

Primary: Most common are extrapyramidal reactions, including but not limited to aching and numbness in the limbs, motor restlessness, dystonia, tight feeling of throat, slurred speech, and ataxia; orthostatic hypotension; blurred vision and other ocular changes; dark urine; bradycardia; dizziness.

Secondary: Jaundice, anemia, agranulocytosis, dermatitis, pain at IM injection site.

Nursing Implications: Monitor vital signs and observe for hypotension or behavioral changes. Monitor level of consciousness. Ongoing assessment should include these observations on a daily basis.

Assess and observe for side effects. The development of extrapyramidal effects can be distressing. Assure client they will subside.

Warn clients on home therapy that care should be used when activities require alertness or coordination. The drowsiness experienced should subside after a period of time.

Warn clients to avoid extended exposure to the sun and to avoid getting drug on skin, since it may cause contact dermatitis.

Dry mouth may be a side effect. Gum or candy may relieve the discomfort.

Generic Name: PHENOBARBITAL SODIUM

Trade Name: LUMINAL SODIUM

Classification: Anticonvulsant, sedative, hypnotic, barbiturate

Actions: Long-acting central nervous system depressant, hypnotic, and anticonvulsant. Barbiturates act at the level of the thalamus to depress cortex functioning, which decreases motor activity and produces sedation.

Indications: For sedation and relief of anxiety; hypertension; as an antispasmotic; acute labyrinthitis; pylorospasm in infants; cardiac failure; in children, preoperative and postoperative sedation; for symptomatic control of acute seizures such as tetanus, eclampsia, status epilepticus, and cerebral hemorrhage.

Dosage:
Neonatal: 3–6 mg/kg. Status epilepticus loading dose: 5 mg/kg followed by 2.5 mg/kg every 5 minutes until seizure stops.
Pediatric: See neonatal dosage.
Adult: Sedative: 100–320 mg/day. Maximum dosage: 600 mg in 24 hours. Dosage should be determined by client response and indication.

Preparation: Supplied in ampules of 120 mg. Reconstitute each 125 mg with 10 ml of sterile water for injection. Also available in prefilled syringes and vials of 30, 60, 65, and 130 mg/ml. Protect ampules from light. Dispose of powder or solution that has been exposed to air for 30 minutes.

Home Stability: Not indicated.

Compatibilities: Do not mix with any other medication.

Administration:
Neonatal: Inject at IV site at a rate not to exceed 60 mg/minute. Injection exceeding 60 mg/minute may result in apnea or hypotension.
Pediatric: See neonatal administration.
Adult: See neonatal administration.

Contraindications: Hypersensitivity, impaired renal function, family or client history of porphyria, impaired respiratory function, history of sedative/hypnotic addiction. Safety in pregnancy has not been established. May cause respiratory depression in the infant if used during labor.

Side Effects:
Primary: Somnolence, agitation, ataxia, central nervous system depression, anxiety, dizziness, respiratory depression, hypotension, bradycardia.
Secondary: Skin rashes, constipation, nausea, vomiting, tissue necrosis from extravasation, headache, fever.

Nursing Implications: Monitor vital signs every 5 minutes for 1 hour after injection. Do not leave patient unattended.

Have supportive equipment available in case of respiratory depression.

Maintain a safe environment for client because of depressant effects. Raise side rails of bed and assist with ambulation.

Do not administer closely with a narcotic analgesic.

Generic Name: PHENTOLAMINE MESYLATE

Trade Name: REGITINE

Classification: Antihypertensive

Actions: Alpha-adrenergic blocking agent

Indications: Diagnosis and treatment of hypertension associated with pheochromocytoma, especially before or during pheochromocytomectomy; prevention and treatment of dermal sloughing and necrosis related to extravasation.

Dosage:
Neonatal: Not applicable.
Pediatric:
Diagnostic Dose: 0.1 mg/kg or 3 mg/m² (average: 1 ml).
Before and During Pheochromocytomectomy: 1 mg.
Adult: 5 mg before and during pheochromocytomectomy.

Preparation: 5-mg vials containing powder for reconstitution. Dilute each 5 mg with 1 ml of sterile water for injection. May be further diluted with 5–10 ml of sterile water for injection.

Home Stability: Not recommended for home use.

Compatibilities: Sodium chloride 0.9% has been recommended for the dilution of phentol-amine. Solution should be used soon, but may be stored for 48 hr at room temperature.

Administration:
Neonatal: Not applicable.
Pediatric: Administer by IV push at the IV site at a rate not to exceed 5 mg/minute.
Adult: See pediatric administration.

Contraindications: Hypersensitivity, history of myocardial infarction, coronary insufficiency, angina. Safe use during pregnancy and lactation has not been established.

Side Effects:
Primary: Cardiac arrhythmias, cerebrovascular occlusion, cerebrovascular spasm, severe hypotension, myocardial infarction, shock, tachycardia, vomiting under anesthesia.
Secondary: Diarrhea, dizziness, nasal stuffiness, nausea, tachycardia, tingling of skin, weakness, vomiting.

Nursing Implications: Monitor vital signs every 2 minutes.
Monitor for cardiac arrhythmias via EKG monitor. Have lidocaine and atropine at the bedside.
Client may ambulate after 1 hour of bedrest. Assess for orthostatic hypotension.

Generic Name: PHENYLEPHRINE HYDROCHLORIDE

Trade Name: NEO-SYNEPHRINE

Classification: Adrenergic (sympathomimetic)

Actions: Produces vasoconstriction causing a rise in systolic and diastolic pressures with little chronotropic or inotropic effect on the heart.

Indications: Hypotensive emergencies during spinal anesthesia, mild to moderate hypotension, paroxysmal supraventricular tachycardia, prolongation of spinal anesthesia, severe hypotension and shock (including drug-induced).

Dosage:
Neonatal: Not applicable.
Pediatric: Not applicable.
Adult:
Hypotensive Emergencies During Spinal Anesthesia: Initially 0.1 mg IV, followed by doses not to exceed the preceding dose by more than 0.1–0.2 mg and not to exceed 0.5 mg per single dose.
Mild to Moderate Hypotension: 0.1–0.5 mg IV; repeat no sooner than in 10–15 minutes.
Paroxysmal Supraventricular Tachycardia: 0.5 mg, followed by doses not to exceed the preceding dose by more than 0.1–0.2 mg and not to exceed 1 mg per single dose.
Prolongation of Spinal Anesthesia: 2–5 mg added to anesthetic solutions.
Severe Hypotension and Shock: Begin an infusion of 10 mg in 500 ml of solution at a rate of 100–180 µg/minute; then decrease to 40–60 µg/minute and titrate.

Preparation: 10 mg/ml in 1-ml ampules or 1-mg cartridge-needle units.

Home Stability: Not applicable.

Compatibilities: Compatible with 5% dextrose or saline.

Administration:
Neonatal: Not applicable.
Pediatric: Not applicable.
Adult: Dilute each 1 mg with 9 ml of sterile water for injection and give over 1 minute, except when treating supraventricular tachycardia, give undiluted over 20–30 seconds. Titrate continuous infusions to blood pressure response.

Contraindications: Hypersensitivity, severe hypertension, ventricular tachycardia, halothane anesthesia. Use with extreme caution in patients with hyperthyroidism, bradycardia, heart block, myocardial disease, severe arteriosclerosis, narrow-angle glaucoma, diabetes, in the elderly, and with concurrent use of oxytoxic drugs, monoamine oxidase inhibitors, or tricyclic antidepressants.

Side Effects:
Primary: Trembling, sweating, pallor, tingling in extremities.
Secondary: Dizziness, sleeplessness, weakness, lightheadedness, palpitations, bradycardia, tachycardia, extrasystoles, short paroxysms of ventricular tachycardia, hypertension, angina, blurred vision, gooseflesh, feelings of coolness.

Nursing Implications: Record baseline heart rate and rhythm, blood pressure, quality of pulses, and color, temperature, and capillary refill of extremities before beginning infusion.

Monitor blood pressure every 2 minutes until stabilized, then every 15 minutes.

Monitor heart rhythm and rate continuously. Document and report any changes to physician.

Assess pulse quality, color, temperature, and capillary refill of extremities.

Infuse continuous drips via automatic infusion pump. Titrate according to physician's guidelines, avoiding an excessive blood pressure response.

Monitor blood sugar levels in diabetics for possible adjustment of insulin requirements.

Phentolamine will decrease vasopressor effects.

Infuse via largest vein possible and assess IV site frequently for signs of infiltration or blanching along course of infused vein. If extravasation occurs, infiltrate site with 5–10 mg of phentolamine within 12 hours.

Generic Name: PHENYTOIN

Trade Name: DILANTIN

Classification: Anticonvulsant of hydantoin family. Prevents spread of seizure activity at level of motor cortex. Seizure activity is limited by the stabilization of neuronal membranes, by the increased efflux or decreased influx of sodium ions across the cell membranes during nerve impulses. As an antiarrhythmic, suppresses atrial and ventricular automaticity without slowing A-V conduction.

Indications: Treatment of grand mal and psychomotor seizures, prevention and treatment of seizures during neurosurgical procedures. Often used in combination with other anticonvulsants in treatment of grand mal and petit mal epilepsy.

Dosage:

Neonatal and Pediatric: Loading dose of 10–15 mg/kg/day with maintenance of 5–7 mg/kg/day. This will produce, in most cases, a therapeutic plasma concentration of 10–20 mcg/ml.

Adult: Loading dose of 10–15 mg/kg/day. Maintenance dose is 100 mg IV or by mouth every 6–8 hours.

Preparation: Injectable form available as 50 mg/ml in 2- and 5-ml ampules and preloaded syringes.

Home Stability: When diluted for administration, solution is stable for 1 hour.

Compatibilities: Because phenytoin is highly alkaline, do not mix with other parenteral medications.

Administration: Only administer a clear solution. Monitor patient for arrhythmias during IV administration. Avoid IM route, because it can cause pain and necrosis at the injection site and the drug is absorbed erratically from muscle.

Neonatal and Pediatric: When administering parenterally to pediatric patients, do not exceed 1–3 mg/kg/minute. Push slowly at this rate. Do not infuse over a period of time because of the chance of precipitation.

Adult: IV administration should not exceed 50 mg/minute.

Contraindications: Hypersensitivity to phenacemide or hydantoin medications, bradycardia, sinoatrial and A-V block, Stokes-Adams syndrome.

Nursing Implications: *Do not exceed* recommended rate of administration. Monitor patient closely during parenteral administration for hypotension and cardiac arrhythmias. Do not administer if solution is hazy. Faint yellow coloration has no effect on potency.

Assess patient for signs of toxicity, which include cardiovascular collapse, central nervous system depression, drowsiness, and circumoral tingling. Monitor plasma levels—toxic symptoms are most likely to occur when concentrations are above 20 μg/ml.

Observe and document any seizure activity. Obtain a history of any previous activity.

Warn patient to avoid activities that require alertness and motor coordination until central nervous system response is known.

Do not mix drug with any solution but normal saline, as a precipitate may form.

Instruct patient to maintain good oral hygiene because of the chance of gingival hyperplasia.

Observe closely for signs of a rash. Notify physician if one develops.

If patient is on long-term oral therapy, the following precautions must be taken. Patient should carry identification that he or she is taking the drug. Doses taken with or after meals may decrease gastrointestinal side effects. Use of alcohol can decrease effectiveness of drug. There are several oral forms of phenytoin, and brands should not be changed once patient is stabilized on therapy. Differentiation must be made between the forms taken, as some are taken once a day or less.

Generic Name: PHYSOSTIGMINE SALICYLATE

Trade Name: ANTILIRIUM

Classification: Cholinergic

Actions: Drugs in this classification act to facilitate transmission of impulses across the myoneural junction and to inhibit the destruction of acetylcholine. This member of the family is easily absorbed, and its duration of action is 45–60 minutes. Antilirium will cross the blood-brain barrier, so it may be used to counteract toxicity to the central nervous system.

Indications: Treatment and diagnosis of myasthenia gravis. Also used to treat the effects of tricyclic antidepressants.

Dosage:

Pediatric (Emergency Use Only): 0.02 or 0.5 mg/kg by *slow* IV injection (over at least 1 minute). May repeat dose every 5–10 minutes until desired outcome is observed or until 2 mg has been given.

Adult: 0.5–1.0 mg IV. Give no faster than 1 mg/minute. May repeat every 10–30 minutes until desired outcome is observed. Maximum: 4 mg.

Preparation: Available as 2-ml ampules, 1 mg/ml, injectable. Use only clear, colorless solution. Discard any tinged solution.

Administration: Must be given IV very slowly (over at least 1 minute).

Contraindications: Hypersensitivity, obstructions (mechanical intestinal and urinary), bradycardia, hypotension. Use with caution in patients with bronchial asthma or cardiac dysrhythmias. Atropine and epinephrine should be available in case of hypersensitivity reaction.

Side Effects: The following side effects may occur but have not been observed with each agent.

Primary: Ocular changes; convulsion; dysphonia; dysphagia; respiratory changes including increased secretions, paralysis, and laryngospasm; arrhythmias; gastrointestinal disturbances; muscle weakness.

Secondary: Urinary frequency, incontinence, thrombophlebitis with IV use.

Nursing Implications: Do a complete assessment of patient and symptoms observed.

Emergency equipment should be readily available in case of hypersensitivity reaction.

Observe myasthenic patient for any exacerbation of symptoms.

If drug is administered as curare antagonist, observe patient for return of muscle movement.

If patient has myasthenia gravis, determine if in a crisis or in a cholinergic crisis. Because symptoms are so similar, it may be necessary to do an edrophonium test.

Monitor vital signs closely.

Patient teaching should include spacing activities to avoid fatigue, signs of drug overdosage or underdosage, and need for follow-up care and close medical supervision.

Physostigmine is also available in an ophthalmic ointment used in the treatment of glaucoma.

May cause temporary blurring of vision. Warn patient to take necessary safety precautions.

Observe for excessive salivation, emesis, frequent urination, or diarrhea. This may indicate a need to discontinue drug.

Generic Name: PHYTONADIONE (VITAMIN K$_1$)

Trade Name: AQUAMEPHYTON

Classification: Vitamin

Actions: Essential for hepatic synthesis of clotting factors II, VII, IX, and X. Used to treat coagulation disorders caused by faulty formation of these factors. Vitamin K does not negate the pharmacologic effects of heparin.

This form of vitamin K has been found safer than others in treating hemorrhagic disease of the newborn.

The action of phytonadione is observable within an hour of IV administration. Hemorrhage can usually be controlled in 3–6 hours.

Indications: Any coagulation disorder due to a defect in formation of clotting factors II, VII, IX, and X (e.g., hemorrhagic disease of the newborn, hypoprothrombinemia due to antibacterial therapy); any condition that limits or interferes with vitamin K absorption or metabolism.

Dosage:
Neonatal: For prophylaxis and treatment of hemorrhagic disease of the newborn.
Prophylaxis: Single IM dose of 0.5–2.0 mg.
Treatment: 1–2 mg SC or IM daily. Treatment also includes laboratory evaluation of coagulation factors to determine cause.
Pediatric: 5–10 mg orally or parenterally.
Adult: 2–25 mg (depending on severity of symptoms) orally or parenterally.

Preparation: Injectable forms available in aqueous colloidal solution (2 and 5 mg/ml) and aqueous dispersion (2 mg/ml and, for IM only, 10 mg/ml).

Home Stability: Unused portions of drug should be discarded immediately—it contains no preservative and is unstable. Protect from light—drug is photosensitive.

Compatibilities: Compatible with 0.9% NaCl, 5% dextrose, and 5% dextrose with NaCl. Preservatives such as benzyl alcohol should be avoided because of toxic reactions in the newborn.

Administration:
Neonatal: IM, SC, or IV. IV rate should not exceed 1 mg/minute.
Pediatric: See neonatal administration.
Adult: See neonatal administration.

Side Effects:
Primary: Transient hypotension can occur with IV administration; cardiac irregularities; dizziness; bronchospasm; anaphylaxis reactions possible after rapid IV administration.
Secondary: Sweating, flushing, nausea and vomiting.

Nursing Implications: Observe patient for signs of bleeding. Monitor laboratory work such as prothrombin time, bleeding time, hemoglobin, and complete blood count.

Monitor for signs and symptoms of anaphylaxis during and after administration. Anaphylaxis is most likely to occur during rapid IV administration.

Emergency equipment should be available during IV administration in case of severe reaction. Vital signs should be monitored every 5 minutes during infusion and every 10–15 minutes for 1 hour thereafter.

Warn patient that pain, swelling, or tenderness at injection site is possible.

During severe bleeding, it may still be necessary to administer blood or blood components.

Generic Name: PIPERACILLIN SODIUM

Trade Name: PIPRACIL

Classification: Antibiotic (penicillin)

Actions: Extended-spectrum penicillin with microbial action against gram-negative and gram-positive anaerobes and aerobes including Clostridium, Bacteroides, Klebsiella, Enterobacter, Pseudomonas, Proteus, Serratia, and anaerobic and aerobic cocci.

Indications: Infections caused by the above-stated organisms, including those of lower respiratory tract, skin, intra-abdomen, bone structures, and joints; gynecologic, gonococcal, and streptococcal infections; septicemia; urinary tract infections. Also indicated for prophylactic treatment for granulocytopenic clients undergoing surgery.

Dosage:
Neonatal: Dosage has not been established.
Pediatric: 76–100 mg/kg/day.
Adult: 12–18 g/day divided into equal doses every 4–6 hours. Maximum dosage: 24 g/day.

Preparation: Supplied as a powder. Dilute each g of drug with at least 5 ml of sterile water or normal saline for injection. Further dilute in 50–100 ml for IV infusion.

Home Stability: After reconstitution, stable for 24 hours at room temperature, for up to 1 week in refrigerator, for 1 month frozen.

Compatibilities: Compatible with solutions containing dextrose, saline, KCl, Ringer's, or lactated Ringer's and with total parenteral nutrition. Do not mix with any other antibiotic unless first consulting with a pharmacist.

Administration:
Neonatal: Administer by IV push over 5–10 minutes.
Pediatric: Administer by IV push or IV Y-site over 5–10 minutes.

Adult: Dilute in IV solution and administer by IV piggyback over 30 minutes.

Contraindications: Hypersensitivity to penicillin derivatives or cephalosporins, use in sodium-restricted clients. Individuals with a history of allergic problems are more susceptible to untoward reactions. Safe use in children under 12 years, lactating mothers, and during pregnancy has not been established.

Side Effects:
Primary: Hypersensitivity reactions such as skin rash, itching palms or axilla, anaphylaxis, urticaria, and febrile reactions; superinfections; pain and thrombosis of the IV site; electrolyte imbalance: hypokalemia, alkalosis, hypernatremia, congestive heart failure, diarrhea.
Secondary: Bone marrow depression: granulocytopenia, abnormal aggregation, prolonged prothrombin time, seizures, neuromuscular hyperirritability, Jarisch-Herxheimer reaction (syphilis).

Nursing Implications: Prior to and during therapy, culture and sensitivity tests should be completed.
Monitor for allergic reactions.
Monitor baseline and periodic renal, hepatic, and hematologic and hepatic functions, especially in long-term therapy.
Monitor for superinfections. Assess for the onset of black, hairy tongue; oral lesions (stomatitis, glossitis); rectal or vaginal itching; vaginal discharge; loose, foul-smelling stools; unusual odor to urine.
Monitor infusion site hourly for signs of thrombophlebitis.
Sodium concentration must be taken into consideration in clients on a sodium-restricted diet.
Observe clients closely for the first half-hour of initial dose for a wheal or redness at IV site for potential allergic reaction.
Monitor intake-output ratio. Report oliguria, hematuria, and changes in intake-output ratio.

Use glucose oxidase reagents to check urine glucose. False positive reactions can occur with Clinitest.

Monitor for signs of neurotoxicity when high doses of piperacillin therapy are being administered.

Monitor for signs of electrolyte imbalance and congestive heart failure.

Generic Name: PLASMA PROTEIN FRACTION

Trade Name: PLASMANATE, PLASMA-PLEX, PROTENATE

Classification: Volume expander

Actions: Expands intravascular volume, maintains colloid osmotic pressure, and maintains appropriate electrolyte balance in cases of burns.

Indications: Shock, hypoproteinemia.

Dosage:
Neonatal: 20 to 30 ml/kg.
Pediatric: 20–30 ml/kg.
Adult: Varies depending on patient's condition. Range: 250–1500 ml/day. Initial doses are usually 250–1000 ml for burns and shock; 1000–1500 ml/24 hours for hypoproteinemia. Dosage should not exceed 250 g in 48 hours.

Preparation: Available in 250- and 500-ml bottles (25 g/500 ml) with injection sets.

Home Stability: Not applicable.

Compatibilities: Infuse through IV line by itself. Infuse saline before and after plasma infusion to clear tubing of maintenance IV fluid.

Administration:
Neonatal: 5 to 10 ml/minute, not to exceed 10 ml/minute.

Pediatric: See neonatal administration.
Adult: Ranges from 1 ml/minute to 500 ml/hour depending on patient condition and response.

Contraindications: Cardiac failure, history of allergic reactions to albumin, normal or increased intravascular volume, severe anemia.

Side Effects:
Primary: Allergic reactions, nausea.
Secondary: Hypotension if infused too rapidly.

Nursing Implications: May be given without regard to blood group or type.

Adjust rate to patient response and blood pressure. Obtain baseline vital signs and check frequently during and after therapy until stable. Monitor hourly urine output.

Assess for jugular venous distension, peripheral edema, dyspnea, wheezing, rales, and rhonchi during therapy.

Monitor daily weights, intake/output, and skin turgor.

Monitor hemoglobin, hematocrit, electrolytes, and serum protein levels during therapy.

Assess for signs of bleeding during and after therapy.

Assess for signs of allergic reactions 5 and 15 minutes after initiation of therapy.

Generic Name: PLICAMYCIN

Trade Name: MITHRACIN

Classification: Antineoplastic antibiotic

Actions: Binds to DNA and inhibits DNA, protein, and especially RNA synthesis; blocks the action of parathyroid hormone and reduces serum calcium.

Indications: Testicular cancers; glioblastoma multiforme; hypernephromas; breast, thyroid, and stomach cancers; Paget's disease of the bone; hypoglycemia secondary to malignant insulinoma.

Dosage:
Neonatal: Not applicable.
Pediatric: 25–30 µg/kg IV every day for 8–10 days (for testicular cancer every 4–6 weeks); or every 3–4 days or every week to decrease calcium, which lowers in 24–72 hours, lasting several days to a week; or 25–50 µg IV every other day for 3–8 days (associated with reduced toxicity).
Adult: See pediatric dosage.

Preparation: Available in 2500-µg vials that should be diluted with 4.9 ml of sterile water and shaken gently to obtain a clear yellow solution.

Home Stability: Unopened vials are stable for 2 years in the refrigerator. Prepared solutions are stable for 48 hours if refrigerated or for 24 hours if diluted in 1 liter of D_5W.

Compatibilities: D_5W should not be the initial diluent. Plicamycin is unstable in acidic solutions and reacts with hyperalimentation, blood, iron infusions, zinc, and calcium. As with most antineoplastic agents, it is advisable not to administer plicamycin with other admixture solutions, especially those with trace elements.

Administration:
Neonatal: Not applicable.
Pediatric: Infuse by IV drip in 1 L of D_5W over 4–6 hours or by IV push over 20–30 minutes.
Adult: See pediatric administration.

Contraindications: Nosebleeding, bruising, facial flushing, or signs of hemorrhage; coagulation disorders; decreased platelets; liver or renal dysfunction.

Side Effects:
Primary:
Hematopoietic: Nosebleeds, bruises, and sudden facial flushing are early signs of a blood dyscrasia that is like disseminated intravascular coagulation (DIC) and is evidenced by decreased clotting factors II, V, VII, and X, decreased platelets, and increased prothrombin and clotting times. The drug must be stopped immediately.
Gastrointestinal: Anorexia, moderate nausea, and vomiting within 6 hours, lasting 12–14 hours; stomatitis; diarrhea.
Hepatoxicity: Increased liver function tests, LDH and SGOT; discontinue drug if LDH greater than 2000.
Neurotoxicity: Severe headache, irritability, depression, lethargy.
Cutaneous: Gradual blushing of the face, with facial skin appearing thickened and more coarse, sometimes with increased pigmentation and temporary disquamation.
Nephrotoxicity: Increased serum creatinine, azotemia, BUN, and proteinuria require discontinuing the drug; decreased serum phosphate, magnesium, calcium, and potassium.
Secondary: Mild bone marrow depression, metallic taste in the mouth, possible alopecia, transient increase in calcium levels for 2–4 days after treatment is discontinued, fever, acnelike skin rash, muscle aches, drowsiness, depression, weakness. Risk of teratogenesis, infertility, and secondary malignancy is unknown.

Nursing Implications: Stop drug and notify physician immediately if patient experiences nosebleed, sudden facial flushing, or marked bruising.

Monitor clotting factors II, V, VII, X; prothrombin times; platelets; LDH and SGOT; serum creatinine; phosphate, magnesium, calcium, and potassium; and BUN.

Premedicate with antiemetics and continue giving them for 14 hours after the drug has been infused.

Emphasize good oral hygiene with a soft-bristled toothbrush.

Assess patient for complaints of headache, irritability, and lethargy and report these changes to physician promptly.

Inform patient of possible facial skin changes.

Check urine protein every shift.

Continue safe-handling precautions for 4 days after last dose of drug.

Generic Name: POLYMYXIN B SULFATE

Trade Name: AEROSPORIN

Classification: Antibiotic

Actions: Polypeptide antibiotic with neuro-muscular blocking action, bactericidal against gram-negative organisms *Pseudomonas aeruginosa, Hemophilus influenzae, Escherichia coli, Aerobacter aerogenes,* and *Klebsiella pneumoniae.* Poorly absorbed into serum and tissues; does not pass the blood-brain barrier.

Indications: Treatment of infections caused by susceptible gram-negative organisms, especially *Pseudomonas aeruginosa.* Not for treatment of meningeal infections unless administered intrathecally.

Dosage:
Neonatal: 15,000–25,000 u/kg/day divided into 2 equal doses and administered every 12 hours.
Pediatric: In the presence of normal renal function, 15,000–25,000 u/kg/day divided into 2 equal doses and administered every 12 hours.
Adult: See pediatric dosage.
General: In the presence of renal failure, adjust dose to the following for children and adults.
Mild Renal Impairment: Maximum dosage: 25,000 u/kg the first day, then 10,000 u/kg every third day divided into 2 equal doses and administered 12 hours apart.
Uremia: Maximum dosage: 25,000 u/kg the first day, then 10,000 u/kg every 5–7 days divided into 2 equal doses and administered 12 hours apart.

Preparation: Supplied as a powder. Each 500,000 u of powder must be initially diluted with 5 ml of sterile water for injection or normal saline for injection. Each single dose must be further diluted in 300–500 ml of 5% dextrose in water.

Home Stability: In reconstituted form, stable in refrigerator for 72 hours.

Compatibilities: Compatible only with 5% dextrose in water or normal saline.

Administration:
Neonatal: Administer via infusion pump over 60–90 minutes.
Pediatric: See neonatal administration.
Adult: Administer via continuous drip over 60–90 minutes.

Contraindications: Hypersensitivity to the drug; pregnancy.

Side Effects:
Primary:
Nephrotoxicity: Albuminuria, cellular casts in the urine, increased BUN.
Neurotoxicity: Irritability, weakness, drowsiness, ataxia, numbness of the extremities, blurring of vision, respiratory paralysis.
Secondary: Rash, drug fever, anaphylaxis, thrombophlebitis.

Nursing Implications: Prior to and during therapy, culture and sensitivity tests should be completed.
Monitor for allergic reactions.
Monitor baseline and periodic renal, hepatic, and hematologic functions for long-term therapy.
Monitor for superinfection as evidenced by fever and increasing malaise; redness, soreness, and drainage of a localized infection; cough; diarrhea; monilial rash in the perineal area; and thrush due to *Candida albicans.*
Monitor intake-output ratio. Notify physician if intake-output ratio changes.
Monitor for signs of neurotoxicity and notify physician. Monitor respiratory function if neurotoxicity occurs.

Generic Name: POTASSIUM CHLORIDE

Trade Name: POTASSIUM CHLORIDE

Classification: Electrolyte

Actions: Potassium is a principal intracellular cation of body tissue and an important component of many physiologic processes, including cellular metabolism, transmission of nerve impulses, muscle contraction, acid-base balance, and normal renal function. A normal plasma concentration of 3.5–5.0 mEq/L is maintained through renal excretion. Any change in plasma concentration usually reflects a change in intracellular concentration.

Indications: Hypokalemia caused by a variety of conditions including metabolic alkalosis, some drug therapies, and chronic physical conditions (congestive heart failure).

Dosage: All ages: *Do not exceed* a concentration of 40 mEq/500 ml.
   Neonatal and Pediatric: Up to 3 mEq/kg/24 hours.
   Adult: Infusion: 40 mEq/L of IV fluid.

Preparation: Injectable form supplied as 2 mEq/ml in 10-, 15-, and 20-ml vials. Also available in premixed bags of IV solution.

Compatibilities: Compatible with dextrose, saline, and multiple electrolyte solutions.

Administration: *Must be diluted* prior to administration. *Do not exceed 20 mEq/hour.* Usually given by slow infusion over 24 hours.

Contraindications: Any condition that increases a patient's chance of high serum levels of potassium (e.g., renal impairment, hyperkalemia).

Side Effects:
Primary: Hyperkalemia and changes in EKG pattern are a sign of poisoning. Muscle weakness, paresthesias, listlessness, mental confusion, cold skin, vascular collapse.
Secondary: Flaccid paralysis, hypotension.

Nursing Implications: Observe for signs of hypo- or hyperkalemia.
   Monitor infusion closely. Insure that ordered rate is maintained. Too rapid administration may cause side effects and cardiac arrhythmias.
   Monitor IV site closely for signs of extravasation.
   Monitor vital signs and urine output as necessary. Monitor serum potassium levels.

Generic Name: PRALIDOXIME CHLORIDE

Trade Name: PROTOPAM

Classification: Antidote

Actions: Reactivates cholinesterase after poisoning by an organophosphate; reverses paralysis of skeletal and respiratory muscles. Administered with atropine to correct depression of the respiratory center. Oral doses are incompletely absorbed, so parenteral administration is suggested. Most effective when administered 24–36 hours after exposure.

Indications: Adjunct in treatment of poisonings with organophosphate anticholinesterase pesticides, chemicals, and drugs. (Check manufacturer's literature for substances that may be treated with this drug.)

Dosage:
Pediatric: 20–40 mg/kg IV over 15–30 minutes. A more rapid effect will be seen by injection of 50 mg/ml over 5–10 minutes. Pediatric dose: 1 mg.
Adult: 1–2 g in IV infusion with 100 ml of saline. Administer over 15–30 minutes. May be given as injection if necessary: 5% solution in water over at least 5 minutes. After 1 hour, if muscle weakness persists, dose is repeated.
Administer IV atropine at the same time in cases where no cyanosis is present. The dose is usually 2–4 mg. When cyanosis is present, give atropine IM while ventilatory assistance is provided, every 5–10 minutes until signs of toxicity appear.

Preparation: Injectable form available in 1-g vial (20 ml).

Administration: See Dosage.

Contraindications: Concurrent use with theophylline, succinylcholine, or respiratory depressants; poisoning with carbaryl.

Side Effects:
Primary: Dizziness, diplopia, blurred vision, headache, drowsiness, nausea, tachycardia.
Secondary: Nausea, hyperventilation, rash, muscular weakness.

Nursing Implications: Obtain the name or product responsible for the poisoning, along with amount ingested and time elapsed since ingestion.
Assess all body systems for signs of toxicity (e.g., vital signs, respiratory effort, secretions), amount of muscular changes, and bowel and bladder control.
Document all initial observations and any changes. Note responses to therapy.
Obtain necessary laboratory work.
Monitor intake and output.

Generic Name: PREDNISOLONE

Trade Name:

Classification: Corticosteroid

Actions: The members of this family have many and varied effects because they influence almost every cell in the body. Some of these actions are accelerated protein metabolism, which results in muscle weakness and wasting; suppression of immune response and impaired wound healing; redistribution of fat; and increased formation of adipose tissue. The levels of blood glucose are increased because it is utilized less. This increases the release of insulin. Steroids suppress the body's immune response by affecting histamine release and inhibit the chain of events that leads to the inflammatory response. They also have an effect on reabsorption and distribution of some electrolytes and other elements necessary for normal body function. Any patient who has been on long-term therapy should have steroids withdrawn slowly to prevent development of acute adrenal insufficiency.

Indications: Steroids are indicated in the treatment of many disorders, including but not limited to inflammatory, endocrine, collagen, dermatologic, rheumatic, allergic, respiratory, hematologic, and gastrointestinal diseases and nervous system disorders.

Dosage: As with other steroids, dose is highly dependent on condition under treatment. With this agent, dose also depends on the form used.

Administration:
All Ages: IM or IV. Check label carefully; some forms should not be given IV.

Contraindications: Hypersensitivity, systemic fungal infections. Smallest dose for shortest period of time should be used because of the chance of side effects. May stunt growth in children. Do not give immunizations during therapy. Use with caution in patients with active infections, congestive heart failure, hypertension, or osteoporosis. May aggravate diabetes mellitus, Cushing's syndrome, and optic nerve damage.

Side Effects: Many effects are dependent on dose or length of therapy. The following side effects are related to the drug itself.
Primary: Fluid and electrolyte disturbances, osteoporosis, long bone fractures, effects on the central nervous system, increased incidence of infections, impaired wound healing, ocular effects, endocrine effects.
Secondary: Abrupt withdrawal may lead to withdrawal syndrome or adrenal insufficiency.

Nursing Implications: Obtain baseline information—height, weight, vital signs, physical assessment, and laboratory results.

Check label carefully—some solution should not be administered IV, only IM.

Any patient who has been on long-term therapy *must* have dose tapered. Observe for clinical symptoms of withdrawal.

Continuing assessment includes weight, vital signs, and laboratory follow-up. Assess for side effects.

Because of decreased resistance, patient at home should be instructed to avoid contact with any person having an active infection.

Dietary adjustments may be necessary in the diabetic patient. Any patient on long-term therapy may need to increase protein intake.

Monitor patient for improvement in condition under therapy. Document observations.

Additional patient teaching may include discussion of side effects such as diarrhea, tarry stools; avoid exposure to infection; report any possible infections or unhealed cuts; have eye examinations periodically as well as routine laboratory tests.

Generic Name: PROCAINAMIDE HYDROCHLORIDE

Trade Name: PRONESTYL INJECTION

Classification: Antiarrhythmic

Actions: Decreases sodium transport through myocardium, slowing conduction through the A-V node, prolonging effective refractory period, and decreasing automaticity.

Indications: Treatment of ventricular extrasystoles and tachycardia, atrial fibrillation, paroxysmal atrial tachycardias.

Dosage:
Neonatal: Not applicable.
Pediatric: Not applicable.
Adult: 100 mg every 5 minutes up to 1 g, then continuous infusion of 2–6 mg/minute.

Preparation: Supplied as sterile aqueous solution in 10-mg vials (100 mg/ml) and 2-ml vials (500 mg/ml).

Home Stability: Not applicable.

Compatibilities: Compatible with solutions containing dextrose or saline.

Administration:
Neonatal: Not applicable.
Pediatric: Not applicable.
Adult: Dilute 100 mg in 10 ml of 5% dextrose or sterile water for injection and give no faster than 25–50 mg/minute. For infusion, dilute 1 g in 250–500 ml of 5% dextrose in water.
General: Decrease dose in cases of hepatic and renal dysfunction and give over 6 hours. In congestive heart failure, smaller doses are also recommended because of lower volume of distribution.

Contraindications: Hypersensitivity, second or third degree heart block unassisted by pacemaker, myasthenia gravis. Use with caution in patients with congestive heart failure, conduction disturbances, digitalis intoxication, or hepatic or renal failure. Cimetidine may increase procainamide blood levels.

Side Effects:
Primary: Severe hypotension, bradycardia, agranulocytosis, increased ANA titer, neutropenia, nausea, vomiting, diarrhea, anorexia, maculopapular rash, fever, lupus erythematosus syndrome.
Secondary: A-V block, ventricular fibrillation, hallucination, confusion, convulsions, depression, thrombocytopenia, myalgia.

Nursing Implications: Continuous cardiac monitoring is essential. Closely observe PR, QRS, and QT intervals. If these intervals widen, or if heart block or increased arrhythmias occur, notify physician immediately, discontinue administration, and document rhythm changes.

Monitor blood pressure and pulse frequently: obtain a baseline, then every 5 minutes during bolus and initiation of continuous drip, then every 15 minutes until stable.

Infuse via automatic infusion pump.

Keep patient supine during IV administration.

If used to convert long-standing atrial fibrillation, anticoagulation is usually advised before restoring sinus rhythm to prevent thromboembolism.

Generic Name: PROCHLORPERAZINE

Trade Name: COMPAZINE

Classification: Antipsychotic, antiemetic

Actions: Mechanism of action not completely understood, but agents in this classification block postsynaptic dopamine receptors in the brain. By inhibiting or altering dopamine release and increasing the firing rate of neuronal cells in the midbrain, antipsychotic drugs suppress the clinical signs of schizophrenia. These medications may also depress control of basic body functions such as metabolism, body temperature, level of consciousness, and hormonal balance. These drugs are widely distributed and stored in the tissues and may be eliminated in the urine for up to 6 months after therapy is discontinued. These drugs differ in the severity of side effects. Major side effects are sedation, extrapyramidal effects, and orthostatic hypotension. These can be minimized by changing from one drug to another.

Indications: Treatment and management of psychotic disorders; may be used in treatment of severe nausea and vomiting.

Dosage:
Neonatal: Not recommended.
Pediatric:
Under 9 kg: Not recommended.
Over 9 kg: IM: 0.06 mg/pound of body weight.
Ages 2–5: Do not exceed 20 mg/day.
Ages 6–12: Do not exceed 25 mg/day.
Adult: IM: 5–10 mg every 3–4 hours.

Preparation: Injectable form available as 5 and 10 mg/ml.

Compatibilities: Administer IV in an isotonic solution.

Administration: May be administered orally, IM, or IV, but oral administration is used for maintenance therapy. Parenteral administration provides more active drug than oral doses.

Neonatal: Not recommended.
Pediatric:
Under 9 kg: Not applicable.
Over 9 kg: Deep IM injection.
Adult: Deep IM injection. Administer by IV method no faster than 5 mg/ml/minute.

Contraindications: Patients who are comatose or experiencing central nervous system depression; blood dyscrasias; hepatic disease; coronary artery disease; convulsive disorders.

Side Effects: All side effects listed have not been observed in the use of this drug, but because of the similarities of the phenothiazines, they are listed for all drugs in this group.
Primary: Most common are extrapyramidal reactions, which include but are not limited to aching and numbness in the limbs, motor restlessness, dystonia, tight feeling of throat, slurred speech, and ataxia. Other reactions include orthostatic hypotension, blurred vision and other ocular changes, dark urine, bradycardia, and dizziness.
Secondary: Jaundice, anemia, agranulocytosis, dermatitis, pain at IM injection site.

Nursing Implications: Monitor vital signs, and observe for hypotension or behavioral changes. Monitor level of consciousness. Ongoing assessments should include these observations on a daily basis.

Assess and observe for side effects. The development of extrapyramidal effects can be distressing—assure client they will subside.

Warn clients on home therapy that care should be used when activities require alertness or coordination. The drowsiness experienced should subside after a period of time.

Warn clients to avoid extended exposure to the sun and to avoid getting drug on skin, since it may cause contact dermatitis.

Dry mouth may be a side effect. Gum or candy may relieve the discomfort.

Generic Name: PROMAZINE HYDROCHLORIDE

Trade Name: NORAZINE, PROZINE, SPARINE

Classification: Antipsychotic, phenothiazine, antianxiety, weak antiemetic

Actions: Inhibits or alters dopamine release and increases firing rate of neuronal cells in the midbrain, which decreases anxiety and tension, relaxes muscles, produces sedation, and tranquilizes. Phenothiazine derivatives depress various components of the reticular activating system. This system is involved in the control of basal metabolism and body temperature, wakefulness, vasomotor tone, emesis, and hormonal balance.

Indications: Control of nausea, vomiting, retching, hiccups, and hyperexcitability before, during, and after surgery; treatment of withdrawal symptoms from alcohol, barbiturates, or narcotics.

Dosage:
Neonatal: Not recommended for children under 12 years of age.
Pediatric (Over 12 Years): 10–25 mg every 4–6 hours for acute episodes of chronic psychotic disease.
Adult: 25–50 mg. May repeat as needed depending on symptoms. Use with caution if repeated within 1 hour.

Preparation: Supplied in injectable form in concentrations of 25 and 50 mg/ml.

Home Stability: Not recommended for home administration in IV form.

Compatibilities: Do not administer with other medications.

Administration:
Neonatal: Not applicable.
Pediatric (Over 12 Years): Dilute each 25–50 mg with 9 ml of normal saline for injection for a final concentration of 2.5 or 5.0 mg/ml. Never administer concentrations greater than 25 mg/ml. Administer at a rate not to exceed 25 mg/minute.
Adult: See pediatric administration.

Contraindications: Hypersensitivity to phenothiazines; children under 12 years of age; pregnancy (except labor and delivery) or lactation; bone marrow depression; comatose or severely depressed clients.

Side Effects:
Primary: Extrapyramidal reactions: aching and numbness in the limbs, motor restlessness, dystonia, tight feeling of throat, slurred speech and ataxia; orthostatic hypotension; blurred vision and other ocular changes; dark urine; bradycardia and dizziness.
Secondary: Jaundice, anemia, agranulocytosis, dermatitis with extravasation.

Nursing Implications: Monitor vital signs frequently and observe for hypotension or behavioral changes.
Monitor level of consciousness.
Assess and observe for side effects. The development of extrapyramidal effects can be distressing—assure client they will subside.
Assist client with ambulation; orthostatic hypotension and drowsiness are side effects.
Instruct client to chew gum or candy to relieve the discomfort of dry mouth.
Assess IV site for extravasation.
May potentiate central nervous system depressant effects of narcotics, barbiturates, alcohol, and anesthetics.

Generic Name: PROMETHAZINE HYDROCHLORIDE

Trade Name: PHENERGAN

Classification: Antihistamine

Actions: Antiemetic, antihistaminic, anticholinergic, and sedative. Antagonizes histamine but does not block its release. Because of antiemetic effects, may be used in treatment of nausea, vomiting, and motion sickness. Phenothiazine derivative and may have similar effects and side effects.

Indications: Despite potent antihistaminic properties, used mostly as antiemetic in motion sickness and for nausea and vomiting with surgery. Sedative action makes it useful as a preoperative medication but limits its use as an antihistaminic in ambulatory patients.

Dosage:
Neonatal and Pediatric: 0.5 mg/kg/dose every 4–6 hours IM.
Antiemetic: 0.25–0.5 mg/kg/dose every 4–6 hours IM.
Adult: Average dose is 25 mg IM twice daily. Amount and frequency may vary depending on condition under treatment.

Preparation: Injectable form available as 25 and 50 mg/ml (IM only).

Administration: Route of choice is deep IM; IV route may cause more side effects; SC will cause tissue necrosis. IV: 25 mg/ml, not to exceed 25 mg/minute. If barbiturates or narcotics are administered to the same patient, dosages must be decreased.

Contraindications: Hypersensitivity, newborns or premature infants, patients on monoamine oxidase therapy or receiving large doses of other central nervous system depressants. Use with caution in patients with cardiovascular disease, hepatic dysfunction, asthmatic attacks, narrow-angle glaucoma, and in children with acute or chronic respiratory impairment.

Side Effects:
Primary: Sedation, confusion, drowsiness, tremors, extrapyramidal effects.
Secondary: Cardiovascular effects, hypersensitivity, photosensitivity, dry mouth.

Nursing Implications: Obtain symptoms of allergy if that is what is under treatment.
   History of motion sickness, nausea, and vomiting should be obtained, if appropriate.
   Give by deep IM injection whenever possible.
   Document response to drug therapy.
   Warn patient to avoid activities requiring alertness. Assist with ambulation.
   Observe for extrapyramidal effects or paradoxical effects. Notify physician as appropriate.

Generic Name: PROPIOMAZINE HYDROCHLORIDE

Trade Name: LARGON

Classification: Sedative, hypnotic

Actions: Phenothiazine compound with sedative, antihistaminic, and antiemetic effects. Will potentiate the effects of other central nervous system depressants. Duration of action much shorter than in other drugs of this type.

Indications: Relief of restlessness preoperatively and during surgery. Also decreases apprehension. Useful during labor.

Dosage:
Neonatal and Pediatric (Under 60 Pounds): 0.25–0.5 mg/pound.
Adult: 20 mg of propiomazine given with 50 mg of meperidine.

Preparation: Injectable form available as 20 mg/ml.

Administration: IM or IV.

Contraindications: Intra-arterial injection may cause arteriospasm.

Side Effects:
Primary: Moderate increase in blood pressure; dizziness; confusion.
Secondary: Dry mouth, rashes, vein irritation.

Nursing Implications: Monitor vital signs closely. Give by deep IM injection. When administering IV, watch closely for extravasation—it may cause chemical irritation.
Monitor for signs of excessive sedation. Warn client that dizziness may occur.

Generic Name: PROPRANOLOL HYDROCHLORIDE

Trade Name: INDERAL

Classification: Beta blocker, antihypertensive, antiarrhythmic

Actions: Beta-adrenergic receptor blocking agent that exerts a negative chronotropic and inotropic effect on the myocardium.

Indications: IV administration reserved for treatment of life-threatening arrhythmias or those occurring under anesthesia. These arrhythmias may include paroxysmal atrial tachycardia, persistent sinus tachycardia, atrial fibrillation, atrial flutter, ventricular tachycardia, and tachycardias resulting from digitalis intoxication, thyrotoxicosis, and catecholamine actions during anesthesia.

Dosage:
Neonatal: Not applicable.
Pediatric: Not applicable.
Adult: 1–3 mg IV; a second dose after 2 minutes; subsequent doses after 4 hours.

Preparation: Available in 1-ml ampules.

Home Stability: Not applicable.

Compatibilities: Compatible with 5% dextrose or normal saline.

Administration:
Neonatal: Not applicable.
Pediatric: Not applicable.
Adult: Dilute drug in 10 ml of 5% dextrose and give no faster than 1 mg/minute. May dilute in 50 ml of normal saline and infuse at a rate of 1 mg over 10–15 minutes.

Contraindications: Cardiogenic shock, sinus bradycardia, heart block greater than first de-gree, bronchial asthma, ethyl ether anesthesia, right ventricular failure secondary to pulmonary hypertension. Use with caution in patients with congestive heart failure, diabetes mellitus, and respiratory disease. Use with insulin and oral hypoglycemics may alter requirements for control of blood sugar. May cause severe bradycardia and increased depressant effect on myocardium if used with cardiac glycosides. Aminophylline, isoproterenol, and glucagon antagonize effects of propranolol, Cimetidine inhibits mechanism of action of propranolol. Epinephrine may cause severe vasoconstriction if administered concurrently.

Side Effects:
Primary: Bradycardia, hypotension, congestive heart failure, increased airway resistance, fatigue, lethargy.
Secondary: Nausea, vomiting, diarrhea, hypoglycemia without tachycardia, rash, fever, vivid dreams, hallucination.

Nursing Implications: Continuous cardiac monitoring is essential; document changes in heart rate and rhythm; notify physician.

Continuous blood pressure monitoring is preferred; if not possible, obtain baseline vital signs and check every 3–5 minutes during administration of the bolus and until stabilized. Frequent checks should then be continued.

Continuous hemodynamic monitoring is advisable, especially for central venous pressure and pulmonary arterial wedge pressure.

Assess heart tones, jugular venous distension, peripheral edema, lung sounds, dyspnea, pulse quality, and color, temperature, and capillary refill of extremities every 4 hours and as needed to ascertain effectiveness of treatment.

Monitor intake and output and daily weights to ascertain fluid status.

Monitor serum electrolytes including glucose levels; adjust insulin dosage accordingly.

Generic Name: PROTAMINE SULFATE

Trade Name: PROTAMINE SULFATE

Classification: Anticoagulant

Actions: Alone, protamine is an anticoagulant. Administered with heparin, protamine forms a stable salt that neutralizes the anticoagulant actions of both drugs.

Indications: To neutralize the anticoagulant action of heparin.

Dosage:
Neonatal: 1 mg per 100 USP u of heparin. May repeat in 10–15 minutes if needed, not to exceed 50 mg per 10-minute period.
Pediatric: See neonatal dosage.
Adult: See neonatal dosage.

Preparation: Supplied as 50 mg of powder.

Home Stability: Not applicable.

Compatibilities: Compatible with dextrose or saline.

Administration: Dilute 50 mg in 5 ml of sterile water. May further dilute with saline or dextrose. Give 20 mg over 1 minute, not to exceed 50 mg in 10 minutes. May infuse over 2–3 hours.
Pediatric: See neonatal administration.
Adult: See neonatal administration.

Contraindications: None if used as directed.

Side Effects:
Primary: With rapid injection, anaphylaxis, bradycardia, dyspnea, feeling of warmth, flushing, severe hypertension or hypotension.
Secondary: None.

Nursing Implications: Dose is effective for approximately 2 hours.
Monitor coagulation studies; dosage is adjusted according to results.
Assess patient for signs of bleeding; estimate amount. Monitor vital signs during and after administration until stable. Be prepared to treat shock if it occurs.

Generic Name: PROTIRELIN

Trade Name: RELEFACT TRH

Classification: Thyroid function (diagnostic agent)

Actions: Synthetic tripeptide identical in structure to naturally occurring thyrotropin-releasing hormone produced by the hypothalamus. Increases release of thyroid-stimulating hormone from the anterior pituitary. Release of prolactin is also increased.

Indications: In combination with other diagnostic agents, to assess thyroid functions; assessment of pituitary and hypothalamic dysfunction; in patients with modular or diffuse goiter, to evaluate effectiveness of a dose of T_4 on thyrotropin suppression; adjustment of thyroid hormone dosage in patients with primary hypothyroidism.

Dosage:
Neonatal: 3–7 ug/kg, although experience is limited in this age group.
Pediatric: 3–7 ug/kg to a maximum dose of 400 ug.
Adult: 200–500 ug.

Preparation: Supplied in 1-ml ampules, each containing 500 ug of drug in an isotonic saline solution.

Home Stability: Stable as prepared by manufacturer until labeled expiration date. The pH must be maintained at approximately 6.5.

Compatibilities: Compatible with dextrose and saline solutions.

Administration:
Neonatal: Give as a bolus over 15–30 seconds.
Pediatric: Give as a bolus over 15–30 seconds.
Adult: Give as a bolus over 15–30 seconds.

Contraindications: Any condition in which marked and rapid changes in blood pressure would be dangerous.

Side Effects:
Primary: Sudden transient increases or decreases in blood pressure; syncope.
Secondary: Breast enlargement, leakage in lactating women for 2–3 days, headaches, nausea, abdominal discomfort, dry mouth, bad taste, lightheadedness, urge to urinate, flushing, anxiety, sweating, drowsiness, tingling sensation, pressure in chest, tight feeling in throat.

Nursing Implications: Plasma T_4, T_3, and/or thyroid stimulating hormone levels should be taken prior to administration of protirelin and 20, 30, and 60 minutes afterward.

Patient's blood pressure should be monitored immediately prior to administration of drug and every 3–5 minutes during the first 15 minutes afterward. Usually increases are seen, but patient may experience hypotension.

When drug is being administered, patient should remain supine throughout blood sampling and until blood pressure is maintained at baseline levels.

If protirelin is being used as a diagnostic agent, thyroid hormones should be discontinued 7–14 days prior to testing, as they will reduce the thyroid stimulating hormone response. Chronic administration of levodopa and acetylsalicylic acid may have the same effect.

Patient should fast overnight or at least have a low-fat meal, as serum lipids may interfere.

If test must be repeated, 7 days should elapse between tests, as thyroid stimulating hormone response is reduced with repetitive administration.

Generic Name: PYRIDOSTIGMINE BROMIDE

Trade Name: MESTINON

Classification: Cholinergic

Actions: Drugs in this classification act to facilitate transmission of impulses across the myoneural junction and to inhibit destruction of acetylcholine. Pyridostigmine bromide has a longer duration of action than neostigmine and has been reported to produce less gastrointestinal irritation.

Indications: This family of drugs is indicated in treatment and diagnosis of myasthenia gravis. This drug is used to improve muscle strength in myasthenia gravis. When given parenterally, it reverses the effects of neuromuscular blockers.

Dosage:

Myasthenia Gravis: 1/30 of oral dose (oral dose range: 60 mg–1.5 g daily) IM or by *slow* IV. Neonates of myasthenic mothers may have transient difficulty with sucking, swallowing, or breathing and may require treatment. An edrophonium chloride test may be done, and minute doses of pyridostigmine bromide may be administered: 0.05–0.15 mg/kg given IM.

Reversal of Nondepolarizing Muscle Relaxants: Usual dose is 10–20 mg. It is recommended that 0.6–1.2 mg of atropine sulfate be administered prior to pyridostigmine bromide to decrease the side effects.

Pediatric: 7 mg/kg/day in 5–6 doses.

Preparation: Supplied in 2-ml ampules for injection.

Compatibilities: Compatible with normal saline.

Administration: By mouth, IM, or *slow* IV push.

Contraindications: Hypersensitivity, obstructions (mechanical, intestinal, and urinary), bradycardia, hypotension. Use with caution in patients with bronchial asthma or cardiac dysrhythmias. Atropine and epinephrine should be available in case of hypersensitivity reaction. Do not use neostigmine bromide or pyridostigmine bromide in patients with a history of hypersensitivity to bromides or urinary tract infections. Safe use in women of childbearing potential or during pregnancy has not been established.

Side Effects:

Primary: Nausea, vomiting, diarrhea, abdominal cramps, increased secretions, diaphoresis. Muscle cramps, fasciculation, and weakness may also be observed.

Secondary: Skin rash, thrombophlebitis.

Nursing Implications: Do a complete assessment of patient and symptoms observed.

Emergency equipment should be readily available in case of hypersensitivity reaction, as well as for infants of myasthenic mothers.

Observe myasthenic patient for any exacerbation of symptoms.

If patient has myasthenia gravis, determine if in a crisis or in a cholinergic crisis. Because symptoms are so similar, it may be necessary to do an edrophonium test.

Monitor vital signs closely.

Patient teaching should include spacing activities to avoid fatigue, signs of drug over- or underdosage, and need for follow-up care and close medical supervision.

Observe patient closely if used as a muscle relaxant antagonist. Maintain ventilator support until normal respiration returns.

Have atropine available—administration of pyridostigmine bromide may cause bradycardia.

Generic Name: PYRIDOXINE HYDROCHLORIDE (VITAMIN B$_6$)

Trade Name: HEXA-BETALIN

Classification: Vitamin

Actions: Water-soluble B-complex vitamin, essential in maintaining health and normal metabolic functioning. Used in metabolism of amino acids, lipids, and carbohydrates. Although vitamins are necessary for normal growth and development, they do not serve as sources of energy. Vitamins must be obtained from sources outside of the body. A dietary deficiency in vitamin B$_6$ is rarely observed in adults but may be found in infants. Signs and symptoms include nausea, vomiting, abdominal distress, ataxia, and convulsions.

Indications: Treatment of deficiency (may include patients taking isomazid or oral contraceptives, patients with metabolic disorders, and infants, who require large amounts of this vitamin); treatment of convulsions.

Dosage: Dose varies with condition under treatment.
Neonatal and Pediatric: 100 mg orally, IM, or IV to correct the deficiency. Then a diet with doses to prevent recurrence of deficiency.
Adult: 10–20 mg orally, IM, or IV daily for 3 weeks. As further supplement to diet, 2–5 mg daily.

Preparation: Injectable form available as 50 and 100 mg/ml.

Home Stability: Protect solution from direct sunlight.

Compatibilities: When given IV, dilute with D$_5$W or normal saline. Do not mix with sodium bicarbonate.

Administration:
Neonatal and Pediatric: Small doses can be given IV over several minutes. Larger doses should be infused over several hours.
Adult: Give by slow IV injection.

Contraindications: Sensitivity to pyridoxine hydrochloride.

Side Effects: Nontoxic in most patients even in large doses.
Primary: Nausea, headache, paresthesias.
Secondary: Allergic reactions, burning at IM injection site.

Nursing Implications: Assess patient's nutritional status. Because pyridoxine hydrochloride deficiency alone is rare in adults, signs and symptoms of other vitamin deficiencies may be present. Signs of vitamin B$_6$ deficiency include nausea and vomiting, abdominal distress, and ataxia.
Warn patient that there is a possibility of pain at the injection site.
Monitor patient daily for improvement in physical symptoms. Document noted changes in condition.
Provide nutritional counseling as necessary to patient and family.

Generic Name: **QUINIDINE GLUCONATE**

Trade Name: **QUINIDINE GLUCONATE**

Classification: Antiarrhythmic

Actions: Exerts depressing antiarrhythmic action on the heart, slowing rate and conduction, reducing myocardial contractility, and prolonging refractory period. Also increases potassium level within the cell and decreases sodium level.

Indications: Premature atrial and ventricular contractions, paroxysmal atrial tachycardia, paroxysmal atrioventricular junctional tachycardia, atrial flutter, paroxysmal atrial fibrillation, paroxysmal ventricular tachycardia when not associated with complete heart block and maintenance therapy after electrical conversion of atrial fibrillation and/or flutter.

Dosage:
Neonatal: Safety has not been established for use in children.
Pediatric: Safety has not been established for use in children.
Adult: Usual dose: 200–330 mg but may be repeated to control arrhythmia. Up to 1 g has been required.

Preparation: Injectable form supplied in concentration of 200 mg/ml.

Compatibilities: Do not administer with other medications. Infuse in 5% dextrose for injection.

Administration:
Neonatal: Not applicable.
Pediatric: Not applicable.
Adult: Dilute 800 mg in at least 40 ml of 5% dextrose for injection. Administer via infusion pump at a rate of 16 mg/minute. Maintenance dose is oral.

Contraindications: Hypersensitivity or idiosyncrasy to quinidine; myasthenia gravis; history of thrombocytopenic purpura associated with previous quinidine administration; digitalis intoxication manifested by arrhythmias or A-V conduction disorders; partial A-V or complete heart block; complete bundle branch block or other severe intraventricular conduction defects exhibiting marked QRS widening or bizarre complexes; complete A-V block with an A-V nodal or idioventricular pacemaker; ectopic impulses due to excapte mechanisms; azotemia from significant renal disease; marked cardiac enlargement, particularly with congestive heart failure; poor renal function and renal tubular acidosis; lactation; in children.

Side Effects:
Primary: Atrioventricular heart block, cardiac standstill, hypotension (acute), tachycardia, thrombocytopenic purpura, urticaria, ventricular fibrillation.
Secondary: Apprehension, cramps, diaphoresis, fever, headache, nausea, rash, tinnitus, urge to defecate, urge to void, vertigo, visual disturbances, vomiting.

Nursing Implications: Monitor continuous EKG. Discontinue administration immediately if signs of cardiotoxicity occur.
Monitor vital signs continuously, especially blood pressure and pulse.
Monitor intake-output ratio. Notify physician of any changes.
Monitor quinidine plasma concentration. Therapeutic levels are 2–6 ug/ml.
Monitor renal, hepatic, and hematologic laboratory values.
Observe closely for bleeding if coumarin anticoagulants are administered concurrently.
Observe for quinidine syncope, exhibited by sudden loss of consciousness and ventricular arrhythmias that have bizarre QRS complexes.
Quinidine gluconate is potentiated or potentiates neuromuscular blocking antibiotics, anticholinergics, thiazide diuretics, antihypertensive agents, muscle relaxants, and anticoagulants.

Generic Name: RITODRINE HYDROCHLORIDE

Trade Name: YUTOPAR

Classification: Beta-adrenergic agonist

Actions: Stimulates beta-2 receptors in uterine smooth muscle, inhibiting contractility, thereby decreasing intensity and frequency of uterine contractions.

Indications: Management of preterm labor.

Dosage:
Neonatal: Not applicable.
Pediatric: Not applicable.
Adult: Continuous infusion begun at 0.1 mg/minute, increasing every 10 minutes by 0.05 mg/minute. Desired effects are usually seen between 0.15 and 0.35 mg/minute. Continue infusion for 12 hours after contractions cease. Then begin oral ritodrine therapy. IV infusion may be discontinued 30 minutes after oral administration.

Preparation: Supplied as 50 mg in 5-ml ampules (10 mg/ml).

Home Stability: Not applicable.

Compatibilities: Infuse with 5% dextrose solutions unless patient is diabetic, in which case saline solutions may be used.

Administration:
Neonatal: Not applicable.
Pediatric: Not applicable.
Adult: Dilute 150 mg in 500 ml of fluid. May concentrate solution further if indicated.

Contraindications: Hypersensitivity, use before 20th week of pregnancy, conditions in which continuation of pregnancy is hazardous such as antepartum hemorrhage requiring immediate delivery, eclampsia, severe preeclampsia, intrauterine fetal death, chorioamnionitis, maternal cardiac disease, pulmonary hypertension, maternal hyperthyroidism, uncontrolled maternal diabetes mellitus, hypovolemia, cardiac arrhythmias, uncontrolled hypertension, pheochromocytoma, bronchial asthma. Use cautiously with corticosteroids, beta blockers, sympathomimetics, magnesium sulfate, diazoxide, meperidine, and potent general anesthetic agents.

Side Effects:
Primary: Dose-related alterations in blood pressure, palpitations, tachycardia, pulmonary edema, nervousness, restlessness, anxiety, hyperglycemia.
Secondary: Nausea, vomiting, erythema, EKG changes, hypokalemia.

Nursing Implications: Monitor uterine contractions, maternal pulse rate and blood pressure, and fetal heart rate every 5 minutes initially, every 15–30 minutes until stable, and every hour until drug is discontinued.

Obtain a baseline EKG. If patient complains of chest pain, obtain EKG and temporarily discontinue drug.

Assess for signs of pulmonary edema frequently.

Monitor intake-output carefully for fluid overload. Monitor serum electrolytes and blood sugar for hyperglycemia and hypokalemia.

Maintain patient in left lateral position during infusion to minimize hypotension.

Infuse via automatic infusion pump.

Generic Name: SECOBARBITAL SODIUM

Trade Name: SECONAL

Classification: Sedative, hypnotic

Actions: Members of the barbiturate family can produce a variety of effects on the central nervous system, from excitation to sedation to deep coma. They act at the level of the thalamus to depress cortex functioning, which decreases motor activity and produces sedation. Barbiturates also produce respiratory depression, but the severity is dose dependent. Barbiturates have limited usefulness as sedatives. They decrease the amount of time spent in the dreaming stage of sleep. Much of their sleep-producing effect disappears after about 2 weeks, so they are not indicated for long-term treatment of insomnia.

Indications: Short-term treatment of insomnia, preanesthetic medication, treatment of acute convulsive episodes.

Dosage:
Neonatal and Pediatric: 3 mg/kg/dose IM. IV bolus—give no faster than 50 mg/minute.
Adult: 100–200 mg IM. Dose varies with effect desired.

Preparation: Injectable form available as 50 mg/ml.

Compatibilities: Compatible with normal saline and sterile water.

Administration:
Neonatal and Pediatric: IM. Give IV bolus no faster than 50 mg/minute.
Adult: IM. IV rate should not exceed 50 mg in 15 seconds.

Contraindications: Hypersensitivity, hepatic dysfunction, respiratory distress, obstetric delivery, acute or chronic pain.

Side Effects:
Primary: Somnolence, agitation, ataxia, central nervous system depression, anxiety, dizziness, respiratory depression, hypotension, bradycardia.
Secondary: Skin rashes, constipation, nausea, vomiting, tissue necrosis from extravasation, headache, fever.

Nursing Implications: Monitor vital signs.
Have supportive equipment available in case of severe respiratory depression.
Do not administer closely with a narcotic analgesic.
When administering IM, give deep into muscle.
Maintain a safe environment for patient because of depressant effects on the central nervous system. Raise side rails of bed, assist with ambulation, etc.

Generic Name: SODIUM BICARBONATE

Trade Name: SODIUM BICARBONATE

Classification: Electrolyte

Actions: Provides base ions that buffer excess hydrogen ion concentrations. This raises pH of blood and reverses manifestations of acidosis. Action is brief but allows time to correct the metabolic disturbance.

Indications: Emergency treatment of metabolic acidosis. Some causes are cardiac arrest, ketoacidosis, renal insufficiency, lactic acidosis, and severe diarrhea.

Dosage: The following doses are guidelines. Dose required depends on baseline deficit obtained from arterial blood pH and $PaCO_2$. Administer IV over several minutes.
Neonatal: Dilute 1:1, 0.5 mEq/ml can be used. 1 mEq/kg every 10 minutes of arrest.
Pediatric: 1–2 mEq/kg/dose IV every 10 minutes of arrest.
Adult: 1 mEq/kg/dose IV, 0.5 mEq/kg, every 10 minutes of arrest.

Preparation: Injectable form available as 1 mEq/ ml in 10- and 50-ml preloaded syringes, 0.5 mEq/ ml in 10-ml syringes.

Compatibilities: Compatible with normal saline.

Administration: See Dosage.

Contraindications: Respiratory or metabolic alkalosis, hypertension, edema. With these conditions, should still be used in life-threatening situations.

Side Effects:
Primary: Hypernatremia with rapid IV administration, decreased cerebrospinal fluid pressure, intracranial hemorrhage (especially in infants and children), hyperosmolarity.
Secondary: Renal calculi, gastric distension, alkalosis.

Nursing Implications: Have resuscitation equipment available as necessary.
Obtain lab work as necessary.
In an emergency situation, IV doses are administered by IV push. Flush before and after administration with normal saline.
Document response to administration.

Generic Name: SODIUM CHLORIDE

Trade Name: SODIUM CHLORIDE

Classification: Electrolyte

Actions: Primary function of sodium is maintenance of plasma tonicity and normal osmolarity. It does this along with other electrolytes, chloride, and bicarbonate.

Indications: Fluid and electrolyte replacement when levels become depleted due to a variety of conditions.

Dosage: Dosage is highly individualized based on age, weight, and condition under treatment.

Preparation: Available in concentrations of 0.45%, 0.9%, 3%, and 5%.

Administration: Highly individualized based on condition under treatment.

Contraindications: If serum sodium levels are normal, elevated, or slightly decreased, 3% and 5% solutions should not be used. They should be used only in emergency situations and then only when the patient is under constant observation.

Side Effects:
Primary: Fluid overload if too much solution is administered too quickly; hypernatremia; 3% or 5% solutions may precipitate pulmonary edema.

Nursing Implications: Baseline vital signs and laboratory work should be obtained and documented.

Monitor rate of infusion closely to prevent under- or overdosing, especially if 3% or 5% solutions are being administered.

Observe IV site closely for signs of extravasation.

Generic Name: STREPTOKINASE

Trade Name: KABIKINASE, STREPTASE

Classification: Anticoagulant

Actions: Converts plasminogen to plasmin, which degrades fibrin clots, fibrinogen, and other plasma proteins on the surface and within the thrombus.

Indications: For lysis of coronary artery thrombi, pulmonary emboli, and deep vein emboli and to dissolve clots occluding A-V cannulas or central venous catheters.

Dosage:
Neonatal: Not applicable.
Pediatric: Not applicable.
Adult:
Coronary Artery Thrombi: 20,000 IU intracoronary within 6 hours of onset of symptoms, followed by a 2,000-IU/minute infusion IV for 1 hour or 750,000 IU within 3 hours of onset of symptoms, followed by 250,000 in 30–60 minutes.
Thrombi or Emboli: 250,000 IU loading dose, followed by a 100,000-IU/hour infusion IV for 24–72 hours.
Occlusion of Cannula or Catheter: 250,000 IU into catheter or each occluded portion of cannula.

Preparation: Supplied in vials.

Home Stability: Not applicable.

Compatibilities: Infuse with dextrose solutions only.

Administration:
Neonatal: Not applicable.
Pediatric: Not applicable.
Adult:
Coronary Artery Thrombi: Bolus intracoronary dose over 15–30 minutes, followed by 2,000 IU/minute for 1 hour. Bolus IV dose over 5–10 minutes.
Thrombi or Emboli: Bolus dose over 25–30 minutes. Infuse maintenance dose over 24–72 hours.
Occlusion of Cannula or Catheter: Slowly push solution into cannula or catheter, without forc-ing. Clamp for 2 hours, aspirate contents, flush with saline, and reconnect.

Contraindications: Active bleeding, status post-cerebrovascular accident within 2 months, intracranial or intraspinal surgery, intracranial neoplasm, hypersensitivity. Use with extreme caution in patients who have had recent surgery, biopsy, lumbar puncture, thoracentesis, paracentesis, cutdowns, or intra-arterial procedures within 10 days; in patients with ulcerative wounds, trauma with possible internal bleeding, any condition with a possibility of bleeding (e.g., diverticulitis), hypertension, hepatic or renal insufficiency, subacute bacterial endocarditis, rheumatic valvular disease, atrial fibrillation; and in pregnancy and first 10 days postpartum.

Side Effects:
Primary: Allergic reaction, including anaphylaxis, fever, bleeding.

Nursing Implications: Obtain baseline hematocrit, platelet count, partial thromboplastin time, thrombin time, and prothrombin time (also CPK if for coronary artery thrombi), and monitor values every 4 hours during therapy and until stable following discontinuation of the drug. Ascertain coagulation parameters to be used during therapy.

Use extreme care in handling the patient. Avoid unnecessary movement and possible contusions, arterial or venous punctures, and IM injection. If punctures are necessary, apply pressure for 30 minutes or more if needed and use peripheral and superficial vessels.

Assess for bleeding and notify physician of any occurrence. Minor bleeding may occur at streptokinase insertion sites. Apply pressure dressing and monitor. This is not serious unless bleeding is major.

Assist with diagnosis of acute myocardial infarction or emboli and probable use of diagnostic angiography. Inform patient about what the procedure involves, what information it will elicit, sensations to expect, and postangiography routine.

For coronary thrombi, monitor EKG continuously for changes. Assess for level and quality of patient's pain.

Follow streptokinase therapy with heparin infusion, beginning 3–4 hours after completion of streptokinase or when prothrombin time is less than twice the control.

Avoid use of drugs that can alter platelet function.

Obtain blood pressures only in upper extremities; if taken in lower extremities, thrombi may be dislodged.

Prior sensitization to streptokinase increases risk of allergic reaction.

Streptokinase should only be used in lysis of catheter or cannula occlusion after heparin therapy is unsuccessful.

Generic Name: STREPTOZOCIN

Trade Name: ZANOSAR

Classification: Antineoplastic nitrosurea, alkylating agent

Actions: Inhibits DNA synthesis and interferes with enzymes in the glyconeogenesis process and selectively affects pancreatic cells.

Indications: Pancreatic tumors; malignant carcinoid tumors; lung, squamous cell, and oral cancers; synovial sarcoma; adenocarcinoma of the gallbladder; malignant Zollinger-Ellison tumors; and Hodgkin's disease.

Dosage:
Neonatal: Not applicable.
Pediatric: 0.5–1.0 g/m^2 IV daily for 5 days every 4–6 weeks or 1.5 g IV every week.
Adult: See pediatric dosage.

Preparation: Available in 1-g vials which should be mixed with 9.5 ml of normal saline or sterile water.

Home Stability: Unopened vials, refrigerated and protected from light, are stable for 3 years. Unrefrigerated vials are stable for 1 year. Because the prepared solution does not contain a preservative, it should be used within 8 hours after vial is opened. No drug should be left in the vial, since it forms a flammable gas. Extra drug should be injected into a drain or commode, which should be flushed 3 times with the lid down.

Compatibilities: As with most antineoplastic agents, it is advisable not to administer streptozocin with other admixture solutions.

Administration:
Neonatal: Not applicable.
Pediatric: Administer by slow IV push (over 10–20 minutes) into side arm of free-flowing IV, checking patency every 2–3 minutes to avoid extravasation of this severe vesicant and burning and/or pain in the vein at the venipuncture site. Or infuse by IV drip over 6 hours, preferably through a central line.

Adult: See pediatric dosage.

Contraindications: Pregnancy. Use with caution in patients with diabetes or who are receiving other nephrotoxic agents. Corticosteroids may increase hyperglycemia secondary to streptozocin. Dilantin may decrease streptozocin's cytotoxicity in pancreatic beta cells. A dose reduction of 50–75 percent is necessary for a creatinine clearance below 25 mg/minute. Intra-arterial administration is not recommended because of increased renal toxicity.

Side Effects:
Primary:
Gastrointestinal: Severe nausea and vomiting in 1–4 hours, diarrhea, abdominal cramps, hyper- or hypoglycemia (an insulin shock reaction may occur within the first 24 hours after administration).
Cutaneous: Severe tissue damage if extravasated.
Nephrotoxicity: Permanent renal damage, first evidenced by decreased serum phosphorus, proteinuria, azotemia, and/or glycosuria; 1–2 L of pre- and posthydration are necessary to minimize this side effect.
Reproductive: Teratogenetic.
Secondary: Duodenal ulcers; mild bone marrow depression; mild and temporary jaundice and increased SGOT, alkaline phosphatase, and bilirubin; decreased blood counts with prolonged use; dark half-circles in nailbeds. Risk of infertility is unknown. Secondary malignancy is possible.

Nursing Implications: Premedicate with antiemetics and continue them for 24 hours.

Monitor serum glucose, phosphorus, and urea and urine protein and glucose. Maintain IV or oral hydration before and after treatment.

Establish and maintain good venous access, checking for patency every 2–3 minutes during IV push administration and instructing the patient to report any sensations of burning or pain.

Inform patient of the possibility of birth defects if pregnancy occurs while taking streptozocin.

Continue safe-handling precautions for 9 days after the last dose of streptozocin.

Generic Name: SUCCINYLCHOLINE CHLORIDE

Trade Name: ANECTINE

Classification: Neuromuscular blocker

Actions: Depolarizing neuromuscular blocker that mimics acetylcholine, causing flaccid skeletal muscle paralysis by prolonging depolarization of the muscle endplate. Action is short: only about 5 minutes. Like pancuronium bromide, it does not change pain perception; unlike pancuronium bromide, it causes some histamine release. This may be observed in cardiovascular effects such as bradycardia, hypotension, and arrhythmias. Also produces transient apnea but not complete respiratory paralysis. Patient should be observed for need of mechanical ventilation.

Indications: Used when skeletal muscle relaxation is necessary for short periods of time.

Dosage: Dosages are guidelines only and must be individually adjusted.
Neonatal and Pediatric: Test dose: 100 ug/kg. Normal dose (given if no apnea or only transient apnea is present): 1–2 mg/kg IV.
Adult: 2.5–4 mg/kg IV. No more than 150 mg should be administered.

Preparation: Available as 20, 50, and 100 mg/ml injectable.

Administration: IV is route of choice. May be given IM if vein unavailable, but duration of action will be longer.

Contraindications: Hypersensitivity, severe hepatic impairment, anemia, genetic plasma cholinesterase deficiency. Use with caution if history of malignant hyperthermia or hypertension is noted as well as renal, cardiac, or respiratory impairment and in patients with myasthenia gravis, electrolyte imbalances, severe burns, or trauma.

Side Effects:
Primary: Prolonged apnea, muscle weakness, pain, stiffness, ventricular arrhythmias, hypotension.
Secondary: Hyperkalemia, excessive salivation, increased intraocular pressure, histamine release.

Nursing Implications: Before administration, intubation and supportive equipment must be available.
Monitor patient for recovery from anesthesia. Observe for return of muscle movement, swallow and gag reflexes. This drug is usually administered by an anesthesiologist.
Maintain patent airway.

Generic Name: SULFISOXAZOLE DIOLAMINE

Trade Name: GANTRISIN

Classification: Antibiotic (sulfonamide)

Actions: Wide-spectrum sulfonamide bactericidal against the following gram-negative and gram-positive organisms: *Escherichia coli, Staphylococcus aureus,* Klebsiella, Enterobacter, *Proteus mirabilis* and *vulgaris,* and *Hemophilus influenzae.*

Indications: Treatment of urinary tract infections when caused by the above-stated organisms; adjunctive therapy for the following infections: chancroid, inclusion conjunctivitis, trachoma, nocardiosis, toxoplasmosis, malaria, acute otitis media, *H. influenzae* meningitis, and meningococcal meningitis.

Dosage:
Neonatal: Not applicable.
Pediatric: Loading dose of 50 mg/kg, then maintenance dose of 100 mg/kg/day equally divided and administered every 6 hours.
Adult: See pediatric dosage.

Preparation: Supplied as a 40% solution. Add a minimum of 35 ml of sterile water for injection to the 5-ml ampule. Use of diluents other than sterile water may cause precipitation.

Home Stability: Store away from light and heat. Stable at room temperature no longer than 12 hours in its diluted form.

Compatibilities: Do not administer with any IV fluids. Administer by direct IV or flush with sterile water before and after IV Y-site infusion.

Administration:
Neonatal: Not applicable.

Pediatric: Administer at a rate of 1 ml of 5% solution over 1 minute via direct IV or IV Y-site.
Adult: See pediatric administration.

Contraindications: Hypersensitivity, infants under 2 months of age, pregnancy at term, lactation, porphyria.

Side Effects:
Primary: Hypersensitivity reactions, agranulocytosis, aplastic anemia, renal and hepatic damage, irreversible neuromuscular and central nervous system changes, fibrosing alveolitis, photosensitization, systemic moniliasis, thrombophlebitis. Blood disorders may be manifested as sore throat, fever, pallor, purpura, and jaundice in the early stages.
Secondary: Anogenital lesions, anorexia, diarrhea, dysphagia, enterocolitis, nausea, skin rashes, vomiting.

Nursing Implications: Prior to and during therapy, culture and sensitivity tests should be completed.

Monitor for allergic reactions.

Monitor baseline and periodic renal, hepatic, and hematologic functions for long-term therapy.

Monitor for superinfection.

Monitor intake-output ratio. Force fluids to prevent crystalluria and stone formation. Notify physician if intake-output ratio changes.

Assess urinary pH daily; notify physician if urine becomes acidic.

Monitor clients receiving tolbutamide or chlorpropamide for hypoglycemia.

Monitor phenytoin and digoxin levels. Dosage adjustments may be indicated.

Instruct clients to avoid prolonged exposure to sunlight or ultraviolet light to prevent photosensitivity.

Generic Name: TETRACYCLINE HYDROCHLORIDE

Trade Name: ACHROMYCIN

Classification: Antibiotic

Actions: Broad-spectrum antibiotic bactericidal against Rickettsia, *Mycoplasma pneumoniae,* agents of psittacosis and ornithosis, agents of lymphogranuloma venereum and granuloma inguinale, the spirochetal agent of relapsing fever (*Borrelia recurrentis*), and infections caused by the following gram-negative organisms: *Hemophilus ducreyi, Pasteurella pestis* and *tularensis, Bartonella bacilliformis,* Bacteroides, *Vibrio comma* and *fetus,* and Brucella.

Indications: For infections caused by the following gram-negative and gram-positive organisms when sensitivity testing shows susceptibility: gram-negative—*Escherichia coli, Enterobacter aerogenes,* Shigella, *Acinetobacter calcoaceticus, Hemophilus influenzae* (in respiratory infections), Klebsiella (respiratory and urinary infections), Mima, and Herellae; gram-positive—*Streptococcus pneumoniae* (not indicated for rheumatic fever prophylaxis), *Diplococcus pneumoniae.* When penicillin is contraindicated, treatment of infections caused by *Neisseria gonorrhoeae* and *meningitidis, Treponema pallidum* and *pertenue* (syphilis and yaws), *Listeria monocytogenes,* Clostridium, *Bacillus anthracis, Fusobacterium fusiforme* (Vincent's infection), Actinomyces, and amebicides.

Dosage:

Neonatal: Not recommended.

Pediatric: Use of this drug during the years of tooth development can cause permanent discoloration of the teeth and enamel hypoplasia. Do not use tetracyclines in this age group or in pregnancy unless other drugs are ineffective or contraindicated.

8 Years and under: 10–15 mg/kg/day in divided doses every 12 hours.

8 Years and over: 10–20 mg/kg/day in divided doses every 12 hours.

Adult: 250–500 mg every 12 hours. Maximum dosage: 500 mg every 6 hours.

Preparation: Supplied as a powder. Reconstitute with sterile water for injection by adding 5 ml of diluent to the 250-mg vial and 10 ml to the 500-mg vial.

Home Stability: Infuse immediately after preparation of solution. Darkening solution indicates deterioration of the medication; discard the solution.

Compatibilities: Compatible with dextrose, saline, Ringer's, or lactated Ringer's. Do not administer with total parenteral nutrition or any other medication. Infusion must be completed within 6 hours when administered with lactated Ringer's.

Administration: Administration should be continued for at least 24–48 hours after symptoms and fever have subsided.

Neonatal: Not recommended.

Pediatric: Further dilute the drug to a concentration of 0.1–1.0 mg/ml and infuse over 1–2 hours. Infusion must be completed within 12 hours.

Adult: See pediatric administration.

Contraindications: Hypersensitivity. Not recommended in clients with renal insufficiency or in pregnancy or lactation.

Side Effects:

Primary: Hypersensitivity reactions including anaphylaxis; liver damage; photosensitivity; systemic moniliasis; thrombophlebitis; renal toxicity including a rise in BUN.

Secondary: Anorexia, nausea, vomiting, diarrhea, glossitis and dysphagia, enterocolitis, *Candida albicans* overgrowth in the perineal area (Monilia) and mouth (thrush), hemolytic anemia, thrombocytopenia. In infants: bulging fontanels and papilledema, which usually disappears with discontinuation of the drug.

Nursing Implications: Prior to and during therapy, culture and sensitivity tests should be completed.

Monitor for allergic reactions.

Monitor baseline and periodic renal, hepatic, and hematologic functions.

Monitor for superinfections. Assess for the onset of black, hairy tongue; oral lesions (stomati-

tis, glossitis); rectal or vaginal itching; vaginal discharge; loose, foul-smelling stools; unusual odor to urine.

Monitor infusion site for signs of thrombophlebitis.

Clients on anticoagulants may require lower doses of those drugs while on tetracycline.

Monitor intake-output ratio. Notify physician of gastrointestinal disturbance or changes in renal status.

Notify physician of signs of increasing intracranial pressure.

Generic Name: THEOPHYLLINE ETHYLENEDIAMINE

Trade Name: AMINOPHYLLINE

Classification: Xanthine derivative

Actions: Relaxes smooth muscle and bronchial tubes; increases cardiac output, urinary output, and sodium excretion; stimulates skeletal and cardiac muscles; effects peripheral vasodilation.

Indications: Bronchial asthma, bronchospasm.

Dosage:
Neonatal: Not applicable.
Pediatric: 6 mg/kg maximum initial dose, followed by continuous infusion of 1.0–1.2 mg/kg/hour for 12 hours, then 0.8–1.0 mg/kg/hour.
Adult: 6 mg/kg initial dose, followed by continuous infusion of 0.5–0.7 mg/kg/hour for 12 hours, then 0.1–0.5 mg/kg/hour.

Preparation: Supplied in 25-mg/ml vials.

Home Stability: Not applicable.

Compatibilities: May infuse with dextrose or saline. Not compatible with many other drugs—check manufacturer's literature.

Administration:
Neonatal: Not applicable.
Pediatric: Do not infuse bolus doses faster than 25 mg/minute or 15 minutes for total bolus dose.
Adult: See pediatric administration.

Contraindications: Sensitivity to theophylline or ethylenediamine, infants under 6 months of age. Use with caution in patients with coronary occlusion, angina pectoris, peptic ulcer disease, renal or hepatic disease, severe hypertension, myocardial damage, hyperthyroidism, or glaucoma and in children.

Side Effects:
Primary: Anxiety, dizziness, headache, nausea, restlessness, vomiting.
Secondary: Cardiac arrest, convulsion, delirium, peripheral vascular collapse, ventricular fibrillation, temporary hypotension.

Nursing Implications: Monitor serum levels. Therapeutic levels are 10–20 mcg/ml.

Infuse via automatic infusion pump, guarding against overdosage, especially in children.

Assess lung sounds, dyspnea, skin color, respiratory rate, rhythm, and effort before infusion begins and every 4 hours thereafter. Monitor arterial blood gases.

Assess for appearance of side effects and notify physician. Obtain serum theophylline level if indicated.

Switch to oral therapy as soon as possible.

Generic Name: THIAMINE HYDROCHLORIDE (VITAMIN B₁)

Trade Name: BETALIN S

Classification: Vitamin

Actions: Used by the body in formation of a coenzyme that plays an important role in metabolism. Signs of deficiency may include edema, pallor, emaciation, cardiac failure, ataxia, and tachycardia. It is rare to have a dietary deficiency in only one member of the vitamin B complex.

Indications: Treatment of thiamine deficiency. In any case of dietary insufficiency, multiple deficiencies should be suspected.

Dosage: Dosage varies with degree of deficiency. The range is from 10–50 mg for children to 10–500 mg for adults.

Preparation: Injectable form supplied as 100 mg/ml.

Administration: Route of choice is by mouth. Serious sensitivity reactions and deaths have occurred from IV use.

Contraindications: Hypersensitivity.

Side Effects:
Primary: Restlessness, feeling of warmth, pruritus, urticaria, allergic reaction, pulmonary edema.
Secondary: Sweating, nausea.

Nursing Implications: Complete health and dietary history is necessary. Document signs of the deficiency—edema, pallor, cardiac failure, and signs of other vitamin B complex deficiencies.

Provide dietary instruction and counseling for patient and family when appropriate.

Document improvement in health status.

Generic Name: TICARCILLIN DISODIUM

Trade Name: TICAR

Classification: Antibiotic (penicillin)

Actions: Extended-spectrum semisynthetic penicillin bactericidal against gram-positive and gram-negative organisms: *Pseudomonas aeruginosa*, Proteus, *Escherichia coli*, Enterobacter, Hemophilus, and *Bacteroides fragilis*.

Indications: For severe infections such as septicemia, genitourinary infection, acute and chronic respiratory infections, infections of the soft tissue, abdominal cavity, skin, and female pelvis.

Dosage:
Neonatal:

Under 1 Week: Under 2000 g: Loading dose: 100 mg/kg. Maintenance dose: 75 mg/kg every 8 hours.

Over 2000 g: Loading dose: 100 mg/kg. Maintenance dose: 75 mg/kg every 4–6 hours.

Over 1 Week: 100 mg/kg every 4 hours.

Pediatric: 200–300 mg/kg/day divided every 4–6 hours.

Adult: See pediatric dosage.

Preparation: Supplied as a powder. Reconstitute with sterile water or normal saline. Do not use bacteriostatic diluent if drug is being administered to a neonate. Reconstitute as follows:

VIAL SIZE	VOLUME DILUENT	CONCENTRATION
1 g	2 ml	400 mg/ml
3 g	6 ml	400 mg/ml
6 g	12 ml	400 mg/ml

Home Stability: Reconstituted solutions are stable for 36 hours in the refrigerator.

Compatibilities: Compatible with dextrose, saline, KCl, Ringer's, or lactated Ringer's. Do not mix with any other antibiotic. Not compatible with total parenteral nutrition.

Administration:
Neonatal: For doses less than 250 mg, dilute to 50 mg/ml and administer by IV push slowly over 5–10 minutes.

Pediatric: Dilute to 50 mg/ml and administer slowly by IV Y-site over 5–10 minutes.

Adult: Dilute to 50 mg/ml and administer by IV piggyback over 30–60 minutes.

Contraindications: Hypersensitivity to penicillin derivatives or cephalosporins. Individuals with a history of allergic problems are more susceptible to untoward reactions. Safety in pregnancy has not been established.

Side Effects:
Primary: Hypersensitivity reactions such as skin rash, pruritus, anaphylaxis, urticaria, and febrile reactions; superinfections; pain and thrombosis of the IV site.

Secondary: Neutropenia; leukopenia; hemolytic anemia; hemorrhagic manifestations; thrombocytopenia; hypernatremia; hypokalemia; increase in alkaline phosphatase, SGOT, SGPT, nausea; vomiting; diarrhea.

Nursing Implications: Prior to and during therapy, culture and sensitivity tests should be completed.

Monitor for allergic reactions.

Monitor baseline and periodic renal, hepatic, and hematologic functions, especially in longterm therapy.

Monitor for superinfections. Assess for the onset of black, hairy tongue; oral lesions (stomatitis, glossitis); rectal or vaginal itching; vaginal discharge; loose, foul-smelling stools; unusual odor to urine.

Monitor infusion site hourly for signs of thrombophlebitis.

Sodium concentration must be taken into consideration in clients on a sodium-restricted diet.

Observe clients closely for the first half-hour after initial dose for a wheal or redness at IV site or other signs of allergic reaction.

Monitor intake-output ratio. Report oliguria, hematuria, and changes in intake-output ratio.

Use glucose oxidase reagents to check urine glucose. False positive reactions can occur with Clinitest.

Monitor for signs of neurotoxity when high doses of ticarcillin therapy are being administered.

Monitor for signs of electrolyte imbalance and congestive heart failure.

Generic Name: TOBRAMYCIN SULFATE

Trade Name: NEBCIN

Classification: Antibiotic (aminoglycoside)

Actions: Semisynthetic aminoglycoside, derived from *Streptomyces tenebrarius,* with neuromuscular blocking action. Inhibits protein synthesis in bacterial cell and is bactericidal against a wide variety of gram-negative bacilli, including *Escherichia coli,* Enterobacter, *Klebsiella pneumoniae,* and most strains of *Pseudomonas aeruginosa,* Proteus, Serratia, Providencia stuartii, Citrobacter, Salmonella, and Shigella. Also effective against staphylococci, including penicillin- and methicillin-resistant strains.

Indications: Bacteremia and septicemia, including neonatal sepsis; serious infections such as those of the urinary or respiratory tract, bones, joints, or central nervous system, including meningitis; burns and postoperative infections.

Dosage:
Premature or Full-Term Neonates (1 Week or Less): 4 mg/kg/day divided into equal doses every 12 hours.
Neonatal: 7.5 mg/kg/day divided into equal doses every 8 hours.
Pediatric: 6.0–7.5 mg/kg/day divided into equal doses every 8 hours.
Adult: Dosage is based on ideal body weight. Usual dose: 3–5 mg/kg/day divided into equal doses every 8 hours.
General: Dosage is highly individualized and should be based on therapeutic drug monitoring. Therapeutic serum level: 4–8 ug/ml. Toxic serum level (peak): over 12 ug/ml.
Duration of therapy: 7–10 days.

Preparation: Supplied as a colorless solution, which does not require refrigeration, in 10- and 40-mg/1-ml vials.

Home Stability: Stable at room temperature as prepared by manufacturer for at least 2 years.

Compatibilities: Compatible with dextrose, saline, KCl, Ringer's, or lactated Ringer's and with total parenteral nutrition.

Administration:
Neonatal: Infuse over 1–2 hours. Administer at appropriate IV site based on infusion rate. Dilution should be based on fluid volume needs.
Pediatric: Infuse over 30–60 minutes. Administer at appropriate IV site based on infusion rate. Dilution should be based on fluid volume needs.
Adult: Dilute in 50–200 ml (1 mg/ml) of IV solution and administer over 30–120 minutes.

Contraindications: Sensitivity. Use with caution in clients with impaired renal function, eighth cranial nerve impairment, dehydration, fever, myasthenia gravis, parkinsonism, or hypocalcemia. Do not administer concurrently with penicillins. If concurrent administration is prescribed, give the drugs 2 hours apart. The neuromuscular blockade effects are enhanced by combined administration of decamethonium, ether, succinylcholine, tubocurarine, and related anesthetics. Cephalosporins may potentiate the nephrotoxic effects of tobramycin. Concurrent administration of other aminoglycosides, ethacrynic acid, and furosemide may enhance the ototoxic effects.

Side Effects:
Primary:
Neophrotoxicity: Proteinurea, presence of red and white blood cells in the urine; granular casts; azotemia; oliguria; urinary frequency; frank hematuria; increase in BUN and serum creatinine; decrease in creatinine clearance and specific gravity; renal damage and failure.
Ototoxicity: Auditory: high-frequency hearing loss; complete hearing loss (occasionally permanent); tinnitus; fullness, ringing, or buzzing in ears. Vestibular: dizziness and vertigo, ataxia, nausea and vomiting, nystagmus.
Neurotoxicity: Drowsiness, headache, unsteady gait, weakness, clumsiness, paresthesias, tremors, muscle twitching and weakness, convulsions, neuromuscular blockade with respiratory depression.
Secondary: Nausea, vomiting, stomatitis, skin rash, urticaria, pruritus, generalized burning sensation, drug fever, arthralgia, eosinophilia, anemia, leukopenia, granulocytopenia, thrombocytopenia, unusual thirst, difficult breathing, superinfections, peripheral neuritis.

Nursing Implications: Monitor serum blood levels initially and throughout therapy.

Document the *exact* time of medication administration for determination of blood levels.

Assess renal function prior to initial administration via baseline BUN, creatinine and creatinine clearance, specific gravity, and urine analysis.

Monitor renal function throughout therapy via assessment of BUN, creatinine and creatinine clearance, specific gravity, urine analysis, and strict intake and output.

Encourage hydration of client to reduce chemical irritation to renal tubules.

Assess eighth cranial (vestibulocochlear) nerve function prior to initial administration, throughout therapy, and upon discharge via audiometric tests and assessment of vestibular disturbance.

Monitor for overgrowth infection as evidenced by diarrhea, anogenital itching, vaginal discharge, stomatitis, or glossitis.

Antidote: Peritoneal dialysis or hemodialysis will assist in removal of the drug from the bloodstream.

Generic Name: TOLAZOLINE HYDROCHLORIDE

Trade Name: PRISCOLINE

Classification: Adrenergic blocker

Actions: Increases blood flow by dilation of vessel wall, sympathetic block, and blocking vasoconstrictive action of epinephrine and levarterenol.

Indications: Spastic peripheral vascular disorders, Buerger's and Raynaud's disease, diabetic arteriosclerosis, gangrene, endarteritis, frostbite, and postthrombotic conditions.

Dosage:
Neonatal: Not applicable.
Pediatric: Investigational use.
Adult: 10–50 mg 4 times a day.

Home Stability: Not applicable.

Compatibilities: Compatible with dextrose or saline solutions.

Administration:
Neonatal: Not applicable.

Pediatric: Investigational use.
Adult: 10 mg/minute IV.

Contraindications: Cerebrovascular accident, coronary artery disease. Use with caution in patients with gastritis, gastric ulcer, or mitral stenosis and in pregnancy and lactation.

Side Effects:
Primary: Chilliness, diarrhea, epigastric discomfort, flushing, increased pilomotor activity, nausea, blood pressure changes, tachycardia, tingling, vomiting.
Secondary: Overdose: Anginal pain, cardiac arrhythmias, exacerbation of peptic ulcer, severe hypotension or hypertension.

Nursing Implications: Observe closely for flushing, which indicates that optimal dose has been achieved.

Keep patient warm to facilitate effects of the drug.

Monitor vital signs during and after administration until stable.

Generic Name:
TRIETHYLENETHIOPHOSPHORAMIDE

Trade Name: THIOTEPA

Classification: Antineoplastic alkylating agent

Actions: Inhibits DNA synthesis and other cellular functions. Considered cell-cycle nonspecific.

Indications: Hodgkin's disease; breast, ovarian, and bladder cancers; malignant pleural effusions; malignant disease of the central nervous system.

Dosage:
Neonatal: Not applicable.
Pediatric: Safety in children has not been established.
Adult: 0.5 mg/kg IV every 1–4 weeks; or 6 mg/m^2 (0.2 mg/kg) IM, IV, or SC daily for 4 days every 2–4 weeks; or 45–60 mg/10–20 ml intraperitoneally, intrapleurally, or intrapericardially or into the bladder in 30–60 ml and retained for 2 hours every 1–4 weeks; or 1–10 mg/m^2 intrathecally 1–2 times a week.

Preparation: Supplied in 15-mg vials that should be mixed with 1.5 or 15 ml of sterile water and should appear clear or slightly opaque. If the solution looks dense, it should be thrown away. It can be given with D_5W or normal saline.

Home Stability: Unopened vials should be stored at 35–46°F. Mixed solutions should be discarded after 24 hours, since they contain no preservatives.

Compatibilities: Compatible with procaine 2% and epinephrine 1:1000. Increases neuromuscular blockade of some muscle relaxants. As with most antineoplastic agents, it is advisable not to administer this drug with other admixture solutions.

Administration:
Neonatal: Not applicable.

Pediatric: Safety in children has not been established.
Adult: Administer by IV push or continuous IV drip at a reasonable rate. Give IM or SC as ordered. Instill into the bladder after dilution with sterile water up to 30–60 ml. Intratumor doses have been given into vaginal and cerebral sites.

Contraindications: Reduce doses for patients with decreased bone marrow, hepatic, and renal functions and those who are on radiation therapy or receiving other myelosuppressive agents.

Side Effects:
Primary:
Hematopoietic: Decreased WBCs, platelets and RBCs starting 2–3 weeks after therapy and lasting 5–7 weeks, especially in combination chemotherapy with other alkylating agents or with concurrent or prior radiation.
Reproductive: Teratogenetic.
Secondary: Nausea, vomiting, headache, lightheadedness, fever, allergic reactions, decreased healing of radiated areas, dermatitis, increased uric acid levels, renal failure, reversible sterility and amenorrhea (usually in 6–8 months). Inflammatory reactions at sites of intratumor injections have occurred. Paresthesias may occur after intrathecal administration. Pain, nausea and vomiting, dizziness, and headache may occur with intracavity use. Risk of secondary malignancy is relatively high.

Nursing Implications: Monitor complete blood count.

Instruct patient and family on infection and bleeding precautions during the second to the third weeks after treatment is given.

Instruct patient to have nothing by mouth for 12 hours before bladder instillation. Once the drug has been inserted into the bladder, instruct the patient to try to retain it for 2 hours, changing position every 15 minutes for 1 hour.

Inform patient of the possibility of birth defects if pregnancy occurs while taking drug.

Continue safe-handling precautions for 6 weeks after the last dose of drug.

Generic Name: TRIFLUOPERAZINE HYDROCHLORIDE

Trade Name: STELAZINE

Classification: Antipsychotic

Actions: Mechanism of action not completely understood, but agents in this classification block postsynaptic dopamine receptors in the brain. By inhibiting or altering dopamine release and increasing the firing rate of neuronal cells in the midbrain, antipsychotic drugs suppress the clinical symptoms of schizophrenia. These medications may also depress control of basic body functions such as metabolism, body temperature, level of consciousness, and hormonal balance. These drugs are widely distributed and stored in the tissues and may be eliminated in the urine for up to 6 months after therapy is discontinued. These drugs differ in the severity of side effects. Major side effects are sedation, extrapyramidal effects, and orthostatic hypotension. These can be minimized by changing from one drug to another.

Indications: Treatment and management of psychotic disorders; may be used in treatment of severe nausea and vomiting.

Dosage:
Neonatal: Not recommended.
Pediatric (6–12 Years): Child should be hospitalized or under close observation. 1 mg by mouth once or twice a day. Used very little in injectable form in children.
Adult: 1–2 mg deep IM every 4–6 hours.

Preparation: Injectable form available as 2 and 10 mg/ml.

Administration: May be administered orally, IM, or IV, but oral administration is used for maintenance therapy. Parenteral administration provides more active drug than oral doses.
Neonatal: Not recommended.

Pediatric (6–12 Years): Should be hospitalized or under close observation. By mouth is recommended route.
Adult: Deep IM injection. Should not exceed 10 mg in 24 hours. Do not give any closer together than 4 hours to prevent cumulative effect.

Contraindications: In patients who are comatose or experiencing central nervous system depression; blood dyscrasias; presence of hepatic disease, coronary artery disease, or convulsive disorders.

Side Effects: All side effects listed have not been observed in the use of this drug, but because of the similarities of the phenothiazines, they are listed for all drugs in this group.
Primary: Most common are extrapyramidal reactions, which include but are not limited to aching and numbness in the limbs, motor restlessness, dystonia, tight feeling of throat, slurred speech, and ataxia. Other reactions include orthostatic hypotension, blurred vision and other ocular changes, dark urine, bradycardia, and dizziness.
Secondary: Jaundice, anemia, agranulocytosis, dermatitis, pain at IM injection site.

Nursing Implications: Monitor vital signs and observe for hypotension or behavioral changes. Monitor level of consciousness. Ongoing assessments should include these observations on a daily basis.

Assess and observe for side effects. The development of extrapyramidal effects can be distressing—assure client they will subside.

Warn clients on home therapy that care should be used when activities require alertness or coordination. The drowsiness experienced should subside after a period of time.

Warn clients to avoid extended exposure to the sun and to avoid getting drug on skin—it may cause contact dermatitis.

Dry mouth may be a side effect. Gum or candy may relieve the discomfort.

Generic Name: TRIMETHAPHAN CAMSYLATE

Trade Name: ARFONAD

Classification: Antihypertensive, ganglionic blocking agent

Actions: Competes with acetylcholine for receptor sites on postganglionic membranes in both adrenergic and cholinergic ganglia. This results in vasodilation and hypotension.

Indications: For controlled hypotension during surgery; hypertensive crisis.

Dosage: For short-term therapy only.
Neonatal: Not applicable.
Pediatric: 50–150 ug/kg/minute.
Adult: Initial dose of 1–2 ug/minute; titrate to achieve desired hypotensive effect.

Preparation: Supplied in ampules containing 500 mg in 10 ml.

Home Stability: Not applicable.

Compatibilities: Dilute and infuse only with 5% dextrose solution.

Administration:
Neonatal: Not applicable.
Pediatric: Dilute 500 mg (10 ml) in 500 ml of 5% dextrose in water to yield concentration of 1 mg/ml. Administer only as a continuous infusion.
Adult: See pediatric administration.

Contraindications: Uncorrected anemia, hypovolemia, shock, asphyxia, uncorrected respiratory insufficiency, pregnancy. Use with caution in the elderly, in children, and in patients with arteriosclerosis, cardiac disease, hepatic or renal system disease, degenerative disorders of the central nervous system, Addison's disease, or diabetes and with concurrent steroid therapy.

Side Effects:
Primary: Tachycardia, severe hypotension, nausea, vomiting, dry mouth, urinary retention, extreme weakness.
Secondary: Dilated pupils, anorexia, respiratory depression.

Nursing Implications: Drug is a potent hypotensive agent. Effects are seen almost immediately and last 10 minutes following discontinuation of infusion.

Monitor blood pressure and vital signs every 2 minutes until stabilized, then every 5 minutes.

Watch for respiratory depression and distress. Facilities for resuscitation and maintenance of oxygenation and ventilation should be immediately available.

Medication should only be infused via infusion pump.

Intensity of hypotensive effect is dependent on positioning. If hypotension fails to occur in the supine position, the physician may order elevation of the head of the bed (no more than 30 degrees to avoid cerebral anoxia).

Discontinue drug before wound closure in surgery to allow blood pressure to return to normal.

Use phenylephrine or mephentermine to counteract hypotension.

Generic Name:
TRIMETHOPRIM-SULFAMETHOXAZOLE

Trade Name: BACTRIM-SEPTRA, CO-TRIMOXAZOLE

Classification: Combination antibacterial agent

Actions: Synthetic broad-spectrum antibiotic that prevents the formation of folic acid and reduction of folates essential for organisms to grow. Bactericidal against the following gram-positive and gram-negative species: *Escherichia coli*, Proteus, Klebsiella, Enterobacter, Staphylococcus, Streptococcus, *Hemophilus influenzae*, Shigella, and pneumocystis.

Indications: Treatment of urinary tract infections due to susceptible organisms; pneumocystis; shigellosis enteritis; prophylaxis in neutropenic clients.

Dosage:
Neonatal: Not recommended.
Pediatric: 8 mg/kg/day (based on trimethoprim component) or 40 mg/kg/day (based on sulfamethoxazole component) every 12 hours for 10 days in urinary tract infections and for 5 days in shigellosis.
Adult: 8–10 mg/kg/day (based on trimethoprim component) every 6, 8, or 12 hours for up to 14 days in urinary tract infections and 5 days in shigellosis; 15–20 mg/kg/day (based on trimethoprim component) every 6–8 hours for up to 14 days in *Pneumocystis carinii* pneumonia; 800 mg of sulfamethoxazole and 160 mg of trimethoprim every 12 hours for prophylactic treatment of neutropenic clients.

Preparation: Supplied in 5-ml ampules containing 80 mg of trimethoprim and 400 mg of sulfamethoxazole. Dilute each 5 ml with 125 ml of 5% dextrose and water only. Use within 6 hours of preparation. Minimum dilution is 75 ml of 5% dextrose and water for fluid-restricted patients. Reconstitute concentrated form immediately prior to administration.

Home Stability: Store at room temperature—do not refrigerate. Use within 6 hours.

Compatibilities: Compatible with 5% dextrose and water only.

Administration:
Neonatal: Not applicable.
Pediatric: Infuse via intermittent infusion over 60–90 minutes.
Adult: See pediatric administration.

Contraindications: Hypersensitivity to either component of the drug, neonates under the age of 2 months, documented megaloblastic anemia due to folate deficiency, creatinine clearance below 15 ml/minute, streptococcal pharyngitis, pregnancy at term and during nursing period (the sulfamethoxazole component crosses the placenta and is excreted in milk, which may cause kernicterus in the infant).

Side Effects:
Primary: Nausea, vomiting, thrombocytopenia, rash, thrombophlebitis at the infusion site.
Secondary: Indications of major toxicity include ataxia, convulsions, tremors, and respiratory depression. Prolonged therapy can result in bone marrow depression (leukopenia, megaloblastic anemia, and thrombocytopenia).

Nursing Implications: Prior to and during therapy, culture and sensitivity tests should be completed.

Obtain baseline and periodic renal, hepatic, and hematologic functions, especially in long-term therapy.

Assess closely for presence of sore throat, fever, pallor, purpura, or jaundice. Notify physician immediately of these early indicators of severe blood disorders.

Monitor renal function and intake-output ratio closely. Maintain a high fluid intake to prevent crystalluria or stone formation unless otherwise contraindicated.

Monitor infusion site hourly for signs of thrombophlebitis.

Generic Name: TUBOCURARINE CHLORIDE

Trade Name: TUBOCURARINE CHLORIDE

Classification: Curare preparation

Actions: Curare preparations differ from other neuromuscular blockers in that they compete for receptor sites at the myoneural junction and actually block the impulses. Cumulative effects may occur from numerous doses. Certain conditions and other medications may potentiate these effects. As with other neuromuscular blockers, pain perception is not altered. Flaccid paralysis occurs a few minutes after administration and may continue for 90 minutes or longer.

Indications: When skeletal muscle relaxation is required; may be used to control artificially induced convulsions or assist with artificially ventilated patients.

Dosage: Highly variable, based on individual needs and patient response.

Preparation: Injectable form available as 3 mg/ml.

Administration:
All ages: IV or IM.

Contraindications: Hypersensitivity, conditions in which histamine release would be hazardous. Use with caution in patients with renal, cardiovascular, hepatic, or pulmonary impairment, myasthenia gravis, or electrolyte disorders.

Side Effects:
Primary: Prolongation of drug action, histamine release, hypersensitivity reactions.
Secondary: Muscle weakness.

Nursing Implications: Before administration, intubation and supportive equipment must be available.

Monitor patient for recovery from anesthesia. Observe for return of muscle movement, swallow and gag reflexes. This drug is usually administered by an anesthesiologist.

Maintain a patent airway.

Patient will require sedation, as this agent has no sedative effects.

Observe for signs and symptoms of histamine release.

Generic Name: UREA-STERILE USP

Trade Name: UREAPHIL, UREVERT

Classification: Diuretic

Actions: Hypertonic urea in the blood absorbs fluid from extravascular tissue, brain, and intraocular and cerebrospinal fluid into the blood. Increased urea in the glomerular filtrate inhibits reabsorption of water.

Indications: For reduction of intracranial pressure, cerebrospinal fluid pressure, and intraocular pressure.

Dosage:
Neonatal: 0.1 g/kg.
Pediatric: 0.5 g/kg.
Adult: 1–1.5 g/kg, not to exceed total dose of 120 g/day.

Preparation: Supplied in vials; diluent provided by some manufacturers.

Home Stability: Not applicable.

Compatibilities: May infuse with dextrose. Not compatible with alkaline solutions.

Administration:
Neonatal: Dilute to 4% solution and infuse at rate not to exceed 1200 mg/minute.
Pediatric: Dilute to 30% solution and infuse at rate not to exceed 1200 mg/minute.
Adult: 100 ml of a 30% solution is usually given over 1–2 hours. Do not exceed infusion rate of 1200 mg/minute.

Contraindications: Severe renal failure, active intracranial, liver failure, congestive heart failure, dehydration.

Side Effects:
Primary: Hyponatremia, hypokalemia, thrombophlebitis, nausea.
Secondary: Disorientation, syncope, vomiting.

Nursing Implications: Because of potential for volume and electrolyte depletion, leading to profound water loss, dehydration, reduction in blood volume, and circulatory collapse, monitor intake and output, serum electrolytes, blood pressure, and pulse rate frequently.

Assess for signs of hypokalemia (muscle weakness and cramping). Be especially careful in patients receiving digitalis because of the increased risk of digitalis toxicity.

Assess for signs of congestive heart failure during treatment.

Caution patient to change position slowly because of orthostatic hypotension.

Monitor BUN and creatinine for signs of deteriorating renal function.

Administer in the morning to prevent nocturia.

Elderly patients are especially susceptible to excessive diuresis.

Mannitol is usually the preferred osmotic diuretic.

Observe IV site frequently; infiltration can cause necrosis; phlebitis and thrombosis occur frequently.

Generic Name: UROKINASE

Trade Name: ABBOKINASE, BREOKINASE

Classification: Anticoagulant

Actions: Converts plasminogen to plasmin, which degrades fibrin clots, fibrinogen, and other plasma proteins on the surface and within the thrombus.

Indications: Lysis of pulmonary and deep vein emboli and to dissolve clots occluding intravenous catheters.

Dosage:
Neonatal: Not applicable.
Pediatric: Not applicable.
Adult:
Thrombi or Emboli: 4400 IU/kg loading dose, followed by a 4400-IU/kg/hour infusion for 12 hours, total volume not to exceed 200 ml.
Occlusion of Catheter: 5000 IU into catheter.

Preparation: Supplied in vials.

Home Stability: Not applicable.

Compatibilities: Compatible with dextrose or saline solutions.

Administration:
Neonatal: Not applicable.
Pediatric: Not applicable.
Adult:
Thrombi or Emboli: Dilute 250,000-IU vial with 5.2 ml of sterile water without preservatives, then further dilute to administer a total infusion of 195 ml. Loading dose is administered over 10 minutes, followed by infusion.
Occlusion of Catheter: Add 1 ml of the initially reconstituted drug (5000 IU) to 9 ml of sterile water without preservatives. Confirm occlusion by aspiration. Then slowly inject urokinase into the catheter. Connect a 5-ml syringe and wait 5 minutes. Attempt aspiration every 5 minutes until clot clears or 30 minutes have passed. If unsuccessful, wait for 30–60 minutes and attempt aspiration again. A second dose may be required.

Contraindications: Active bleeding, status post-cerebrovascular accident within 2 months, intracranial or intraspinal surgery, intracranial neoplasm, hypersensitivity. Use with extreme caution in patients who have had recent surgery, biopsy, lumbar puncture, thoracentesis, paracentesis, cutdowns, or intra-arterial procedures within 10 days and in patients with ulcerative wounds, trauma with possible internal bleeding, any condition with a possibility of bleeding (e.g., diverticulitis), hypertension, hepatic or renal insufficiency, subacute bacterial endocarditis, rheumatic valvular disease, atrial fibrillation and in pregnancy and first 10 days postpartum.

Side Effects:
Primary: Allergic reaction including bronchospasm, skin rash, fever, bleeding.
Secondary: None.

Nursing Implications: Obtain baseline hematocrit, platelet count, partial thromboplastin time, thrombin time, and prothrombin time (also creatinine phosphokinase if for coronary artery thrombi) and monitor values every 4 hours during therapy and until stable following discontinuation of the drug. Ascertain coagulation parameters to be used during therapy.

Use extreme care in handling the patient. Avoid unnecessary movement and possible contusions, arterial or venous punctures, and IM injection. If punctures are necessary, apply pressure for 30 minutes or more if needed and use peripheral and superficial vessels.

Assess for bleeding and notify physician of any occurrence. Minor bleeding may occur at urokinase insertion sites. Apply pressure dressing and monitor. This is not serious unless bleeding is major.

Assist with diagnosis of emboli and probable use of diagnostic angiography. Inform patient about what the procedure involves, what information it will elicit, sensations to be expected, and postangiography routine.

Follow urokinase therapy with heparin infusion, beginning 3–4 hours after completion of urokinase or when prothrombin time is less than twice the control.

Avoid use of drugs that can alter platelet function.

Obtain blood pressures only in upper extremities; if taken in lower extremities, thrombi may be dislodged.

Urokinase has less potential for allergic reaction than streptokinase.

Urokinase will not dissolve drug precipitate, only blood product occlusions.

Generic Name: VANCOMYCIN HYDROCHLORIDE

Trade Name: **VANCOCIN**

Classification: Antibiotic

Actions: Glycopeptide antibiotic, derived from *Streptomyces orientalis,* that inhibits bacterial cell wall synthesis.

Indications: Treatment of life-threatening infections caused by gram-positive bacteria such as streptococci and staphylococci that cannot be treated by less toxic drugs. These include staphylococcal (including methicillin-resistant) and streptococcal endocarditis, osteomyelitis, pneumonia, septicemia, and soft-tissue infections.

Dosage:
Neonatal: 10 mg/kg/day in divided doses every 12 hours.
Pediatric: 44 mg/kg/day every 6–12 hours or by continuous infusion.
Adult: 2 g/day every 6 hours or by continuous infusion.
General: Decreased dosage may be indicated in renal-impaired clients.

Preparation: Available in 500-mg vials. Reconstitute with 10 ml of sterile water per 500-mg vial.

Home Stability: Refrigerate and discard after 96 hours.

Compatibilities: Compatible with solutions containing dextrose and saline. Do not mix with any other drug or with total parenteral nutrition. Avoid concurrent or sequential use with other neurotoxic or nephrotoxic antibiotics.

Administration:
Neonatal: Dilute dosage to 5 mg/ml using 5% dextrose or normal saline and infuse over 20–30 minutes using a syringe infusion pump.
Pediatric: Dilute dosage to 5 mg/ml using 5% dextrose or normal saline and infuse over 20–30 minutes using a syringe infusion pump or dilute 24-hour dosage to at least 5 mg/ml and infuse continuously by infusion pump.
Adult: Dilute 12- or 24-hour dose in 1000 ml and infuse via infusion pump over 12 or 24 hours. Smaller or larger doses may be indicated based on client's fluid balance.

Contraindications: Hypersensitivity, renal insufficiency, hearing loss.

Side Effects:
Primary: Ototoxicity, nephrotoxicity, severe hypotension with rapid infusion, extravasation, anaphylaxis, eosinophilia, hearing loss, thrombophlebitis.
Secondary: Nausea, chills, fever, urticaria, macular rashes.

Nursing Implications: Monitor for allergic reactions.

Monitor baseline and periodic serum drug levels and renal, hepatic, and hematologic functions. In renal insufficiency there may be an accumulation of the drug, and the dosage may need to be adjusted.

Monitor for ototoxicity: dizziness, vertigo, tinnitus, roaring in the ears, and hearing loss. Hearing loss may not halt when drug is discontinued.

Monitor urine output. Notify physician of urine output less than 30 ml/hour.

Monitor blood pressure and pulse every 5 minutes during infusions of less than 30–60 minutes. Monitor blood pressure, pulse, and infusion rate every half-hour for continuous infusion.

Monitor infusion site for signs of complications with blood pressure and pulse assessment. If extravasation occurs, apply a warm compress for 2 hours and then for 20 minutes every 4 hours.

Monitor for superinfection. Assess for the onset of fever, increasing malaise, localized infection, cough, diarrhea, or oral lesions.

Generic Name: VERAPAMIL HYDROCHLORIDE

Trade Name: CALAN, ISOPTIN

Classification: Antiarrhythmic

Actions: Inhibits influx of calcium ions into myocardial and vascular smooth muscle cells, thereby slowing A-V conduction and prolonging refractory period within A-V node.

Indications: Treatment of paroxysmal supraventricular tachyarrhythmias, including Wolff-Parkinson-White and Lown-Ganong-Levine syndromes; temporary control of rapid ventricular responses in atrial flutter or atrial fibrillation.

Dosage:
Neonatal: 0.1–0.2 mg/kg; repeat in 30 minutes if first dose is not adequate.
Pediatric: 0.1–0.3 mg/kg; repeat in 30 minutes if first dose is not adequate.
Adult: 5–10 mg; repeat with 10 mg in 30 minutes if first dose is not adequate.

Preparation: Supplied in 5- and 10-mg ampules, vials, and syringes.

Home Stability: Not applicable.

Compatibilities: Compatible with dextrose, saline, or lactated Ringer's.

Administration:
Neonatal: Give as an intravenous bolus over 2 minutes.

Pediatric: See neonatal administration.
Adult: Give as an intravenous bolus over 2 minutes. Give over 3 minutes for elderly clients.

Contraindications: Severe hypotension or cardiogenic shock, second- or third-degree A-V block, sick sinus syndrome, severe congestive heart failure, hypersensitivity. Do not give concurrently with intravenous beta-adrenergic blocking drugs or disopyramide. Carefully monitor concurrent use with digitalis preparations, quinidine, procainamide, and oral beta-adrenergic blocking agents.

Side Effects:
Primary: Transient hypotension, heart failure, bradycardia.
Secondary: Dizziness, headache, fatigue, A-V block, ventricular asystole, peripheral edema, constipation, nausea, elevated liver enzymes.

Nursing Implications: Continuous cardiac monitoring is essential. Document heart rate and rhythm before and after verapamil dose; immediately notify physician of patient's response.
Obtain baseline vital signs before dose, then 2–3 minutes after dose until stable.
Assess level of consciousness, capillary refill, and skin color and temperature along with vital signs.
Assess for signs of congestive heart failure with repeated doses.

Generic Name: VIDARABINE

Trade Name: ARA-A, VIRA-A

Classification: Antiviral agent

Actions: Antiviral agent effective against herpes simplex types 1 and 2. Exact mechanism has not been established, but it may interfere with viral DNA synthesis.

Indications: Treatment of herpes simplex encephalitis. This antiviral agent may reduce mortality but not morbidity and neurologic sequelae in the comatose client.

Dosage: 15 mg/kg/day for 10 days.

Preparation: Supplied in vials of 200 mg/ml. Reconstitute with any IV solution except biologic and colloidal fluids such as blood products or protein solutions. Dilute 1 mg of vidarabine with 2.22 ml of solution (1 L of fluid will provide a maximum of 450 mg of drug). Warm diluent to 35–40°C (95–100°F) and thoroughly agitate solution until clear.

Home Stability: Dilute just prior to administration and use within 48 hours. Do not refrigerate.

Compatibilities: Compatible with dextrose, saline, KCl, Ringer's, or lactated Ringer's. Do not mix with any other drug or with total parenteral nutrition.

Administration: Infuse total daily dose via infusion pump at a constant rate over 12–24 hours.

Final filtration with a 0.45-micron or smaller filter is necessary.

Contraindications: Hypersensitivity. Safety in pregnancy and lactation has not been established. Use should be limited to life-threatening illnesses where the benefits outweigh the potential risks.

Side Effects:
Primary: Fluid overload, tremor, dizziness, hallucinations, confusion, psychosis, ataxia, decreased hemoglobin, hematocrit, white cell and platelet count, increase in SGOT and total bilirubin.
Secondary: Anorexia, nausea, vomiting, hematemesis, diarrhea, weight loss, malaise, pruritus, rash, pain at the infusion site.

Nursing Implications: Prior to initiation of therapy, the diagnosis should be confirmed by a cell culture from a brain biopsy.
Monitor for allergic reactions.
Monitor baseline and periodic renal, hepatic, and hematologic functions. In renal insufficiency there may be an accumulation of the drug, and the dosage may need to be adjusted.
Monitor the client's fluid balance: Measure urine output to assure an average output of 30 ml/hour. Weigh every 24 hours and monitor for signs of fluid overload.
Monitor infusion site hourly for signs of pain or thrombophlebitis.

Generic Name: VINBLASTINE SULFATE

Trade Name: VELBAN

Classification: Antineoplastic plant alkaloid

Actions: Affects mitosis by stopping the cell cycle at metaphase as a result of interference with spindle proteins. Although cell-cycle specific at the M phase, at high doses it may affect RNA synthesis and be active in other phases of the cell cycle.

Indications: Breast cancer, choriocarcinoma, Hodgkin's disease, testicular tumors, renal cell carcinoma, chronic myelocytic leukemia.

Dosage:
Neonatal: Not applicable.
Pediatric: 0.1–0.5 mg/kg (4–20 mg/m^2) IV every week or 1.5–2.0 mg/m^2 by continuous IV drip every day for 5 days. Usual maximum dose is 12.5 mg/m^2.
Adult: Same as pediatric dosage, except maximum dose is 18.5 mg/m^2.

Preparation: Supplied in 10-mg vials to be mixed with 10 ml of normal saline.

Home Stability: Unopened vials should be refrigerated and protected from light. Prepared solution is stable for 30 days if refrigerated and protected from light.

Compatibilities: Vinblastine may increase the accumulation of methotrexate in tumor cells. Mitomycin increases the risk of acute shortness of breath and severe bronchospasm with vinblastine administration. Vinblastine decreases the effects of phenytoin. As with most antineoplastic agents, it is not advisable to administer drug with other admixture solutions.

Administration:
Neonatal: Not applicable.
Pediatric: Administer by slow IV push into side arm of free-flowing IV, checking patency every 2–3 minutes to avoid extravasation of this vesicant. Infuse continuous IV drip solutions through a central line only.
Adult: See pediatric administration.

Contraindications: Pregnancy. Reduced dose with liver dysfunction (50 percent dose reduction if bilirubin greater than 1.5). Neurotoxicity may be increased in patients who are cachectic or who already have neurologic deficits. Use with caution in patients with infections or open wounds.

Side Effects:
Primary:
Hematopoietic: Decreased WBCs, with a nadir in 5–9 days and recovery in 14–21 days.
Gastrointestinal: Constipation, abdominal cramping, paralytic ileus, stomatitis, anorexia, gastrointestinal bleeding.
Neurotoxicity: Peripheral neuropathy, paresthesias, jaw pain, headache, depression, urinary retention, loss of deep tendon reflexes (foot and wrist drop).
Reproductive: Possibly teratogenetic.
Secondary: Decreased platelets and red blood cells, mild nausea and vomiting, malaise, urinary retention, increased heart rate, decreased blood pressure, seizures, partial alopecia, rashes, photosensitivity reactions, temporary hepatitis, a Raynaud's-like phenomenon, inappropriate ADH secretion, burning and pain at the tumor site. Acute shortness of breath and severe bronchospasm have occurred within minutes or hours of administration. Convulsions and severe, permanent brain damage may occur with prolonged use. Risk of infertility is high. Risk of secondary malignancy is unknown. (*Note:* Corneal ulceration if splashed into the eye.)

Nursing Implications: Monitor WBC.

Instruct patient and family on infection precautions during second and third weeks after treatment is given.

Instruct patient to report to physician symptoms of constipation. Recommend high-fiber/bulk diet and/or stool softeners. Guaiac all stools.

Instruct patient to report to physician changes in sensation—numbness and tingling in fingers and toes, inability to button clothes, or tendency to drop objects. Warn patient against handling heavy objects.

Instruct patient to report jaw or abdominal pain, urinary retention, or headache to physician.

Emphasize good oral hygiene with a soft-bristled toothbrush.

Establish and maintain good venous access, checking for patency every 2–3 minutes during IV push administration and instructing the patient to report any sensations of burning or pain.

Inform patient of the possibility of birth defects if pregnancy occurs while taking drug.

Continue safe-handling precautions for 6 days after the last dose of drug.

Generic Name: VINCRISTINE SULFATE

Trade Name: ONCOVIN

Classification: Antineoplastic plant alkaloid

Actions: Affects mitosis by stopping the cell cycle at metaphase as a result of interference with spindle proteins. Also binds to proteins in the S phase, thereby interrupting DNA and RNA synthesis. Considered cell-cycle specific at the M phase.

Indications: Acute lymphoblastic leukemia, breast cancer, sarcomas, Wilms' tumor, Hodgkin's disease, non-Hodgkin's lymphoma.

Dosage:
Neonatal: Not applicable.
Pediatric: 2 mg/m^2 IV every week.
Adult: 0.4–2.0 mg/m^2 IV every week.

Preparation: Available in 1- and 5-mg vials to be mixed with 10 ml of copackaged diluent, sodium chloride and benzyl alcohol.

Home Stability: Both unopened vials and prepared solution should be protected from light and refrigerated. Unopened vials are stable at room temperature for 6 months. Prepared solutions are stable for 15 days if refrigerated and protected from light.

Compatibilities: The synchronization of bleomycin 6–12 hours after vincristine may be effective. Vincristine given 8–48 hours after methotrexate may increase cellular uptake of methotrexate by malignant cells. Other neurotoxic drugs may increase vincristine's peripheral neuropathy. Vincristine decreases effectiveness of oral digoxin. As with most antineoplastic agents, it is not advisable to administer drug with other admixture solutions.

Administration:
Neonatal: Not applicable.
Pediatric: Administer by slow IV push into side arm of free-flowing IV, checking patency every 2–3 minutes to avoid extravasation of this vesicant. Do not give intrathecally.
Adult: See pediatric administration.

Contraindications: Pregnancy, in patients with demyelinating Charcot-Marie-Tooth disease, preexisting neuromuscular disease, presence of neurotoxicity, or who are receiving other neurotoxic drugs. Reduce dose by 50 percent with liver dysfunction or a bilirubin greater than 1.5 mg/dl. Neurotoxicity may be increased in patients who are cachectic or who already have neurological deficits. Mitomycin increases the risk of acute shortness of breath and severe bronchospasm with vincristine administration.

Side Effects:
Primary:
Neurotoxicity: Jaw pain, peripheral neuropathy, numbness, weakness, muscle pain, loss of deep tendon reflexes (foot and wrist drop), impotence. All occur more often in the elderly and bedridden and are reversible except for possible permanent motor deficits.
Gastrointestinal: Constipation, abdominal cramping, paralytic ileus (especially in children).
Reproductive: Teratogenesis, infertility that may be permanent.
Secondary: Seizures, often with increased blood pressure; bladder atony; mild bone marrow depression; central nervous system depression; cranial and vocal chord nerve paralysis (hoarseness, diplopia, or facial palsies); dysphagia; metallic taste; partial alopecia that is reversible; dermatitis; possible Raynaud's phenomenon; acute shortness of breath with severe bronchospasm; increased uric acid levels; decreased serum sodium secondary to syndrome of inappropriate antidiuretic hormone secretion. Secondary malignancies are possible, especially with combination therapy. (*Note:* Avoid splashing in eyes, which results in severe irritation and possible ulceration.)

Nursing Implications: Instruct patient to report to physician any symptoms of constipation. Recommend high-fiber/bulk diet and/or stool softeners or laxatives.

Instruct patient to report to physician changes in sensation—numbness and tingling in fingers and toes, inability to button clothes or tendency to drop objects. Warn patient against handling heavy objects.

Instruct patient to report jaw, muscle, or abdominal pain to physician.

Establish and maintain good venous access, checking for patency every 2–3 minutes during IV push administration. Instruct patient to report any sensations of burning or pain.

Inform patient of possibility of birth defects if pregnancy occurs while taking vincristine.

Continue safe-handling precautions for 18 days after the last dose of vincristine (70 percent is excreted in feces).

Generic Name: WARFARIN SODIUM

Trade Name: COUMADIN

Classification: Anticoagulant

Actions: Depresses formation of prothrombin and other coagulation factors in the liver.

Indications: Prevention and/or treatment of thromboses and emboli.

Dosage:
Neonatal: Not applicable.
Pediatric: Not applicable.
Adult: 40–60 mg (0.75–1.0 mg/kg) initially, with a maintenance dose of 2–10 mg, depending on prothrombin time.

Preparation: Supplied as 50 mg of powder with diluent.

Home Stability: Not applicable.

Compatibilities: Compatible with dextrose.

Administration:
Neonatal: Not applicable.
Pediatric: Not applicable.
Adult: 25 mg (1 ml) over 1 minute IV.

Contraindications: Active bleeding, anesthesia, blood dyscrasias, continuous gastrointestinal suctioning, history of bleeding, pregnancy and lactation, recent surgery (especially neurosurgical, ophthalmic, or traumatic procedures), subacute bacterial endocarditis, threatened abortion, vitamin C deficiency. Use cautiously with other drugs; numerous drug interactions are possible, potentiating or inhibiting actions of coumadin.

Side Effects:
Primary: Bruising, epistaxis, hematuria, prothrombin time less than 20 percent of normal activity, signs of bleeding.
Secondary: Allergic reaction, alopecia.

Nursing Implications: Obtain baseline prothrombin time and daily thereafter during therapy. Dosage adjusted daily based on value with a goal of 20 percent of normal activity (21–35 seconds, control 14 seconds).

Switch to oral therapy as soon as possible.

Observe for signs of bleeding. Use care in handling patient. Hold pressure on puncture sites 5–30 minutes depending on prothrombin time.

Index

Drug Index